Cardiac Resynchronization Therapy: State of the Art

Editors

LUIGI PADELETTI
MARTINA NESTI
GIUSEPPE BORIANI

CARDIAC ELECTROPHYSIOLOGY CLINICS

www.cardiacEP.theclinics.com

Consulting Editors
RANJAN K. THAKUR
ANDREA NATALE

December 2015 • Volume 7 • Number 4

ELSEVIER

1600 John F. Kennedy Boulevard • Suite 1800 • Philadelphia, Pennsylvania, 19103-2899

http://www.theclinics.com

CARDIAC ELECTROPHYSIOLOGY CLINICS Volume 7, Number 4
December 2015 ISSN 1877-9182, ISBN-13: 978-0-323-40238-5

Editor: Lauren Boyle
Developmental Editor: Susan Showalter

Cardiac Electrophysiology Clinics (ISSN 1877-9182) is published quarterly by Elsevier Inc., 360 Park Avenue South, New York, NY 10010-1710. Months of issue are March, June, September, and December. Subscription prices are $200.00 per year for US individuals, $293.00 per year for US institutions, $105.00 per year for US students and residents, $225.00 per year for Canadian individuals, $331.00 per year for Canadian institutions, $285.00 per year for international individuals, $354.00 per year for international institutions and $150.00 per year for Canadian and international students/residents. To receive student/resident rate, orders must be accompanied by name of affilliated institution, date of term, and the signature of program/residency coordinator on institution letterhead. Orders will be billed at individual rate until proof of status is received. Foreign air speed delivery is included in all Clinics subscription prices. All prices are subject to change without notice. **POSTMASTER:** Send address changes to Cardiac Electrophysiology Clinics, Elsevier Health Sciences Division, Subscription Customer Service, 3251 Riverport Lane, Maryland Heights, MO 63043. **Customer Service: 1-800-654-2452 (US and Canada). From outside of the US and Canada, call 314-477-8871. Fax: 314-447-8029. E-mail: JournalsCustomerService-usa@elsevier.com (for print support); JournalsOnlineSupport-usa@elsevier.com (for online support).**

Reprints. For copies of 100 or more of articles in this publication, please contact the Commercial Reprints Department, Elsevier Inc., 360 Park Avenue South, New York, NY 10010-1710. Tel.: 212-633-3874; Fax: 212-633-3820; E-mail: reprints@elsevier.com.

Cardiac Electrophysiology Clinics is covered in *MEDLINE/PubMed (Index Medicus).*

Contributors

CONSULTING EDITORS

RANJAN K. THAKUR, MD, MPH, MBA, FACC, FHRS
Professor of Medicine and Director, Arrhythmia Service, Thoracic and Cardiovascular Institute, Sparrow Health System, Michigan State University, Lansing, Michigan

ANDREA NATALE, MD, FACC, FESC, FHRS
Texas Cardiac Arrhythmia Institute, St. David's Medical Center; Dell Medical School, University of Texas, Austin, Texas; MetroHealth Medical Center, Case Western Reserve University School of Medicine, Cleveland, Ohio; Division of Cardiology, Stanford University, Stanford, California; Electrophysiology and Arrhythmia Services, California Pacific Medical Center, San Francisco, California; Division of Cardiovascular Diseases, Scripps Clinic, La Jolla, California

EDITORS

LUIGI PADELETTI, MD
Chair of Cardiology, Director of the Specialty School in Cardiovascular Diseases, University of Firenze, Firenze, Italy

MARTINA NESTI, MD
Electrophysiology and Pacing Centre, Heart and Vessels Department, University of Firenze, Firenze, Italy

GIUSEPPE BORIANI, MD, PhD
Professor of Cardiology, Institute of Cardiology, Department of Experimental, Diagnostic and Specialty Medicine, University of Bologna, S. Orsola-Malpighi University Hospital, Bologna, Italy

AUTHORS

AMIN AL-AHMAD, MD, FACC, FHRS, CCDS
Texas Cardiac Arrhythmia Institute, St. David's Medical Center, Austin, Texas

ADVAY G. BHATT, MD
Arrhythmia Institute, The Valley Health System, Ridgewood, New Jersey

RASMUS BORGQUIST, MD, PhD
Cardiology Division, Cardiac Arrhythmia Service, Massachusetts General Hospital, Boston, Massachusetts; Lund University, Skane University Hospital, Lund, Sweden

GIUSEPPE BORIANI, MD, PhD
Professor of Cardiology, Institute of Cardiology, Department of Experimental, Diagnostic and Specialty Medicine, University of Bologna, S. Orsola-Malpighi University Hospital, Bologna, Italy

FRIEDER BRAUNSCHWEIG, MD, PhD
Department of Cardiology, Karolinska
University Hospital, Karolinska Institutet,
Stockholm, Sweden

VENUGOPAL BRIJMOHAN BHATTAD, MD
Department of Medicine, Saint Vincent
Hospital, University of Massachusetts Medical
School, Worcester, Massachusetts

J. DAVID BURKHARDT, MD, FACC, FHRS
Texas Cardiac Arrhythmia Institute, St. David's
Medical Center, Austin, Texas

LOVELY CHHABRA, MD
Department of Cardiovascular Medicine,
Hartford Hospital, University of Connecticut
School of Medicine, Hartford, Connecticut

DANIEL B. COBB, MD
Division of Cardiology, Department of
Medicine, Medical University of South
Carolina, Charleston, South Carolina

**MARIA ROSA COSTANZO, MD, FACC,
FAHA, FESC**
Advocate Heart Institute, Edward Heart
Hospital, Naperville, Illinois

**EDMOND M. CRONIN, MB BCh BAO,
FHRS, CCDS**
Attending Electrophysiologist, Hartford
Hospital, Hartford, Connecticut; Assistant
Professor, University of Connecticut School of
Medicine, Farmington, Connecticut

JAMES P. DAUBERT, MD
Clinical Cardiac Electrophysiology, Cardiology
Division, Department of Medicine, Duke
Clinical Research Institute, Duke University
Medical Center, Durham, North Carolina

JEAN-CLAUDE DAUBERT, MD
Professor, University of Rennes, Rennes,
France

LUIGI DI BIASE, MD, PhD, FHRS
Texas Cardiac Arrhythmia Institute, St. David's
Medical Center, Austin, Texas; Arrhythmia
Services, Department of Medicine, Montefiore
Medical Center, Albert Einstein College of
Medicine, Bronx, New York; Department of
Biomedical Engineering, University of Texas,
Austin, Texas; Department of Cardiology,
University of Foggia, Foggia, Italy

DOMENICO FACCHIN, MD
Cardiology Unit, University Hospital Santa
Maria della Misericordia, Udine, Italy

YALÇIN GÖKOĞLAN, MD
Texas Cardiac Arrhythmia Institute, St. David's
Medical Center, Austin, Texas

MAHMUT FATIH GÜNEŞ, MD
Texas Cardiac Arrhythmia Institute, St. David's
Medical Center, Austin, Texas

MAURIZIO GASPARINI, MD
Chief, EP and Pacing Unit, Humanitas
Research Hospital, Rozzano, Milano, Italy

CAROLA GIANNI, MD
Texas Cardiac Arrhythmia Institute, St. David's
Medical Center, Austin, Texas; Department of
Clinical Sciences and Community Health,
University of Milan, Milan, Italy

MICHAEL R. GOLD, MD, PhD
Division of Cardiology, Department of
Medicine, Medical University of South
Carolina, Charleston, South Carolina

JOHN GORCSAN III, MD
Professor of Medicine, Division of Cardiology,
Heart and Vascular Institute, University of
Pittsburgh, Pittsburgh, Pennsylvania

MARIELL JESSUP, MD
Cardiovascular Division, Department of
Medicine, University of Pennsylvania
Perelman School of Medicine, Philadelphia,
Pennsylvania

DAVID A. KASS, MD
Professor of Medicine, Division of Cardiology,
Department of Medicine, Johns Hopkins
University School of Medicine, Baltimore,
Maryland

JONATHAN A. KIRK, PhD
Research Associate, Division of Cardiology,
Department of Medicine, Johns Hopkins
University School of Medicine, Baltimore,
Maryland

MARIËLLE KLOOSTERMAN, BSc
Department of Cardiology, University of
Groningen, University Medical Center
Groningen, Groningen, The Netherlands

CHRISTOPHE LECLERCQ, MD, PhD
Professor, University of Rennes, Rennes,
France

FRANCISCO LEYVA, MD, FRCP, FACC
Aston Medical Research Institute, Aston
Medical School, Aston University; Department
of Cardiology, University Hospital Birmingham
Queen Elizabeth, Birmingham, United
Kingdom

CECILIA LINDE, MD, PhD
Department of Cardiology, Karolinska
University Hospital, Karolinska Institutet,
Stockholm, Sweden

ALEXANDER H. MAASS, MD, PhD
Department of Cardiology, University of
Groningen, University Medical Center
Groningen, Groningen, The Netherlands

RAPHAËL MARTINS, MD, PhD
Assistant Professor, University of Rennes,
Rennes, France

JEREMY A. MAZUREK, MD
Cardiovascular Division, Department of
Medicine, University of Pennsylvania
Perelman School of Medicine, Philadelphia,
Pennsylvania

SARFARAZ MEMON, MD
Department of Cardiovascular Medicine,
Hartford Hospital, Hartford, Connecticut

SANGHAMITRA MOHANTY, MD, MS
Texas Cardiac Arrhythmia Institute, St. David's
Medical Center, Austin, Texas

LLUÍS MONT, MD, PhD
Hospital Clinic, Universitat de Barcelona,
Barcelona, Catalonia, Spain

DANIELE MUSER, MD
Cardiac Electrophysiology, Hospital of the
University of Pennsylvania, Philadelphia,
Pennsylvania

ANDREA NATALE, MD, FACC, FESC, FHRS
Texas Cardiac Arrhythmia Institute, St. David's
Medical Center; Dell Medical School,
University of Texas, Austin, Texas;
MetroHealth Medical Center, Case Western
Reserve University School of Medicine,
Cleveland, Ohio; Division of Cardiology,
Stanford University, Stanford, California;
Electrophysiology and Arrhythmia Services,
California Pacific Medical Center,
San Francisco, California; Division of
Cardiovascular Diseases, Scripps Clinic,
La Jolla, California

MARTINA NESTI, MD
Electrophysiology and Pacing Centre, Heart
and Vessels Department, University of Firenze,
Firenze, Italy

LUIGI PADELETTI, MD
Chair of Cardiology, Director of the Specialty
School in Cardiovascular Diseases, University
of Firenze, Firenze, Italy

FRITS W. PRINZEN, PhD
Department of Physiology, Cardiovascular
Research Institute Maastricht, Maastricht
University, Maastricht, The Netherlands

ALESSANDRO PROCLEMER, MD
Cardiology Unit, University Hospital Santa
Maria della Misericordia, Udine, Italy

MICHIEL RIENSTRA, MD, PhD
Department of Cardiology, University of
Groningen, University Medical Center
Groningen, Groningen, The Netherlands

ATTILA ROKA, MD, PhD
Cardiology Division, Cardiac Arrhythmia
Service, Massachusetts General Hospital,
Boston, Massachusetts

VAIBHAV SATIJA, MD
Thoracic and Cardiovascular Institute,
Michigan State University, Lansing,
Michigan

RICK SCHREURS, MD
Department of Physiology, Cardiovascular
Research Institute Maastricht; Department of
Cardiothoracic Surgery, Maastricht
University Medical Center, Maastricht, The
Netherlands

JAGMEET SINGH, MD, DPhil
Cardiology Division, Cardiac Arrhythmia
Service, Massachusetts General Hospital,
Boston, Massachusetts

VINI SINGH, MD
Thoracic and Cardiovascular Institute,
Michigan State University, Lansing, Michigan

DWARAKRAJ SOUNDARRAJ, MD, FACC
Liberty Cardiovascular Associates, Liberty
Hospital, Liberty, Missouri

DAVID H. SPODICK, MD, DSc
Department of Medicine, Saint Vincent
Hospital, University of Massachusetts Medical
School, Worcester, Massachusetts

JONATHAN S. STEINBERG, MD
Director, Arrhythmia Institute, The Valley Health
System, Ridgewood, New Jersey; Adjunct
Professor of Medicine, University of Rochester
School of Medicine and Dentistry, Rochester,
New York

EDWARD SZE, MD
Clinical Cardiac Electrophysiology, Cardiology
Division, Department of Medicine, Duke
University Medical Center, Durham, North
Carolina

BHUPENDAR TAYAL, MD
Post-Doctoral Associate, Division of Cardiology,
Heart and Vascular Institute, University of
Pittsburgh, Pittsburgh, Pennsylvania

**RANJAN K. THAKUR, MD, MPH, MBA,
FACC, FHRS**
Professor of Medicine and Director, Arrhythmia
Service, Thoracic and Cardiovascular Institute,
Sparrow Health System, Michigan State
University, Lansing, Michigan

JOSÉ MARÍA TOLOSANA, MD, PhD
Hospital Clinic, Universitat de Barcelona,
Barcelona, Catalonia, Spain

ISABELLE C. VAN GELDER, MD, PhD
Department of Cardiology, University of
Groningen, University Medical Center
Groningen, Groningen, The Netherlands

ROB F. WIEGERINCK, PhD
Department of Physiology, Cardiovascular
Research Institute Maastricht, Maastricht
University, Maastricht, The Netherlands

BRUCE L. WILKOFF, MD, FHRS, CCDS
Director, Cardiac Pacing and Tachyarrhythmia
Devices, Department of Cardiovascular
Medicine, Cleveland Clinic; Professor of
Medicine, Lerner College of Medicine of
Case Western Reserve University,
Cleveland, Ohio

MATTEO ZIACCHI, MD, PhD
Department of Experimental, Diagnostic and
Specialty Medicine, Institute of Cardiology,
S. Orsola-Malpighi University Hospital,
University of Bologna, Bologna, Italy

Contents

Heart Failure

> Heart failure (HF) is a growing global health concern that affects more than 20 million people worldwide. With an ever-growing segment of the population over the age of 65, the prevalence of HF and its associated costs are expected to increase exponentially over the next decade. Advances in the understanding of the pathophysiology and treatment of HF have resulted in the ability to enhance both the quantity and the quality of life of patients with HF. This article reviews the current understanding of the pathophysiology, cause, classification, and treatment of HF and describes areas of uncertainty that demand future study.

Cost of Heart Failure

> Heart failure (HF) consumes a large proportion of the total national health care budget. Incidence and prevalence of HF are increasing and may give rise to an unsustainable increase in health care spending. Hospitalizations account for the vast majority of HF-related expenses, and 20% to 25% of patients discharged with a diagnosis of HF are readmitted within 60 days. Thus, efforts to reduce HF readmissions are a reasonable target for reducing overall expenses. It is to be seen if targeting readmission rates will lead to significant cost savings, and more importantly, to improved patient outcomes.

Ventricular Dyssynchrony and Resynchronization: From Bench to Bedside

> Dyssynchronous contraction of the ventricle significantly worsens morbidity and mortality in patients with heart failure (HF). Approximately one-third of patients with HF have cardiac dyssynchrony and are candidates for cardiac resynchronization

therapy (CRT). The initial understanding of dyssynchrony and CRT was in terms of global mechanics and hemodynamics, but lack of clinical benefit in a sizable subgroup of recipients who appear otherwise appropriate has challenged this paradigm. This article reviews current understanding of these cellular and subcellular mechanisms, arguing that these aspects are key to improving CRT use, as well as translating its benefits to a wider HF population.

Cardiac resynchronization therapy (CRT) is an important therapy for heart failure patients with prolonged QRS duration. In patients with left bundle branch block the altered left ventricular electrical activation results in dyssynchronous, inefficient contraction of the left ventricle. CRT aims to reverse these changes and to improve cardiac function. This article explores the electrophysiologic and hemodynamic changes that occur during CRT in patient and animal studies. It also addresses how novel techniques, such as multipoint and endocardial pacing, can further improve the electromechanical response.

Assessment of Dyssynchrony

Echocardiographic imaging plays a major role in patient selection for cardiac resynchronization therapy (CRT). One-third of patients do not respond; there is interest in advanced echocardiographic imaging to improve response. Current guidelines favor CRT for patients with electrocardiographic (ECG) QRS width of 150 milliseconds or greater and left bundle branch block. ECG criteria are imperfect; there is interest in advanced echocardiographic imaging to improve patient selection. This discussion focuses on newer echocardiographic methods to improve patient selection, improve delivery, and identify patients at risk for poor outcomes and serious ventricular arrhythmias.

Randomized, controlled trials have shown that cardiac resynchronization therapy (CRT) is beneficial in patients with heart failure, impaired left ventricular (LV) systolic function, and a wide QRS complex. Other studies have shown that targeting the LV pacing site can also improve patient outcomes. Cardiovascular magnetic resonance (CMR) is a radiation-free imaging modality that provides unparalleled spatial resolution. In addition, emerging data suggest that targeted LV lead deployment over viable myocardium improves the outcome of patients undergoing CRT. This review explores the role of CMR in the preoperative workup of patients undergoing CRT.

Implantation and Extraction Technique

Although cardiac resynchronization therapy improves morbidity and mortality in patients with cardiomyopathy, heart failure, and electrical dyssynchrony, the rate of nonresponders using standard indications and implant techniques is still high. Optimal coronary sinus lead positioning is important to increase the chance of successful resynchronization. Patient factors such as cause of heart failure, type of dyssynchrony, scar burden, coronary sinus anatomy, and phrenic nerve capture may affect the efficacy of the therapy. Several modalities are under investigation. Alternative left ventricular lead implantation strategies are occasionally required when the transvenous route is not feasible or would result in a suboptimal lead position.

Indication for CRT Implantation

as to defining differentiated approaches according to the forms of atrial fibrillation other than permanent. These recommendations remain unsupported by evidence derived from randomized controlled trials, which are much needed.

Carola Gianni, Luigi Di Biase, Sanghamitra Mohanty, Yalçın Gökoğlan, Mahmut Fatih Güneş, Amin Al-Ahmad, J. David Burkhardt, and Andrea Natale

Although cardiac resynchronization therapy (CRT) is an important treatment of symptomatic heart failure patients in sinus rhythm with low left ventricular ejection fraction and ventricular dyssynchrony, its role is not well defined in patients with atrial fibrillation (AF). CRT is not as effective in patients with AF because of inadequate biventricular capture and loss of atrioventricular synchrony. Both can be addressed with catheter ablation of AF. It is still unclear if these therapies offer additive benefits in patients with ventricular dyssynchrony. This article discusses the role and techniques of catheter ablation of AF in patients with heart failure, and its application in CRT recipients.

Response to CRT

Daniel B. Cobb and Michael R. Gold

Many patients with left ventricular systolic dysfunction may benefit from cardiac resynchronization therapy; however, approximately 30% of patients do not experience significant clinical improvement with this treatment. AV and VV delay optimization techniques have included echocardiography, device-based algorithms, and several other novel noninvasive techniques. Using these techniques to optimize device settings has been shown to improve hemodynamic function acutely; however, the long-term clinical benefit is limited. In most cases, an empiric AV delay with simultaneous biventricular or left ventricular pacing is adequate. The value of optimization of these intervals in "nonresponders" still requires further investigation.

Alessandro Proclemer, Daniele Muser, and Domenico Facchin

This review discusses the state of the art of knowledge to help decision making in patients who are candidates for cardiac resynchronization therapy (CRT) and to analyze the long-term total and cardiac mortality, sudden death, and CRT with a defibrillator intervention rate, as well as the evolution of echocardiographic parameters in patients with a left ventricular (LV) ejection fraction of greater than 50% after CRT implantation. Owing to normalization of LV function in super-responders, the need for a persistent defibrillator backup is also considered.

José María Tolosana and Lluís Mont

Nonresponse to cardiac resynchronization therapy (CRT) is still a major issue in therapy expansion. The description of fast, simple, cost-effective methods to optimize CRT could help in adapting pacing intervals to individual patients. A better understanding of the importance of appropriate patient selection, left ventricular lead placement, and device programming, together with a multidisciplinary approach and an optimal follow-up of the patients, may reduce the percentage of nonresponders.

Follow-up

Cardiac resynchronization therapy (CRT) is increasingly used in heart failure treatment and management of these patients imposes significant challenges. Remote monitoring is becoming essential for CRT follow-up and allows close surveillance of device function and patient condition. It is helpful to reduce clinic visits, increase device longevity and provide early detection of device failure. Clinical effects include prevention of appropriate and inappropriate shocks and early detection of arrhythmias, such as atrial fibrillation. For modification of heart failure the addition of monitoring to CRT by means of device-based multiparameters may help to modify disease progression and improve survival.

CARDIAC ELECTROPHYSIOLOGY CLINICS

THE CLINICS ARE AVAILABLE ONLINE!
Access your subscription at:
www.theclinics.com

Foreword

Cardiac Resysnchronization Therapy: State of the Art

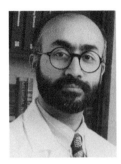　　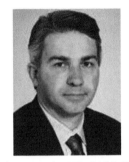

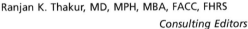

Ranjan K. Thakur, MD, MPH, MBA, FACC, FHRS　　Andrea Natale, MD, FACC, FHRS

Consulting Editors

Although mortality from coronary heart disease has been declining in Western Europe and North America since the 1970s, this is not the case elsewhere in the world. In fact, economic development in the world has led to an increase in global burden of coronary heart disease because rising living standards and increasing lifespans around the world have also been accompanied by increased caloric, fat, and salt intake, cigarette smoking, sedentary lifestyle, and obesity. Diabetes, hypertension, and coronary artery disease follow, and heart failure (HF) is the end product of myocardial damage caused by these disease processes.

HF is an immense global challenge. Just in the United States, the annual incidence has increased from 250,000 in 1970 to 825,000 in 2010; there are now 5.1 million patients with HF in the United States. In an adult, the lifetime risk of developing HF is 1 in 5. HF hospitalizations have tripled, and 50% of hospitalized patients are readmitted within 6 months. The annual cost of HF care in the United States in 2012 exceeded $30 billion, and HF is a major contributor to mortality. These statistics are likely to be worse in less developed economies.

Medical therapy for HF has been established based on large clinical trials. The use of β-blockers, ACE inhibitors, aldosterone receptor blockers, spironolactone, and digoxin, in some circumstances, has become routine. The realization that altered electrochemical substrate and impaired conduction fibers can change the velocity and uniformity of electrical propagation in diseased hearts and lead to areas of activation delay and electrical dyssynchrony paved the way for cardiac resynchronization. Since its inception in the 1990s, we have come a long way in understanding this new intervention, indications and contraindications for its use, as well as development of tools and techniques to accomplish it safely and effectively in a large majority of patients.

We congratulate Drs Padeletti, Nesti, and Boriani for providing the readers with a state-of-the-art summary of this interesting therapy focused on contemporary issues relevant in clinical practice. They have assembled thought-leaders in cardiac resynchronization and covered a wide spectrum of topics from a general discussion of HF and its economic significance to very specific details about cardiac resynchronization, such as the role of echocardiography and cardiac MRI, use of CRT-P and CRT-D, coronary sinus lead placement and extraction, resynchronization therapy in women, what we can learn from superresponders, and how to decrease nonresponders, among others.

Card Electrophysiol Clin 7 (2015) xv–xvi
http://dx.doi.org/10.1016/j.ccep.2015.09.002
1877-9182/15/$ – see front matter © 2015 Published by Elsevier Inc.

We thank Drs Padeletti, Nesti and Boriani for editing this issue and expect that the readership will benefit from reading it.

Ranjan K. Thakur, MD, MPH, MBA, FACC, FHRS
Sparrow Thoracic and
Cardiovascular Institute
Michigan State University
1200 East Michigan Avenue, Suite 585
Lansing, MI 48912, USA

Andrea Natale, MD, FACC, FHRS
Texas Cardiac Arrhythmia Institute
Center for Atrial Fibrillation at
St. David's Medical Center
1015 East 32nd Street, Suite 516
Austin, TX 78705, USA

E-mail addresses:
thakur@msu.edu (R.K. Thakur)
andrea.natale@stdavids.com (A. Natale)

Preface

Cardiac Resynchronization Therapy: State of the Art

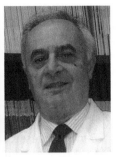 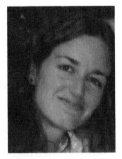 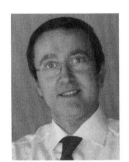

Luigi Padeletti, MD   Martina Nesti, MD   Giuseppe Boriani, MD, PhD

Editors

Heart failure (HF) is a fascinating, complex syndrome, whose treatment continues to be refined and improved. Several decades of research and clinical experience in cardiac care have continuously increased our understanding of the pathophysiology and natural history of HF, allowing the development of targeted medical therapy to improve patient functional status, reduce hospitalizations, and prolong life. Despite the impressive therapeutic armamentarium, patients with HF continue to experience progressive symptoms and shorter life expectancy.

Cardiac resynchronization therapy (CRT) was first described in 1983 at the 7th World Symposium on Cardiac Pacing by de Teresa and colleagues, and the first report on the clinical use in HF was published by Cazeau and colleagues in 1994. In the following 20 years, the scientific community passed from initial feasibility studies to prospective multicenter randomized studies.

We now recognize that CRT has transformed the management of chronic HF, significantly reducing cardiovascular morbidity and mortality in patients with both advanced and mild HF, impaired left ventricular function, and a wide QRS complex.

As editors, we have been privileged to invite internationally recognized experts to contribute to this issue of *Cardiac Electrophysiology Clinics*.

Part 1 of the issue addresses the state of knowledge of pathophysiology, clinics, prognosis, and management of HF.

Part 2 focuses on ventricular dyssynchrony in experimental settings and in man, providing insight into the causes, mechanism, and treatment.

Noninvasive assessment of the patients and of the efficacy of the therapy has been developed in Part 3.

Part 4 addresses CRT from the indications to the implantation and extraction techniques and to the choice of the devices.

Treatment of AF in CRT is a crucial topic and is addressed in Part 5, while Part 6 focuses on

Card Electrophysiol Clin 7 (2015) xvii–xviii
http://dx.doi.org/10.1016/j.ccep.2015.09.001
1877-9182/15/$ – see front matter © 2015 Published by Elsevier Inc.

cardiacEP.theclinics.com

optimization of therapy and follow-up of the patients.

As editors, we would like to express our gratitude to the authors of the individual articles for their dedication to the production of this issue. The donation of their expertise, time, and effort was essential.

This issue also would not have been possible without the dedicated assistance of Susan Showalter. The support and encouragement of Ranjan Thakur and Andrea Natale as consulting editors were also essential.

Luigi Padeletti, MD
Specialty School in Cardiovascular Diseases
University of Firenze
Largo Brambilla 3
50134 Firenze, Italy

Martina Nesti, MD
Electrophysiology and Pacing Centre
Heart and Vessels Department
University of Firenze
Largo Brambilla 3
50134 Firenze, Italy

Giuseppe Boriani, MD, PhD
Institute of Cardiology
Department of Experimental, Diagnostic
and Specialty Medicine
University of Bologna
S.Orsola-Malpighi University Hospital
Via Giuseppe Massarenti 9
40138 Bologna, Italy

E-mail addresses:
luigi.padeletti@unifi.it (L. Padeletti)
martina.nesti@tiscali.it (M. Nesti)
giuseppe.boriani@unibo.it (G. Boriani)

Letter to the Editor:
Arrhythmogenic Potential of Acute Idiopathic Pericarditis

Baksi and colleagues[1] provided a commendable review about the incidence of ventricular and supraventricular arrhythmias in patients with myocarditis and acute pericarditis.[1] The authors described a high incidence of ventricular arrhythmias in viral myocarditis as opposed to those affected with acute pericarditis. Similarly, the authors pointed out that the most common arrhythmia encountered in pericarditis is the supraventricular type (atrial fibrillation [AF] in 7.7% patients and other supraventricular arrhythmias in 9% patients).[1] This conclusion is indeed supported by the reviewed literature; however, it may give a clinical perception that atrial arrhythmias may be of very common occurrence in acute pericarditis.

We want to highlight our clinical perspective on this issue, specifically, pertaining to the fact about the association of supraventricular arrhythmias in acute idiopathic pericarditis. It is a commonly perceived misconception that acute idiopathic pericarditis predisposes to AF due to an accompanying inflammatory state. One, however, must remember that the occurrence of new-onset atrial arrhythmias (especially AF) in acute idiopathic pericarditis is often related to other coexisting comorbidities, such as ventricular dysfunction, aging, myocardial ischemia, as well as other factors predisposing to left atrial abnormality.[2–5] This observation has been supported by the data from multiple prior controlled investigations led by the senior author of this correspondence. Even a very recent randomized controlled study conducted by our Italian colleagues showed that the incidence of AF in lone acute idiopathic pericarditis was only 4% and the only significant risk factor for association with AF was increased age.[6] The mean age of the patient population experiencing AF in that study was 67 years; furthermore, the age-stratified prevalence of AF in that study was nearly comparable to that in the general population of a developed nation, further supporting the fact that acute idiopathic pure pericarditis by itself may not be significantly arrhythmogenic.[6] Stratification of occurrence of arrhythmias is best explained by Imazio and colleagues[7] in one of their cohort studies. They stratified the patient population into myopericarditis, perimyocarditis, and pure pericarditis. Ventricular arrhythmia occurrence was 4.4%, 7.7%, and 0.3% in the above conditions, respectively. Supraventricular arrhythmias incidence was lower in pure pericarditis compared with that in myopericarditis and perimyocarditis, although statistically nonsignificant in this study.[7]

Nonidiopathic forms of pericarditis like suppurative pericarditis and those complicated with effusions and hemodynamic instability may be at a higher risk for developing AF due to sepsis and fluid shifts. This can be attributed to some studies showing exaggerated incidence of AF in patients with pericarditis secondary to nonidiopathic causes, such as tuberculous infections.[8]

Pericardial effusions, postoperative pericarditis, and postpericardiotomy syndrome may have a higher incidence of AF due to the similar reasons associated with any other form of postsurgical AF.[3]

In summary, supraventricular arrhythmias in pure acute pericarditis may be encountered, but the data on their occurrence as a direct result of nonidiopathic pericarditis are not strong. Hence, their co-occurrence should not be perceived as a causal association, and in fact, the presence of a prior underlying risk substrate, such as

Card Electrophysiol Clin 7 (2015) xix–xx
http://dx.doi.org/10.1016/j.ccep.2015.08.021
1877-9182/15/$ – see front matter © 2015 Published by Elsevier Inc.

myocardial involvement, aging, and other such related causes, should be carefully considered.

Lovely Chhabra, MD
Department of Cardiovascular Medicine
Hartford Hospital
University of Connecticut School of Medicine
80 Seymour Street
Hartford, CT 06102, USA

Venugopal Brijmohan Bhattad, MD
Department of Medicine
Saint Vincent Hospital
University of Massachusetts Medical School
Worcester, MA 01608, USA

Sarfaraz Memon, MD
Department of Cardiovascular Medicine
Hartford Hospital
80 Seymour Street
Hartford, CT 06102, USA

David H. Spodick, MD, DSc
Department of Medicine
Saint Vincent Hospital
University of Massachusetts Medical School
Worcester, MA 01608, USA

E-mail address:
lovely.chhabra@hhchealth.org

REFERENCES

1. Baksi AJ, Kanaganayagam GS, Prasad SK. Arrhythmias in viral myocarditis and pericarditis. Card Electrophysiol Clin 2015;7:269–81.

2. Spodick DH. Significant arrhythmias during pericarditis are due to concomitant heart disease. J Am Coll Cardiol 1998;32:551–2.

3. Chhabra L, Bhattad VB, Sareen P, et al. Atrial fibrillation in acute pericarditis: an overblown association. Heart 2015. [Epub ahead of print].

4. Spodick DH. Arrhythmias during acute pericarditis. A prospective study of 100 consecutive cases. JAMA 1976;235:39–41.

5. Lambert CR. The pericardium: a comprehensive textbook by David H. Spodick. New York: Marcel Dekker; 1997. Clin Cardiol 1998;21:311.

6. Imazio M, Lazaros G, Picardi E, et al. Incidence and prognostic significance of new onset atrial fibrillation/flutter in acute pericarditis. Heart 2015. http://dx.doi.org/10.1136/heartjnl-2014-307398.

7. Imazio M, Cecchi E, Demichelis B, et al. Myopericarditis versus viral or idiopathic acute pericarditis. Heart 2008;94:498–501.

8. Syed FF, Ntsekhe M, Wiysonge CS, et al. Atrial fibrillation as a consequence of tuberculous pericardial effusion. Int J Cardiol 2012;158:152–4.

Heart Failure

Understanding Heart Failure

Jeremy A. Mazurek, MD, Mariell Jessup, MD*

KEYWORDS

- Heart failure • HFrEF • Ejection fraction • β-Blockers • ACE inhibitors • Neurohormonal blockade
- Treatment

KEY POINTS

- Heart failure (HF) is a progressive, clinical syndrome hallmarked by the inability of the heart to efficiently fill or provide systemic blood flow, resulting in symptoms of fatigue, dyspnea, and ultimately, significant morbidity and mortality.
- Current guidelines support the use of HF with reduced ejection fraction (HFrEF) and HF with preserved ejection fraction to replace systolic HF and diastolic HF, respectively.
- Although neurohormonal and sympathetic inhibition form the foundation of HFrEF medical therapy, the future role of these and other therapies, such as combined angiotensin-receptor blocker-neprilysin inhibition, implantable cardioverter-defibrillators, and cardiac resynchronization therapy, may be better optimized with more precise subgroup phenotyping within the HFrEF population.

INTRODUCTION

Heart failure (HF) is a significant public health concern, affecting nearly 20 million people worldwide, with a projected 25% increase in prevalence by 2030.[1] Concomitantly, HF-associated health care expenditures are expected to more than double by 2030.[1] For example, current US costs for HF are estimated at $30 billion. More importantly, HF significantly impacts the lives of those suffering from this condition, resulting in significant morbidity and mortality.[2]

HF is a complex clinical syndrome that can result from abnormalities in myocardial function (systolic and diastolic function), valvular or pericardial disease, any of which lead to impaired forward flow of blood with resultant fluid retention, often manifesting as pulmonary congestion, peripheral edema, dyspnea, and fatigue (Box 1).[3] This cycle is fueled by neurohormonal upregulation that initially serves as a compensatory mechanism to maintain Frank-Starling mechanics, but ultimately proves to exacerbate fluid overload and cardiac dysfunction.[2,4]

The HF guidelines on both sides of the Atlantic recommend differentiating between HF with reduced ejection fraction (HFrEF) and HF with preserved ejection fraction (HFpEF).[2,3] Although HFrEF and HFpEF each comprise roughly half of the HF population, they encompass different demographics and are associated with different proportions of comorbidities and responses to medical interventions (Table 1).[2,5–8] In fact, although the exact cutoff for preserved ejection fraction (EF) remains debatable (EF range from >40% to ≥55%), the presence of HFrEF suggests a different trajectory in response to current medical HF therapy as compared with HFpEF, regardless of the exact EF cut-point for HFpEF used. Moreover, the overwhelming majority of treatment approaches for HF, including both medical and device therapy, has targeted or shown benefit specifically in the HFrEF population as opposed to the HFpEF population.

Disclosure Statement: No conflicts of interest.
Cardiovascular Division, Department of Medicine, University of Pennsylvania Perelman School of Medicine, 3400 Civic Center Boulevard, Philadelphia, PA 19104, USA
* Corresponding author. 2 East Perelman Pavilion, 3400 Civic Center Boulevard, Philadelphia, PA 19104.
E-mail addresses: mariell.jessup@uphs.upenn.edu; Jessupm@uphs.upenn.edu

Card Electrophysiol Clin 7 (2015) 557–575
http://dx.doi.org/10.1016/j.ccep.2015.08.001
1877-9182/15/$ – see front matter © 2015 Elsevier Inc. All rights reserved.

This review, in the context of cardiac resynchronization therapy (CRT), primarily focuses on patients with chronic HFrEF.

PATHOPHYSIOLOGY

The syndrome of HF develops from an index event that results in ventricular dysfunction and ultimately HF symptoms. The index event, depending on cause, can be abrupt in onset (ie, myocardial infarction [MI], viral myocarditis) or may be gradual and develop over time (ie, left ventricular [LV] hypertrophy, genetic).[4] This index event results in compensatory mechanisms that at first serve to maintain adequate cardiac output in the face of LV dysfunction. Over time, however, salt and water retention become the predominant feature of HF symptoms. Specifically, the sympathetic nervous system and neurohormonal cascade (including the renin-angiotensin-aldosterone system [RAAS], as well as neprilysin, endothelin, and various inflammatory cytokines), are upregulated after the index event, helping to preserve cardiac output by increasing heart rate and stroke volume.[4,9,10] Eventually, this neurohormonal activation results in deleterious effects, including LV hypertrophy and remodeling, pulmonary edema, and excessive vasoconstriction, all of which serve to promote disease progression.[4,9] Levels of endogenous vasodilatory

peptides, including natriuretic peptides, prostaglandins, and nitric oxide, are increased in this setting to counteract the vasoconstrictive effects of neurohormonal activation, but are often insufficient (**Figs. 1** and **2**).[4,9] Further perturbations include abnormalities in cellular signaling, with increased myocyte apoptosis,[11] fibrosis,[12] necrosis,[13] and inflammation,[14] which contribute to ventricular remodeling. Ventricular interaction and valvular function (ie, mitral or tricuspid regurgitation) are compromised, and a predisposition to the development of supraventricular and ventricular arrhythmias ensues.[9,15]

Thus, the HF syndrome is the following:

- The interaction between hemodynamic dysregulation via alterations in myocardial preload, afterload, and contractility (hemodynamic model), and
- Neurohormonal disarray (neurohormonal model) that results in symptom development and disease progression.[4,15]

Current treatment approaches, as described later, target elements within and across these models to slow disease progression as well as to improve symptoms and outcomes.

CAUSE OF HEART FAILURE

HF often develops from intrinsic myocardial structural or functional abnormalities. This dysfunction, first termed cardiomyopathy in 1957, can result from a myriad of causes; many remain unknown.[16] Clinically, the initial distinction in categorizing a cardiomyopathy, specifically in the setting of HFrEF, is to identify whether the myocardial dysfunction is associated with coronary artery disease (CAD). CAD can be assessed by either invasive or noninvasive means.[2,3,17,18] Treatment of ischemic cardiomyopathy (ICM) with revascularization may improve or resolve the myocardial dysfunction. Next, the identification of an underlying systemic condition or genetic disorder may allow for disease-specific treatment and may also highlight other associated sequelae for which the patient (or relatives) may be at risk. The classification and subclassification of cardiomyopathies will grow in importance as therapies may ultimately be cause-specific, or genetically precise.[19,20]

Proposed by Maron and colleagues[16] and depicted in **Fig. 3**, nonischemic cardiomyopathies (NICM) are classified into genetic, mixed (in which some forms may be genetic in origin), and acquired causes. Within the mixed category, there is a significant proportion (20%–35%) of those diagnosed with dilated cardiomyopathy (DCM) who may have familial cardiomyopathy,

Table 1
Demographic and clinical characteristics in heart failure with reduced ejection fraction versus heart failure with preserved ejection fraction

Demographic and Clinical Characteristics[a]	HFrEF EF <40% (n = 55,083), 50%	HFpEF EF ≥50% (n = 40,354), 36%
Age, y	70 (58–80)	78 (67–85)
Female	36%	63%
African American race	25%	16%
Medical history		
CAD	52%	44%
Pulmonary disease	27%	33%
CKD	48%	52%
Anemia	14%	22%
Diabetes mellitus	22% oral therapy/18% insulin	24% oral therapy/22% insulin
Hypertension	72%	80%
Hyperlipidemia	44%	43%
Atrial fibrillation	28%	34%
CVA/TIA	13%	15%
Obesity (%)	25%	33%
BMI, kg/m^2	27 (23–32)	29 (24–35)
Hemoglobin, g/dL	12.4 (11–13.8)	11.5 (10.2–12.9)
Creatinine, mg/dL	1.3 (1–1.8)	1.3 (1–1.9)

Values are displayed as percentages or median (interquartile range) when appropriate.
Abbreviations: BMI, body mass index; CVA/TIA, cerebrovascular accident/transient ischemic attack.
[a] Data obtained from the "Get with the Guidelines" Registry, comprising acute heart failure admissions in 275 hospitals from 2005 to 2010.
Data from Mentz RJ, Kelly JP, von Lueder TG, et al. Noncardiac comorbidities in heart failure with reduced versus preserved ejection fraction. J Am Coll Cardiol 2014;64:2283; and Steinberg BA, Zhao X, Heidenreich PA, et al. Trends in patients hospitalized with heart failure and preserved left ventricular ejection fraction: prevalence, therapies, and outcomes. Circulation. 2012;126:67.

defined as 2 or more closely related family members with DCM.[20,21] Currently, 33 genes (31 autosomal and 2 X-linked) are identified in non-syndromic DCM.[20] Pathogenic mutations are identified in only 30% to 35% of cases of familial DCM; a negative genetic screen does not rule out the possibility, especially in the setting of a highly suggestive family history.[20] In addition, there are a variety of conditions, many of which that are genetically determined, that can predispose to the development of a secondary NICM, as enumerated in **Box 2**.[16] This list highlights the importance of a thorough past medical and family history to aid in the appropriate classification of NICM. More recently, given the ever-expanding understanding of the genetic basis for cardiomyopathy, and the varied morphofunctional phenotype a given mutation can display, the MOGE(S) classification has been proposed.[22,23] Two increasingly recognized DCMs are briefly discussed later, primarily because it is not clear whether patients with the described phenotypes respond to CRT.

The incidence of chemotherapy-induced cardiomyopathy (CHIC) has increased exponentially over the last decade with the growth in chemotherapeutic options as well as improved long-term survival rates of patients treated with cardiotoxic chemotherapy and radiation.[24,25] Beyond the significant and numerous cardiovascular (CV) effects of chemotherapy and radiation exposure, including premature CAD and peripheral vascular disease, diabetes and metabolic syndrome, hypertension, valvular disease, conduction disease, pericardial disease, and restrictive cardiomyopathy, several chemotherapeutic agents have been implicated in the development of CHIC.[24] As noted in **Table 1**, CHIC is a form of secondary DCM, which occurs in a dose-dependent manner after exposure to chemotherapies, including the following:

- Anthracyclines,
- Cyclophosmamide,
- Monoclonal antibodies, including trastuzumab (monoclonal antibody targeting human

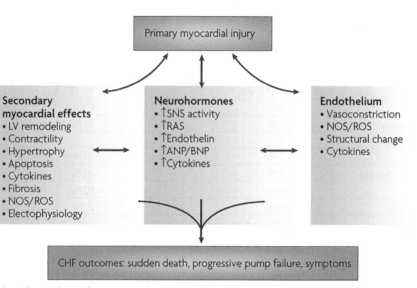

Fig. 1. Pathophysiology of HF. After an initial event resulting in myocardial injury, there are alterations that occur at the myocardial, vascular, and neurohormonal level. These changes initially serve in a compensatory fashion, but over time result in further dysfunction and disease progression. ANP, atrial natriuretic peptide; BNP, B-type natriuretic peptide; CHF, congestive heart failure; NOS, nitric oxide synthase; RAS, renin-angiotensin system; ROS, reactive oxygen species; SNS, sympathetic nervous system. (*From* Kaye DM, Krum H. Drug discovery for heart failure: a new era or the end of the pipeline? Nat Rev Drug Discov 2007;6(2):128; with permission.)

epidermal growth factor receptor 2 [HER2] in HER2+ breast cancer), and
- Proteasome inhibitors, of which the latter 2 are often reversible with discontinuation of

therapy.[2,24–26] Although a proportion of patients can develop HFrEF acutely with initiation of therapy, all those exposed to these agents are at risk for HF for years after

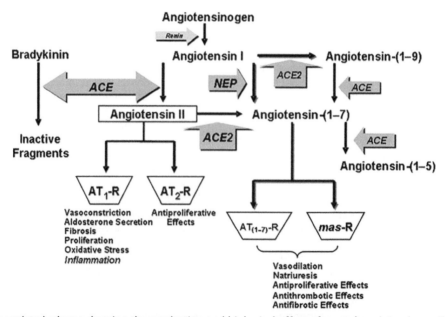

Fig. 2. An updated schema showing the production and biological effect of several angiotensin peptides. AT-R, angiotensin type receptor; mas-R, mas oncogene G protein-couples receptor; NEP, neprilysin. (*From* Ferrario CM, Strawn WB. Role of the renin-angiotensin-aldosterone system and proinflammatory mediators in cardiovascular disease. Am J Cardiol 2006;98(1):122; with permission.)

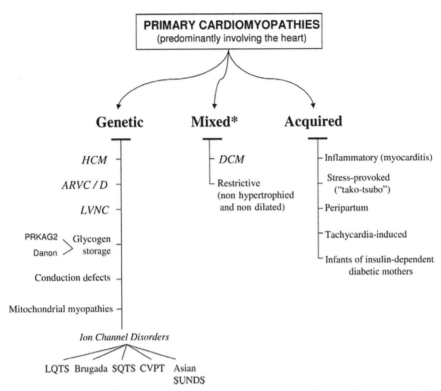

Fig. 3. Proposed classification of primary cardiomyopathies by cause. *May be genetic or nongenetic; familial disease with a genetic origin has been increasingly reported. ARVC/D, arrhythmogenic right ventricular cardiomyopathy/dysplasia; HCM, hypertrophic cardiomyopathy; LQTS, long QT syndrome; LVNC, left ventricular noncompaction; PRKAG2, γ-2-regulatory subunit of the AMP-activated protein kinase; SQTS, short QT syndrome; SUNDS, sudden unexplained nocturnal death syndrome. (*Reprinted with permission from* Maron BJ, Towbin JA, Thiene G, et al. Contemporary definitions and classification of the cardiomyopathies: An American Heart Association Scientific Statement from the Council on Clinical Cardiology, Heart Failure and Transplantation Committee; Quality of Care and Outcomes Research and Functional Genomics and Translational Biology Interdisciplinary Working Groups; and Council on Epidemiology and Prevention. Circulation 2006;113:1810. © 2006, American Heart Association, Inc.)

chemotherapy. The onset and risk of symptomatic HF are ~1% to 2% at 10 years and increase to 10% to 15% at 25 years or more.[24]

Similarly, the exponential increase in the incidence of metabolic syndrome, specifically the obesity and diabetes mellitus (DM) epidemics, has impacted and shaped the trajectory of HF development and progression over the last 2 decades.[2] Both obesity and DM are independent risk factors for the future development of HF,[27,28] with the latter conferring a worse outcome in those with established HF.[29] Several mechanisms describing obesity's role in HF development have been proposed, including the effects of increased circulating blood volume,[30] myocardial lipotoxicity, and myocardial lipid-deposition resulting in myocardial dysfunction.[31,32] Diabetic cardiomyopathy develops via several mechanisms, including increased oxidative stress,[33] endothelial dysfunction,[34] accelerated atherosclerosis,[35] advanced glycation end-products resulting in increased

myocardial stiffness and cellular dysfunction,[36,37] and alterations in myocardial metabolism and inefficient glucose utilization in the setting of insulin resistance.[35,38]

CURRENT APPROACH TO HEART FAILURE STAGING

First described in 1928, the New York Heart Association (NYHA) functional classification remains a commonly used system to describe functional capacity in HF.[2,39] As described in **Table 2**, this system subjectively assesses disease-related symptoms and exercise capacity and stratifies patients into 4 categories ranging from lack of symptoms with ordinary activity (class I) to the inability to perform any physical activity without symptoms and with symptoms at rest (class IV).[2] Although this system is an effective way of communicating symptom severity, it does not identify those who are at risk for the development of HF. In addition, the NYHA classification may downgrade those who are asymptomatic

---

Box 2
Secondary cardiomyopathies

Infiltrative[a]

  Amyloidosis (primary, familial autosomal dominant,[b] senile, secondary forms)

  Gaucher disease[b]

  Hurler disease[b]

  Hunter disease[b]

Storage[c]

  Hemochromatosis

  Fabry disease[b]

  Glycocgn storage disease[b] (type II, Pompe)

  Niemann-Pick disease[b]

Toxicity

  Drugs, heavy metals, chemical agents

Endomyocardial

  Endomyocardial fibrosis

  Hypereosinophilic syndrome (Löeffler endocarditis)

Inflammatory (granulomatous)

  Sarcoidosis

Endocrine

  Diabetes mellitus[b]

  Hyperthyroidism

  Hypothyroidism

  Hyperparathyroidism

  Pheochromocytoma

  Acromegaly

Cardiofacial

  Noonan syndrome[b]

  Lentiginosis[b]

Neuromuscular/neurologic

  Friedreichs ataxia[b]

  Duchenne-Becker muscular dystrophy[b]

  Emery-Dreifuss muscular dystrophy[b]

  Myotonic dystrophy[b]

  Neurofibromatosis[b]

  Tuberous sclerosis[b]

Nutritional deficiencies

  Beriberi (thiamine), pellagra, scurvy, selenium, carnitine, kwashiorkor

Autoimmune/collagen

  Systemic lupus erythematosis

  Dermatomyositis

  Rheumatoid arthritis

  Scleroderma

  Polyarteritis nodosa

Electrolyte imbalance

Consequence of cancer therapy

  Anthracyclines: doxorubicin (adriamycin), daunorubicin

  Cyclophosphamide

  Trastuzumab and other monoclonal antibody-based tyrosine kinase inhibitors

  Radiation

  [a] Accumulation of abnormal substances between myocytes (ie, extracellular).
  [b] Genetic (familial) origin.
  [c] Accumulation of abnormal substances within myocytes (ie, intracellular).
  Reprinted with permission from Maron BJ, Towbin JA, Thiene G, et al. Contemporary definitions and classification of the cardiomyopathies: An American Heart Association Scientific Statement from the Council on Clinical Cardiology, Heart Failure and Transplantation Committee; Quality of Care and Outcomes Research and Functional Genomics and Translational Biology Interdisciplinary Working Groups; and Council on Epidemiology and Prevention. Circulation 2006;113:1814. © 2006, American Heart Association, Inc.

despite significant underlying disease. An alternative was proposed in 2001 by the American College of Cardiology Foundation (ACCF) and American Heart Association (AHA): a staging system to serve in a complementary fashion to the NYHA functional classification.[40] As listed in **Table 2** and depicted in **Fig. 4**, the ACCF/AHA HF staging system ranges from those at risk of HF to those patients with severe HF. This staging system allows for preventative and treatment recommendations that are stage-specific (**Figs. 4** and **5**).

CURRENT APPROACH TO HEART FAILURE TREATMENT

Beyond those with stage A HF, in which the current approach is largely control of modifiable risk factors (for CAD, diabetes, hypertension, and other risk factors), a remarkable evidence base has amassed over the last 3 decades informing the approach to the treatment of stage B HF and beyond (**Figs. 4–6**, **Table 3**). As evident from **Figs. 4–6**, treatment recommendations for chronic HFrEF are largely uniform across the American and European guidelines, although differences exist, including the use of the ACCF/AHA HF staging system, and with regard to the role of second-line agents (ie, ivabradine, hydralazine-isosorbide dinitrate) in the treatment of HFrEF.[2,3]

Table 2
Summary and comparison of the American College of Cardiology Foundation and American Heart Association stages of heart failure and New York Heart Association functional classifications

ACCF/AHA Stages of HF		NYHA Functional Classification	
A	At high risk for HF but without structural heart disease or symptoms of HF	None	—
B	Structural heart disease but without signs or symptoms of HF	I	No limitation of physical activity. Ordinary physical activity does not cause symptoms of HF.
C	Structural heart disease with prior or current symptoms of HF	I	No limitation of physical activity. Ordinary physical activity does not cause symptoms of HF.
		II	Slight limitation of physical activity. Comfortable at rest, but ordinary physical activity results in symptoms of HF.
		III	Marked limitation of physical activity. Comfortable at rest, but less than ordinary activity causes symptoms of HF.
		IV	Unable to carry on any physical activity without symptoms of HF, or symptoms of HF at rest.
D	Refractory HF requiring specialized interventions	IV	Unable to carry on any physical activity without symptoms of HF, or symptoms of HF at rest.

Adapted from Yancy CW, Jessup M, Bozkurt B, et al. 2013 ACCF/AHA guideline for the management of heart failure: a report of the American College of Cardiology Foundation/American Heart Association task force on practice guidelines. J Am Coll Cardiol 2013;62(16):e155; with permission.

PHARMACOLOGIC THERAPY
Angiotensin-Converting Enzyme Inhibitors and Angiotensin II Receptor Blockers

Beginning in the 1980s, and continuing for the better part of a decade, several clinical trials emerged solidifying the beneficial effects of angiotensin-converting enzyme inhibitors (ACEI) in the improvement of mortality as well as symptoms, hemodynamics, and ventricular dysfunction seen in HFrEF (see **Table 3**).[41–44] The aggregate of these trials reveal an ~25% reduction in mortality in those treated with ACEI as compared with controls.[45] Furthermore, ACEI therapy has been shown to be beneficial in those with asymptomatic LV dysfunction (stage B), in both the setting of NICM and after MI.[43,44] Angiotensin-receptor blocker (ARBs), although less extensively and individually studied in large HF trials, seem to display similar favorable effects in HFrEF and are often used if ACEI are not well-tolerated.[2,46,47] In addition, ARBs added to a background of ACEI (especially in the context of aldosterone antagonists) do not confer a mortality benefit in HF and increase the risk of adverse events.[2,3,47–49]

Aldosterone Antagonists

Elevations in aldosterone levels produce negative effects on myocardial and vascular structure and function independent of those induced by angiotensin II.[50] In addition, although initial treatment with ACEI or ARBs reduces aldosterone levels, over time the phenomenon of "aldosterone escape" occurs, resulting in renewed elevations of aldosterone levels.[51] This background led to several studies evaluating the role of aldosterone blockade in HFrEF in those already on standard HF therapy including ACEI/ARB and β-blockers (see **Table 3**). The result was a significant, 30% decrease in the risk of death in patients with a spectrum of symptoms.[50,52,53] Current guidelines recommend consideration of aldosterone antagonists in patients with a serum creatinine less than 2.5 mg/dL (or an estimated glomerular filtration rate >30 mL/min/1.73 m^2), without recent worsening and serum potassium less than 5.0 mEq/L without a history of severe hyperkalemia.[2]

β-Blockers

The sympathetic nervous system activation in HF has many deleterious effects, including the following:

- Increased vasoconstriction and LV afterload,
- Adverse cardiac remodeling and fibrosis,
- Pro-arrhythmic effects,
- Potentiation of the RAAS.

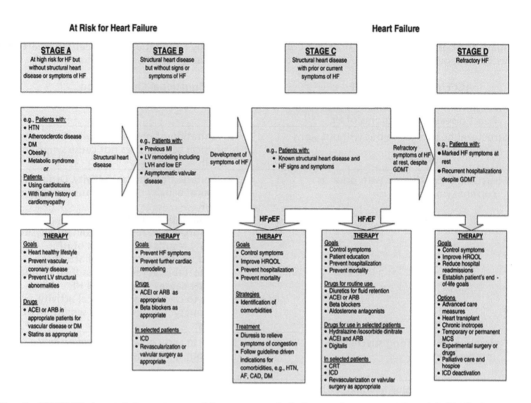

Fig. 4. ACCF/AHA heart failure stages with recommended therapy by stage. AF, atrial fibrillation; GDMT, guideline-directed medical therapy; HRQOL, health-related quality of life; HTN, hypertension; ICD, implantable cardioverter-defibrillator; LVH, left ventricular hypertrophy. (*Adapted from* Yancy CW, Jessup M, Bozkurt B, et al. 2013 ACCF/AHA guideline for the management of heart failure: a report of the American College of Cardiology Foundation/American Heart Association Task Force on Practice Guidelines. J Am Coll Cardiol 2013;62(16):e193; with permission.)

When added to established background HF therapy including ACEI and diuretics, β-blockers result in an ∼30% risk reduction in mortality along with an improvement in HF symptoms, reduced HF hospitalizations, and improvement in clinical status (see **Table 3**).[54–58] These benefits do not seem to be a class effect; studies evaluating bucindolol (vs placebo) and metoprolol tartrate (as compared with carvedilol) did not result in similar improvements.[58,59]

Ivabradine

Ivabradine is a novel I_f current inhibitor in the sinoatrial node. This current, a mixed sodium-potassium inward current, is activated by the sympathetic nervous system, resulting in enhanced pacemaker activity and increased heart rate. Inhibition with ivabradine results in reduction in heart rate and myocardial oxygen demand. Ivabradine was studied in HFrEF in the SHIFT trial, which demonstrated an 18% reduction in the composite of CV death or HF hospitalization (see **Table 3**).[60]

Nearly 90% of patients studied were on background β-blocker therapy, with the effect of ivabradine maintained regardless of β-blocker dose.[61] Although already approved and in use in Europe,[3] ivabradine only recently obtained Food and Drug Administration (FDA) approval in the United States for use in HFrEF to reduce HF hospitalization in patients with resting heart rate of 70 beats per minute or more and on maximally tolerated β-blocker therapy.[62]

Hydralazine and Isosorbide Dinitrate

Initially studied in the V-HeFT I trial (in comparison to prazosin and placebo), combination hydralazine and isosorbide dinitrate (HISDN) therapy resulted in an improvement in left ventricular ejection fraction (LVEF) and exercise capacity, with a mortality reduction that was intermediately significant.[63] Based on subsequent data,[64–66] the A-HeFT trial studied the role of HISDN therapy in African American patients with HFrEF (already on background ACEI/ARBs and β-blockers) and

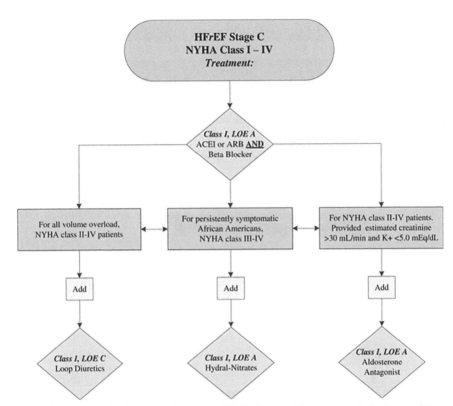

Fig. 5. Guideline-directed medical therapy for stage C HFrEF. Hydral-Nitrates, hydralazine and isosorbide dinitrate; LOE, level of evidence. (*Adapted from* Yancy CW, Jessup M, Bozkurt B, et al. 2013 ACCF/AHA guideline for the management of heart failure: a report of the American College of Cardiology Foundation/American Heart Association Task Force on practice guidelines. J Am Coll Cardiol 2013;62(16):e173; with permission.)

found that compared with placebo, HISDN resulted in significant improvements in survival and HF hospitalization among other endpoints (see **Table 3**).[67] This trial underscores the potential for more precise HF therapy in the future.

Digoxin

Digoxin is a cardiac glycoside that inhibits the sodium-potassium ATPase resulting in increased sodium concentrations, increasing intracellular calcium via the sodium-calcium exchanger. Although digoxin has been used for the treatment of HF for centuries, the DIG trial is the only randomized, placebo-controlled trial powered to assess the effect of digoxin on morbidity and mortality in HF. Overall, digoxin did not reduce mortality, although it led to a reduction in all-cause and HF hospitalization (see **Table 3**).[68] Subanalysis of this trial has revealed increased morbidity and mortality with digoxin levels greater than 0.8 ng/mL,[69,70] as well as in women, the elderly, and those with compromised renal function.[69,71]

DEVICE THERAPY
Implantable Cardioverter-Defibrillators

Patients with HFrEF are at increased risk for ventricular arrhythmias and sudden cardiac death (SCD). For this reason, over the last 20 years, ICDs have been studied for both primary and secondary prevention in the setting of ICM and NICM across several clinical trials and have emerged as extremely effective in reducing SCD in these populations.[2,72–76]

The Multicenter Automatic Defibrillator Implantation Trial (MADIT) was the first to show a mortality benefit of ICD therapy as compared with medical therapy. This study included patients with ICM and LVEF less than or equal to 35% and asymptomatic nonsustained ventricular tachycardia (VT). ICD implantation resulted in a 54% relative risk reduction for mortality over 5 years.[72] The MADIT-II trial evaluated a similar population (LVEF <30%) on more conventional HF therapy, at least 1 month after MI or 3 months after revascularization, but did not require electrophysiology study for study entry. MADIT-II revealed a 31% relative risk reduction in death over 20 months of therapy.[73] The Sudden Cardiac Death

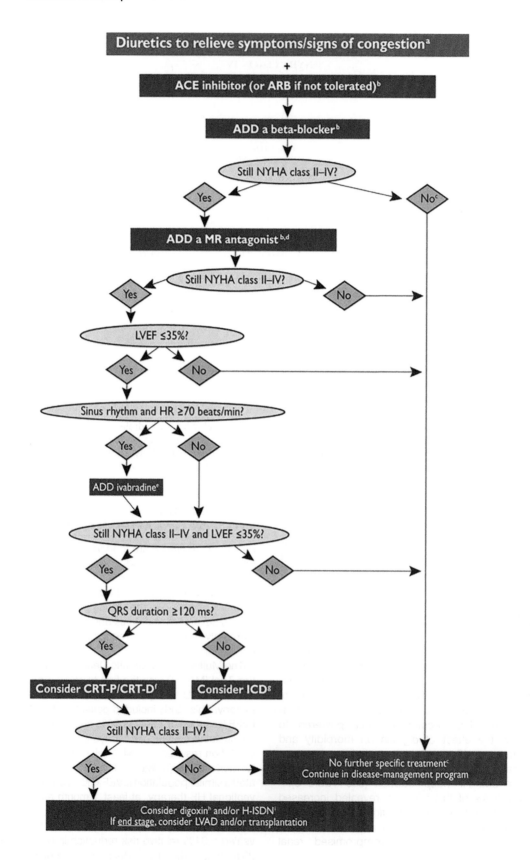

Diuretics to relieve symptoms/signs of congestion[a]
+
ACE inhibitor (or ARB if not tolerated)[b]

ADD a beta-blocker[b]

Still NYHA class II–IV?

Yes   No[c]

ADD a MR antagonist[b,d]

Still NYHA class II–IV?

Yes   No

LVEF ≤35%?

Yes   No

Sinus rhythm and HR ≥70 beats/min?

Yes   No

ADD ivabradine[e]

Still NYHA class II–IV and LVEF ≤35%?

Yes   No

QRS duration ≥120 ms?

Yes   No

Consider CRT-P/CRT-D[f]   Consider ICD[g]

Still NYHA class II–IV?

Yes   No[c]

No further specific treatment[c]
Continue in disease-management program

Consider digoxin[h] and/or H-ISDN[i]
If end stage, consider LVAD and/or transplantation

in Heart Failure Trial (SCD-HeFT) randomized patients with ICM or NICM (LVEF ≤35%) to ICD, amiodarone, or placebo in addition to conventional HF therapy. This trial found a significant, 23% relative risk reduction in death for the ICD arm compared with placebo, with no benefit in the amiodarone arm compared with placebo (see **Table 3**).[74] Data from subanalyses of these[77,78] and other trials,[79,80] as well as from real world registries, highlight the lack of benefit, and even increased risks associated with inappropriate ICD implantation.[81] Furthermore, several patient populations were not included or were underrepresented in these seminal trials, including those with significant chronic kidney disease/end-stage renal disease (CKD/ESRD),[82] as well the elderly[83,84] and those with a host of other life-limiting medical comorbidities.[82,85]

Cardiac Resynchronization Therapy

Fifty percent of patients with HFrEF develop conduction disease from a variety of mechanisms, which can result in electrical dyssynchrony and further compromise ventricular efficiency.[86–88] As highlighted by the contents of this dedicated volume on CRT, restoration of electrical and mechanical coordination with CRT have led to significant improvements in LV structure and function, exercise capacity, and quality of life, with reductions in HF hospitalization and mortality.[89–97] These changes are reflected in improvements in myocyte function as well, with enhanced calcium handling, normalization of the action potential duration, in addition to improved mitochondrial energetics, among others.[98,99]

Although the initial studies evaluated those with more severe and symptomatic HF (NYHA class III–IV),[89–92] more recent studies have further clarified the populations who stand to benefit from CRT, including those with milder HF symptoms.[93–95] Subgroups more likely to improve with CRT include women, those with a left bundle branch block, and those with a QRS duration of 150 ms or more.[76,100–103] More recently, given the increase in recognition of CHIC, the MADIT-CHIC trial is underway to assess the benefit of CRT in this population.[104] Several important CRT trials and their key findings are listed in **Table 3**.

ADVANCED THERAPIES

It is estimated that 5% of patients with HF have end-stage, or stage D disease, carrying 1- and 5-year mortality rates of 28% and 80%, respectively.[105] These patients are characterized by features of worsening symptoms, objective evidence of reduced exercise capacity, fluid retention, recent HF admissions, biomarker and echocardiographic evidence of severe cardiac dysfunction, as well as inability to tolerate standard HF therapy.[106,107] These signs and symptoms should prompt the clinician to consider referral for more advanced HF therapies (**Box 3**).[107] Stage D patients may consider options including mechanical circulatory support (MCS; as destination therapy[108,109] or bridge to transplant),[110,111] cardiac transplantation, or palliative/hospice care. Joint decision-making between the patient, their family, and the care team is necessary in this setting.

Given the scarcity of available hearts suitable for donation, MCS has grown over the last 2 decades, offering the potential for increased quantity and quality of life for patients with end-stage HF. Although left ventricular assist devices are the most common form of MCS, other devices, including the total artificial heart, represent a

◀

Fig. 6. European Society of Cardiology 2012 Guidelines: treatment options for patients with chronic symptomatic HFrEF. CRT-D, cardiac resynchronization therapy defibrillator; CRT-P, cardiac resynchronization therapy pacemaker; H-ISDN, hydralazine and isosorbide dinitrate; HR, heart rate; ICD, implantable cardioverter-defibrillator; LVAD, left ventricular assist device; MR antagonist, mineralocorticoid receptor antagonist. [a]Diuretics may be used as needed to relieve the signs and symptoms of congestion but they have not been shown to reduce hospitalization or death. [b]Should be titrated to evidence-based dose or maximum tolerated dose below the evidence-based dose. [c]Asymptomatic patients with an LVEF less than or equal to 35% and a history of MI should be considered for an ICD. [d]If mineralocorticoid receptor antagonist is not tolerated, an ARB may be added to an ACE inhibitor as an alternative. [e]European Medicines Agency has approved ivabradine for use in patients with a heart rate greater than or equal to 75 bpm. May also be considered in patients with a contraindication to a β-blocker or β-blocker intolerance. [f]See Section 9.2 of the ESC guidelines for details—indication differs according to heart rhythm, NYHA class, QRS duration, QRS morphology, and LVEF. [g]Not indicated in NYHA class IV. [h]Digoxin may be used earlier to control the ventricular rate in patients with atrial fibrillation—usually in conjunction with a β-blocker. [i]The combination of hydralazine and isosorbide dinitrate may also be considered earlier in patients unable to tolerate an ACE inhibitor or an ARB. (*Adapted from* McMurray JJ, Adamopoulos S, Anker SD, et al. ESC guidelines for the diagnosis and treatment of acute and chronic heart failure 2012: the Task Force for the Diagnosis and Treatment of Acute and Chronic Heart Failure 2012 of the European Society of Cardiology. developed in collaboration with the Heart Failure Association (HFA) of the ESC. Eur J Heart Fail 2012;14(8):821; with permission.)

Table 3
Summary of selected landmark trials in heart failure therapy

	Year	Study Title	Study Drug	Key Findings
ACEI	1987	CONSENSUS[41]	Enalapril vs placebo	27% overall RRR death
	1991	SOLVD Treatment[42]	Enalapril vs placebo	16% RRR death
	1992	SOLVD Prevention[43]	Enalapril vs placebo	Asymptomatic HFrEF patients; 29% RRR death or development of HF
	1992	SAVE[44]	Captopril vs placebo	Post-MI, HFrEF; 19% RRR death
ARB	2001	Val-HeFT[48]	Valsartan vs placebo	No mortality benefit but improved CV morbidity, QOL
	2003	VALIANT[47]	Valsartan vs valsartan + captopril vs captopril	HFrEF post-MI; valsartan noninferior to captopril, increased adverse events with valsartan + captopril
	2003	CHARM-Alternative[46]	Candesartan vs placebo	Patients intolerant to ACEI; 23% RRR in CV death or HF hospitalization
	2003	CHARM-Added[49]	Candesartan vs placebo	ARB added to open-label ACEI; 15% RRR CV death and unplanned HF admission
Aldosterone antagonists	1999	RALES[50]	Spironolactone vs placebo	Severe HFrEF (11% on background β-blocker); 30% RRR death
	2003	EPHESUS[52]	Eplerenone vs placebo	HFrEF post-MI (75% on β-blocker); 15% RRR death
	2010	EMPHASIS-HF[53]	Eplerenone vs placebo	Mild HFrEF (87% on β-blocker); 34% RRR death
β-Blockers	1996	US Carvedilol Study[54]	Carvedilol vs placebo	65% RRR death
	1999	CIBIS-II[55]	Bisoprolol vs placebo	32% RRR death
	1999	MERIT-HF[56]	Metoprolol succinate vs placebo	34% RRR death
	2001	COPERNICUS[57]	Carvedilol vs placebo	35% RRR death
	2003	COMET[58]	Carvedilol vs metoprolol tartrate	17% RRR death
I$_f$ current inhibitor	2010	SHIFT[60]	Ivabradine vs placebo	18% RRR CV death and HF hospitalization
HISDN	1986	V-HeFT I[63]	HISDN vs prazosin vs placebo	NS RRR death. Improvements in EF and exercise capacity with HISDN
	1991	V-HeFT II[64]	Enalapril vs HISDN	NS RRR death. Improvements in EF and exercise capacity with HISDN
	2004	A-HeFT[67]	HISDN vs placebo	African Americans with HFrEF; 40% and 33% RRR death and first HF admission, respectively

	Year	Trial	Comparison	Results
Angiotensin-neprilysin inhibitor	2014	PARADIGM-HF[117]	LCZ696 (valsartan + sacubitril) vs enalapril	18% RRR CV death or first HF hospitalization
ICDs	1996	MADIT[72]	ICD vs OMT	ICM (EF 35%), asymptomatic NSVT, inducible VT/VF on EPS. 54% RRR death
	2002	MADIT-II[73]	ICD vs OMT	ICM (EF 30%), no need for VT/VF on EPS, 31% RRR death
	2005	SCD-HeFT[74]	ICD vs amiodarone vs placebo	NICM or ICM (EF <35%), 23% RRR death in ICD vs placebo
CRT	2001	MUSTIC[89]	CRT vs control	Small trial (n = 67), NYHA class III, EF <35%, QRS >150 ms, crossover design, improvements in 6MWD, QOL, peak Vo_2
	2002	MIRACLE[90]	CRT vs control	NYHA class III-IV, EF ≤35%, QRS >130 ms; significant improvement in functional capacity, QOL, echo parameters and death/worsening HF with CRT
	2004	COMPANION[91]	CRT vs CRT-D vs control	ICM or NICM, NYHA III-IV, EF ≤35%, QRS ≥120 ms, 20% RRR combined mortality and hospitalization in CRT or CRT-D vs control; mortality significant in CRT-D vs control only
	2005	CARE-HF[92]	CRT vs control	36% RRR death; improvements in LV size/function, MR, NYHA class, QOL
	2008	REVERSE[93]	CRT (CRT-D or CRT-P) vs ICD	NYHA class I-II, EF ≤40%, QRS ≥ 120 ms Overall, NS 1° end-point (worsened HF), but significant reduction in time-to-first HF hospitalization (hazard ratio: 0.47, $P = .03$) at 12 mo At 24 mo, 44% RRR worsening HF and significant reduction In time-to-first HF hospitalization or death (hazard ratio: 0.38; $P = .003$)
	2009	MADIT-CRT[94]	CRT-D vs ICD	NYHA I-II, EF ≤30%, QRS ≥130 ms, 34% RRR combined death and worsening HF
	2010	RAFT[95]	CRT-D vs ICD	NYHA II-III, EF ≤30%, QRS ≥120 ms, 25% RRR combined death and HF hospitalization and death alone

Abbreviations: 6MWD, 6-min walk distance; CRT-D, cardiac resynchronization therapy-defibrillator; CRT-P, cardiac resynchronization therapy-pacing; EPS, electrophysiology study; ICD, implantable cardioverter-defibrillator; MR, mitral regurgitation; NS, not significant; NSVT, nonsustained ventricular tachycardia; OMT, optimal medical therapy; QOL, quality of life; RRR, relative risk reduction; Vo_2, oxygen consumption.

biventricular MCS option, although they currently comprise less than 5% of all MCS implants.[107] MCS devices, however, are not free of complications, including device malfunction, infection, stroke, bleeding, thrombosis, and death.[112,113]

BIOMARKER ASSESSMENT IN HEART FAILURE

There has been significant growth in the identification and understanding of biomarkers and their role in the diagnosis, management, and prognostication of HF.[114–116] Such molecules, most notably B-type natriuretic peptide (BNP) or NT-proBNP, have been shown to be prognostically powerful, although their role in optimizing HF management and improving survival and readmission rates has been less clear.

THE FUTURE

The publication of the Angiotensin-Neprilysin Inhibition versus Enalapril in HF (PARADIGM-HF) trial, evaluating combined ARB/Neprilysin-inhibition (LCZ696) as compared with enalapril alone in HFrEF

Box 3
Triggers for referral for ventricular assist device evaluation

Inability to wean inotropes or frequent inotrope use

Peak Vo_2 <14 to 16 mL kg^{-1} min^{-1} or less than 50% predicted

Two or more HF admissions in 12 mo

Worsening right HF and secondary pulmonary hypertension

Diuretic refractoriness associated with worsening renal function

Circulatory-renal limitation to ACE inhibition

Hypotension limiting β-blocker therapy

NYHA class IV symptoms at rest on most days

Seattle HF model score with anticipated mortality greater than 15% at 1 y

Six-minute walk distance less than 300 m

Persistent hyponatremia (serum sodium <134 mEq/L)

Recurrent, refractory ventricular tachyarrhythmias

Cardiac cachexia

Abbreviation: Vo$_2$, oxygen consumption.
Adapted from Stewart GC, Givertz MM. Mechanical circulatory support for advanced heart failure: patients and technology in evolution. Circulation 2012;125:1311; with permission.

---

patients may be seen as representative of a new era of HF therapeutic discovery.[117] The new drug resulted in an additional 18% relative risk reduction in the combined primary endpoint (CV death or first HF hospitalization) over those treated with ACEI, with similar significant reductions in the individual components of the primary endpoint (see **Table 3**). Several other promising drugs are in clinical trials as well, including serelaxin,[118] omecamtiv mecarbil,[119,120] and LCZ596 in HFpEF.[121]

Other areas of continued research include the following:

- The role of implantable hemodynamic and biomarker-guided monitoring in HFrEF[122–124]
- Honing the ability to maximize response to both pharmacotherapy[125,126] and device therapy,[98,127] specifically assessing the role/benefit of these therapies in patients with significant comorbidities, (ie, CKD/ESRD)[128]
- Clarifying the role of stem cell therapy in HFrEF[129]
- Expanding the understanding of the genetic and epigenetic factors as well as the identification of potential novel screening, classification, and treatment targets in HFrEF[19,23]
- Assessing the role and methods of rhythm control in patients with HFrEF and atrial fibrillation,[130] given the coexistence of these conditions and their association with worse outcomes[131]

Last, while beyond the scope of this review, there has been increased interest in optimizing the authors' approach and identifying novel treatment targets in acute decompensated HF[118,120] as well as improving MCS decision-making and heart transplant donor allocation in those with advanced disease.[107,132]

SUMMARY

Despite significant advances in the understanding of the pathophysiology and treatment of HF over the last 3 decades, HF is a progressive condition with a rising prevalence, and the primary cause for hospitalization among the elderly. In addition to the current evidence-based treatment approaches, further study is required to improve the ability to identify, treat, and ultimately prevent this condition.

REFERENCES

1. Heidenreich PA, Albert NM, Allen LA, et al. Forecasting the impact of heart failure in the united states: a policy statement from the American Heart Association. Circ Heart Fail 2013;6:606–19.

2. Yancy CW, Jessup M, Bozkurt B, et al. 2013 ACCF/ AHA guideline for the management of heart failure: a report of the American College of Cardiology Foundation/American Heart Association Task Force on Practice Guidelines. J Am Coll Cardiol 2013;62: e147–239.

3. McMurray JJ, Adamopoulos S, Anker SD, et al. ESC guidelines for the diagnosis and treatment of acute and chronic heart failure 2012: the task force for the diagnosis and treatment of acute and chronic heart failure 2012 of the European Society of Cardiology. Developed in collaboration with the Heart Failure Association (HFA) of the ESC. Eur J Heart Fail 2012;14:803–69.

4. Mann DL, Bristow MR. Mechanisms and models in heart failure: the biomechanical model and beyond. Circulation 2005;111:2837–49.

5. Owan TE, Hodge DO, Herges RM, et al. Trends in prevalence and outcome of heart failure with preserved ejection fraction. N Engl J Med 2006;355: 251–9.

6. Mentz RJ, Kelly JP, von Lueder TG, et al. Noncardiac comorbidities in heart failure with reduced versus preserved ejection fraction. J Am Coll Cardiol 2014;64:2281–93.

7. Steinberg BA, Zhao X, Heidenreich PA, et al. Trends in patients hospitalized with heart failure and preserved left ventricular ejection fraction: prevalence, therapies, and outcomes. Circulation 2012;126:65–75.

8. Salamon JN, Kelesidis I, Msaouel P, et al. Outcomes in world health organization group II pulmonary hypertension: mortality and readmission trends with systolic and preserved ejection fraction-induced pulmonary hypertension. J Card Fail 2014;20:467–75.

9. Kaye DM, Krum H. Drug discovery for heart failure: a new era or the end of the pipeline? Nat Rev Drug Discov 2007;6:127–39.

10. Ferrario CM, Strawn WB. Role of the renin-angiotensin-aldosterone system and proinflammatory mediators in cardiovascular disease. Am J Cardiol 2006;98:121–8.

11. Moorjani N, Westaby S, Narula J, et al. Effects of left ventricular volume overload on mitochondrial and death-receptor-mediated apoptotic pathways in the transition to heart failure. Am J Cardiol 2009;103:1261–8.

12. Sundstrom J, Evans JC, Benjamin EJ, et al. Relations of plasma matrix metalloproteinase-9 to clinical cardiovascular risk factors and echocardiographic left ventricular measures: the Framingham Heart Study. Circulation 2004;109: 2850–6.

13. Mann DL, Kent RL, Parsons B, et al. Adrenergic effects on the biology of the adult mammalian cardiocyte. Circulation 1992;85:790–804.

14. Aukrust P, Gullestad L, Ueland T, et al. Inflammatory and anti-inflammatory cytokines in chronic heart failure: potential therapeutic implications. Ann Med 2005;37:74–85.

15. Jessup M, Brozena S. Heart failure. N Engl J Med 2003;348:2007–18.

16. Maron BJ, Towbin JA, Thiene G, et al. Contemporary definitions and classification of the cardiomyopathies: an American Heart Association Scientific Statement from the Council on Clinical Cardiology, Heart Failure and Transplantation Committee; Quality of Care and Outcomes Research and Functional Genomics and Translational Biology Interdisciplinary Working Groups; and Council on Epidemiology and Prevention. Circulation 2006; 113:1807–16.

17. Soman P, Lahiri A, Mieres JH, et al. Etiology and pathophysiology of new-onset heart failure: evaluation by myocardial perfusion imaging. J Nucl Cardiol 2009;16:82–91.

18. Ghostine S, Caussin C, Habis M, et al. Non-invasive diagnosis of ischaemic heart failure using 64-slice computed tomography. Eur Heart J 2008; 29:2133–40.

19. Rau CD, Lusis AJ, Wang Y. Genetics of common forms of heart failure: challenges and potential solutions. Curr Opin Cardiol 2015;30:222–7.

20. Hershberger RE, Siegfried JD. Update 2011: clinical and genetic issues in familial dilated cardiomyopathy. J Am Coll Cardiol 2011;57:1641–9.

21. Petretta M, Pirozzi F, Sasso L, et al. Review and metaanalysis of the frequency of familial dilated cardiomyopathy. Am J Cardiol 2011;108:1171–6.

22. Arbustini E, Narula N, Dec GW, et al. The MOGE(S) classification for a phenotype-genotype nomenclature of cardiomyopathy: endorsed by the World Heart Federation. J Am Coll Cardiol 2013;62: 2046–72.

23. Arbustini E, Narula N, Tavazzi L, et al. The MOGE(S) classification of cardiomyopathy for clinicians. J Am Coll Cardiol 2014;64:304–18.

24. Carver JR, Szalda D, Ky B. Asymptomatic cardiac toxicity in long-term cancer survivors: defining the population and recommendations for surveillance. Semin Oncol 2013;40:229–38.

25. Bovelli D, Plataniotis G, Roila F, ESMO Guidelines Working Group. Cardiotoxicity of chemotherapeutic agents and radiotherapy-related heart disease: ESMO clinical practice guidelines. Ann Oncol 2010;21(Suppl 5):v277–82.

26. Grandin EW, Ky B, Cornell RF, et al. Patterns of cardiac toxicity associated with irreversible proteasome inhibition in the treatment of multiple myeloma. J Card Fail 2015;21:138–44.

27. Kenchaiah S, Evans JC, Levy D, et al. Obesity and the risk of heart failure. N Engl J Med 2002;347: 305–13.

28. Nichols GA, Gullion CM, Koro CE, et al. The incidence of congestive heart failure in type 2 diabetes: an update. Diabetes Care 2004;27:1879–84.

29. Shindler DM, Kostis JB, Yusuf S, et al. Diabetes mellitus, a predictor of morbidity and mortality in the studies of left ventricular dysfunction (SOLVD) trials and registry. Am J Cardiol 1996;77:1017–20.

30. Alpert MA. Obesity cardiomyopathy: pathophysiology and evolution of the clinical syndrome. Am J Med Sci 2001;321:225–36.

31. Marfella R, Di Filippo C, Portoghese M, et al. Myocardial lipid accumulation in patients with pressure-overloaded heart and metabolic syndrome. J Lipid Res 2009;50:2314–23.

32. Schulze PC. Myocardial lipid accumulation and lipotoxicity in heart failure. J Lipid Res 2009;50:2137–8.

33. Bojunga J, Nowak D, Mitrou PS, et al. Antioxidative treatment prevents activation of death-receptor- and mitochondrion-dependent apoptosis in the hearts of diabetic rats. Diabetologia 2004;47:2072–80.

34. Williams SB, Goldfine AB, Timimi FK, et al. Acute hyperglycemia attenuates endothelium-dependent vasodilation in humans in vivo. Circulation 1998;97:1695–701.

35. Karnik AA, Fields AV, Shannon RP. Diabetic cardiomyopathy. Curr Hypertens Rep 2007;9:467–73.

36. van Heerebeek L, Hamdani N, Handoko ML, et al. Diastolic stiffness of the failing diabetic heart: importance of fibrosis, advanced glycation end products, and myocyte resting tension. Circulation 2008;117:43–51.

37. Goldin A, Beckman JA, Schmidt AM, et al. Advanced glycation end products: sparking the development of diabetic vascular injury. Circulation 2006;114:597–605.

38. Fields AV, Patterson B, Karnik AA, et al. Glucagon-like peptide-1 and myocardial protection: more than glycemic control. Clin Cardiol 2009;32:236–43.

39. The Criteria Committee of the New York Heart Association. Nomenclature and criteria for diagnosis of diseases of the heart and great vessels. 9th edition. Boston: Little, Brown & Co; 1994. p. 253–6.

40. Hunt SA, Baker DW, Chin MH, et al. ACC/AHA Guidelines for the Evaluation and Management of Chronic Heart Failure in the Adult: executive summary. A report of the American College of Cardiology/American Heart Association Task Force on Practice Guidelines (Committee to Revise the 1995 Guidelines for the Evaluation and Management of Heart Failure): developed in collaboration with the International Society for Heart and Lung Transplantation; endorsed by the Heart Failure Society of America. Circulation 2001;104:2996–3007.

41. Effects of enalapril on mortality in severe congestive heart failure. Results of the Cooperative North Scandinavian Enalapril Survival Study (CONSENSUS). The CONSENSUS trial study group. N Engl J Med 1987;316:1429–35.

42. Effect of enalapril on survival in patients with reduced left ventricular ejection fractions and congestive heart failure. The SOLVD investigators. N Engl J Med 1991;325:293–302.

43. Effect of enalapril on mortality and the development of heart failure in asymptomatic patients with reduced left ventricular ejection fractions. The SOLVD investigators. N Engl J Med 1992;327:685–91.

44. Pfeffer MA, Braunwald E, Moye LA, et al. Effect of captopril on mortality and morbidity in patients with left ventricular dysfunction after myocardial infarction. Results of the survival and ventricular enlargement trial. The SAVE investigators. N Engl J Med 1992;327:669–77.

45. Deedwania PC, Carbajal E. Evidence-based therapy for heart failure. Med Clin North Am 2012;96:915–31.

46. Granger CB, McMurray JJ, Yusuf S, et al. Effects of candesartan in patients with chronic heart failure and reduced left-ventricular systolic function intolerant to angiotensin-converting-enzyme inhibitors: the CHARM-alternative trial. Lancet 2003;362:772–6.

47. Pfeffer MA, McMurray JJ, Velazquez EJ, et al. Valsartan, captopril, or both in myocardial infarction complicated by heart failure, left ventricular dysfunction, or both. N Engl J Med 2003;349:1893–906.

48. Cohn JN, Tognoni G, Valsartan Heart Failure Trial Investigators. A randomized trial of the angiotensin-receptor blocker valsartan in chronic heart failure. N Engl J Med 2001;345:1667–75.

49. McMurray JJ, Ostergren J, Swedberg K, et al. Effects of candesartan in patients with chronic heart failure and reduced left-ventricular systolic function taking angiotensin-converting-enzyme inhibitors: the CHARM-added trial. Lancet 2003;362:767–71.

50. Pitt B, Zannad F, Remme WJ, et al. The effect of spironolactone on morbidity and mortality in patients with severe heart failure. Randomized Aldactone Evaluation Study Investigators. N Engl J Med 1999;341:709–17.

51. Cicoira M, Zanolla L, Franceschini L, et al. Relation of aldosterone "escape" despite angiotensin-converting enzyme inhibitor administration to impaired exercise capacity in chronic congestive heart failure secondary to ischemic or idiopathic dilated cardiomyopathy. Am J Cardiol 2002;89:403–7.

52. Pitt B, Remme W, Zannad F, et al. Eplerenone, a selective aldosterone blocker, in patients with left ventricular dysfunction after myocardial infarction. N Engl J Med 2003;348:1309–21.

53. Zannad F, McMurray JJ, Krum H, et al. Eplerenone in patients with systolic heart failure and mild symptoms. N Engl J Med 2011;364:11–21.

54. Packer M, Bristow MR, Cohn JN, et al. The effect of carvedilol on morbidity and mortality in patients with chronic heart failure. U.S. Carvedilol Heart Failure Study Group. N Engl J Med 1996;334: 1349–55.

55. The cardiac insufficiency bisoprolol study II (CIBIS-II): a randomised trial. Lancet 1999;353:9–13.

56. Effect of metoprolol CR/XL in chronic heart failure: metoprolol CR/XL randomised intervention trial in congestive heart failure (MERIT-HF). Lancet 1999; 353:2001–7.

57. Packer M, Coats AJ, Fowler MB, et al. Effect of carvedilol on survival in severe chronic heart failure. N Engl J Med 2001;344:1651–8.

58. Poole-Wilson PA, Swedberg K, Cleland JG, et al. Comparison of carvedilol and metoprolol on clinical outcomes in patients with chronic heart failure in the carvedilol or metoprolol european trial (COMET): randomised controlled trial. Lancet 2003;362:7–13.

59. Beta-Blocker Evaluation of Survival Trial Investigators. A trial of the beta-blocker bucindolol in patients with advanced chronic heart failure. N Engl J Med 2001;344:1659–67.

60. Swedberg K, Komajda M, Bohm M, et al. Ivabradine and outcomes in chronic heart failure (SHIFT): a randomised placebo-controlled study. Lancet 2010;376:875–85.

61. Swedberg K, Komajda M, Bohm M, et al. Effects on outcomes of heart rate reduction by ivabradine in patients with congestive heart failure: is there an influence of beta-blocker dose?: findings from the SHIFT (Systolic Heart Failure Treatment with the I(f) Inhibitor Ivabradine Trial) study. J Am Coll Cardiol 2012;59:1938–45.

62. FDA news release: FDA approves corlanor to treat heart failure. 2015. Available at: http://www.fda.gov/ NewsEvents/Newsroom/PressAnnouncements/ucm 442978.htm. Accessed April 30, 2015.

63. Cohn JN, Archibald DG, Ziesche S, et al. Effect of vasodilator therapy on mortality in chronic congestive heart failure. Results of a Veterans Administration Cooperative Study. N Engl J Med 1986;314: 1547–52.

64. Cohn JN, Johnson G, Ziesche S, et al. A comparison of enalapril with hydralazine-isosorbide dinitrate in the treatment of chronic congestive heart failure. N Engl J Med 1991;325: 303–10.

65. Carson P, Ziesche S, Johnson G, et al. Racial differences in response to therapy for heart failure: analysis of the vasodilator-heart failure trials. Vasodilator-Heart Failure Trial Study Group. J Card Fail 1999;5:178–87.

66. Exner DV, Dries DL, Domanski MJ, et al. Lesser response to angiotensin-converting-enzyme inhibitor therapy in black as compared with white patients with left ventricular dysfunction. N Engl J Med 2001;344:1351–7.

67. Taylor AL, Ziesche S, Yancy C, et al. Combination of isosorbide dinitrate and hydralazine in blacks with heart failure. N Engl J Med 2004;351:2049–57.

68. Digitalis Investigation Group. The effect of digoxin on mortality and morbidity in patients with heart failure. N Engl J Med 1997;336:525–33.

69. Rathore SS, Curtis JP, Wang Y, et al. Association of serum digoxin concentration and outcomes in patients with heart failure. JAMA 2003;289:871–8.

70. Ambrosy AP, Butler J, Ahmed A, et al. The use of digoxin in patients with worsening chronic heart failure: reconsidering an old drug to reduce hospital admissions. J Am Coll Cardiol 2014;63:1823–32.

71. Rathore SS, Wang Y, Krumholz HM. Sex-based differences in the effect of digoxin for the treatment of heart failure. N Engl J Med 2002;347:1403–11.

72. Moss AJ, Hall WJ, Cannom DS, et al. Improved survival with an implanted defibrillator in patients with coronary disease at high risk for ventricular arrhythmia. Multicenter automatic defibrillator implantation trial investigators. N Engl J Med 1996; 335:1933–40.

73. Moss AJ, Zareba W, Hall WJ, et al. Prophylactic implantation of a defibrillator in patients with myocardial infarction and reduced ejection fraction. N Engl J Med 2002;346:877–83.

74. Bardy GH, Lee KL, Mark DB, et al. Amiodarone or an implantable cardioverter-defibrillator for congestive heart failure. N Engl J Med 2005;352: 225–37.

75. A comparison of antiarrhythmic-drug therapy with implantable defibrillators in patients resuscitated from near-fatal ventricular arrhythmias. The Antiarrhythmics versus Implantable Defibrillators (AVID) Investigators. N Engl J Med 1997;337:1576–83.

76. Epstein AE, DiMarco JP, Ellenbogen KA, et al. 2012 ACCF/AHA/HRS focused update incorporated into the ACCF/AHA/HRS 2008 guidelines for device-based therapy of cardiac rhythm abnormalities: a report of the American College of Cardiology Foundation/American Heart Association Task Force on practice guidelines and the Heart Rhythm Society. J Am Coll Cardiol 2013;61:e6–75.

77. Daubert JP, Zareba W, Cannom DS, et al. Inappropriate implantable cardioverter-defibrillator shocks in MADIT II: frequency, mechanisms, predictors, and survival impact. J Am Coll Cardiol 2008;51: 1357–65.

78. Barsheshet A, Moss AJ, Huang DT, et al. Applicability of a risk score for prediction of the long-term (8-year) benefit of the implantable cardioverter-defibrillator. J Am Coll Cardiol 2012;59:2075–9.

79. Steinbeck G, Andresen D, Seidl K, et al. Defibrillator implantation early after myocardial infarction. N Engl J Med 2009;361:1427–36.

80. Hohnloser SH, Kuck KH, Dorian P, et al. Prophylactic use of an implantable cardioverter-defibrillator after acute myocardial infarction. N Engl J Med 2004;351:2481–8.

81. Al-Khatib SM, Hellkamp A, Curtis J, et al. Non-evidence-based ICD implantations in the United States. JAMA 2011;305:43–9.

82. Setoguchi S, Nohria A, Rassen JA, et al. Maximum potential benefit of implantable defibrillators in preventing sudden death after hospital admission because of heart failure. CMAJ 2009; 180:611–6.

83. Epstein AE, Kay GN, Plumb VJ, et al. Implantable cardioverter-defibrillator prescription in the elderly. Heart Rhythm 2009;6:1136–43.

84. Santangeli P, Di Biase L, Dello Russo A, et al. Meta-analysis: age and effectiveness of prophylactic implantable cardioverter-defibrillators. Ann Intern Med 2010;153:592–9.

85. Al-Khatib SM, Greiner MA, Peterson ED, et al. Patient and implanting physician factors associated with mortality and complications after implantable cardioverter-defibrillator implantation, 2002-2005. Circ Arrhythm Electrophysiol 2008;1: 240–9.

86. Han W, Chartier D, Li D, et al. Ionic remodeling of cardiac purkinje cells by congestive heart failure. Circulation 2001;104:2095–100.

87. Ghio S, Constantin C, Klersy C, et al. Interventricular and intraventricular dyssynchrony are common in heart failure patients, regardless of QRS duration. Eur Heart J 2004;25:571–8.

88. Liu L, Tockman B, Girouard S, et al. Left ventricular resynchronization therapy in a canine model of left bundle branch block. Am J Physiol Heart Circ Physiol 2002;282:H2238–44.

89. Cazeau S, Leclercq C, Lavergne T, et al. Effects of multisite biventricular pacing in patients with heart failure and intraventricular conduction delay. N Engl J Med 2001;344:873–80.

90. Abraham WT, Fisher WG, Smith AL, et al. Cardiac resynchronization in chronic heart failure. N Engl J Med 2002;346:1845–53.

91. Bristow MR, Saxon LA, Boehmer J, et al. Cardiac-resynchronization therapy with or without an implantable defibrillator in advanced chronic heart failure. N Engl J Med 2004;350:2140–50.

92. Cleland JG, Daubert JC, Erdmann E, et al. The effect of cardiac resynchronization on morbidity and mortality in heart failure. N Engl J Med 2005;352: 1539–49.

93. Linde C, Abraham WT, Gold MR, et al. Randomized trial of cardiac resynchronization in mildly symptomatic heart failure patients and in asymptomatic patients with left ventricular dysfunction and previous heart failure symptoms. J Am Coll Cardiol 2008;52:1834–43.

94. Moss AJ, Hall WJ, Cannom DS, et al. Cardiac-resynchronization therapy for the prevention of heart-failure events. N Engl J Med 2009;361: 1329–38.

95. Tang AS, Wells GA, Talajic M, et al. Cardiac-resynchronization therapy for mild-to-moderate heart failure. N Engl J Med 2010;363:2385–95.

96. Daubert C, Gold MR, Abraham WT, et al. Prevention of disease progression by cardiac resynchronization therapy in patients with asymptomatic or mildly symptomatic left ventricular dysfunction: insights from the European Cohort of the REVERSE (Resynchronization Reverses Remodeling in Systolic Left Ventricular Dysfunction) trial. J Am Coll Cardiol 2009;54:1837–46.

97. St John Sutton M, Ghio S, Plappert T, et al. Cardiac resynchronization induces major structural and functional reverse remodeling in patients with New York Heart Association class I/II heart failure. Circulation 2009;120:1858–65.

98. Chatterjee NA, Singh JP. Cardiac resynchronization therapy: past, present, and future. Heart Fail Clin 2015;11:287–303.

99. Kirk JA, Kass DA. Electromechanical dyssynchrony and resynchronization of the failing heart. Circ Res 2013;113:765–76.

100. Sipahi I, Carrigan TP, Rowland DY, et al. Impact of QRS duration on clinical event reduction with cardiac resynchronization therapy: meta-analysis of randomized controlled trials. Arch Intern Med 2011;171:1454–62.

101. Sipahi I, Chou JC, Hyden M, et al. Effect of QRS morphology on clinical event reduction with cardiac resynchronization therapy: meta-analysis of randomized controlled trials. Am Heart J 2012; 163:260–7.

102. Gold MR, Thebault C, Linde C, et al. Effect of QRS duration and morphology on cardiac resynchronization therapy outcomes in mild heart failure: results from the resynchronization reverses remodeling in systolic left ventricular dysfunction (REVERSE) study. Circulation 2012; 126:822–9.

103. Hsu JC, Solomon SD, Bourgoun M, et al. Predictors of super-response to cardiac resynchronization therapy and associated improvement in clinical outcome: the MADIT-CRT (multicenter automatic defibrillator implantation trial with cardiac resynchronization therapy) study. J Am Coll Cardiol 2012; 59:2366–73.

104. University of Rochester. Multicenter automatic defibrillator implantation trial - chemotherapy-induced cardiomyopathy (MADIT-CHIC). Bethesda (MD): ClinicalTrials.gov; National Library of Medicine

(US); 2000 [April 30, 2015]. Available at: https://clinicaltrials.gov/ct2/show/NCT02164721. NLM Identifier: NCT02164721.

105. Costanzo MR, Mills RM, Wynne J. Characteristics of "stage D" heart failure: insights from the Acute Decompensated Heart Failure National Registry Longitudinal Module (ADHERE LM). Am Heart J 2008;155:339–47.

106. Metra M, Ponikowski P, Dickstein K, et al. Advanced chronic heart failure: a position statement from the Study Group on Advanced Heart Failure of the Heart Failure Association of the European Society of Cardiology. Eur J Heart Fail 2007;9:684–94.

107. Stewart GC, Givertz MM. Mechanical circulatory support for advanced heart failure: patients and technology in evolution. Circulation 2012;125:1304–15.

108. Rose EA, Gelijns AC, Moskowitz AJ, et al. Long-term use of a left ventricular assist device for end-stage heart failure. N Engl J Med 2001;345:1435–43.

109. Slaughter MS, Rogers JG, Milano CA, et al. Advanced heart failure treated with continuous-flow left ventricular assist device. N Engl J Med 2009;361:2241–51.

110. Miller LW, Pagani FD, Russell SD, et al. Use of a continuous-flow device in patients awaiting heart transplantation. N Engl J Med 2007;357:885–96.

111. Aaronson KD, Slaughter MS, Miller LW, et al. Use of an intrapericardial, continuous-flow, centrifugal pump in patients awaiting heart transplantation. Circulation 2012;125:3191–200.

112. Kirklin JK, Naftel DC, Pagani FD, et al. Sixth INTERMACS annual report: a 10,000-patient database. J Heart Lung Transpl 2014;33:555–64.

113. Starling RC, Moazami N, Silvestry SC, et al. Unexpected abrupt increase in left ventricular assist device thrombosis. N Engl J Med 2014;370:33–40.

114. Braunwald E. Biomarkers in heart failure. N Engl J Med 2008;358:2148–59.

115. Bayes-Genis A, de Antonio M, Vila J, et al. Head-to-head comparison of two myocardial fibrosis biomarkers for long-term heart failure risk stratification: ST2 vs. galectin-3. J Am Coll Cardiol 2014;63:158–66.

116. van Veldhuisen DJ, Linssen GC, Jaarsma T, et al. B-type natriuretic peptide and prognosis in heart failure patients with preserved and reduced ejection fraction. J Am Coll Cardiol 2013;61:1498–506.

117. McMurray JJ, Packer M, Desai AS, et al. Angiotensin-neprilysin inhibition versus enalapril in heart failure. N Engl J Med 2014;371:993–1004.

118. Teerlink JR, Cotter G, Davison BA, et al. Serelaxin, recombinant human relaxin-2, for treatment of acute heart failure (RELAX-AHF): a randomised, placebo-controlled trial. Lancet 2013;381:29–39.

119. Cleland JG, Teerlink JR, Senior R, et al. The effects of the cardiac myosin activator, omecamtiv mecarbil, on cardiac function in systolic heart failure: a double-blind, placebo-controlled, crossover, dose-ranging phase 2 trial. Lancet 2011;378:676–83.

120. Givertz MM, Teerlink JR, Albert NM, et al. Acute decompensated heart failure: update on new and emerging evidence and directions for future research. J Card Fail 2013;19:371–89.

121. Novartis Pharmaceuticals. Efficacy and safety of LCZ696 compared to valsartan, on morbidity and mortality in heart failure patients with preserved ejection fraction (PARAGON-HF). Bethesda (MD): ClinicalTrials.gov; National Library of Medicine (US); 2000 [April 30, 2015]. Available at: https://clinicaltrials.gov/ct2/show/NCT01920711. NLM Identifier: NCT01920711.

122. Bourge RC, Abraham WT, Adamson PB, et al. Randomized controlled trial of an implantable continuous hemodynamic monitor in patients with advanced heart failure: the COMPASS-HF study. J Am Coll Cardiol 2008;51:1073–9.

123. Abraham WT, Adamson PB, Bourge RC, et al. Wireless pulmonary artery haemodynamic monitoring in chronic heart failure: a randomised controlled trial. Lancet 2011;377:658–66.

124. Felker GM, Ahmad T, Anstrom KJ, et al. Rationale and design of the GUIDE-IT study: guiding evidence based therapy using biomarker intensified treatment in heart failure. JACC Heart Fail 2014;2:457–65.

125. Pereira NL, Weinshilboum RM. The impact of pharmacogenomics on the management of cardiac disease. Clin Pharmacol Ther 2011;90:493–5.

126. Liggett SB, Mialet-Perez J, Thaneemit-Chen S, et al. A polymorphism within a conserved beta(1)-adrenergic receptor motif alters cardiac function and beta-blocker response in human heart failure. Proc Natl Acad Sci U S A 2006;103:11288–93.

127. Pezzali N, Curnis A, Specchia C, et al. Adrenergic receptor gene polymorphism and left ventricular reverse remodelling after cardiac resynchronization therapy: preliminary results. Europace 2013;15:1475–81.

128. Damman K, Tang WH, Felker GM, et al. Current evidence on treatment of patients with chronic systolic heart failure and renal insufficiency: practical considerations from published data. J Am Coll Cardiol 2014;63:853–71.

129. Patel AN, Silva F, Winters AA. Stem cell therapy for heart failure. Heart Fail Clin 2015;11:275–86.

130. Aagaard P, Di Biase L, Natale A. Ablation of atrial arrhythmias in heart failure. Heart Fail Clin 2015;11:305–17.

131. Khazanie P, Liang L, Qualls LG, et al. Outcomes of Medicare beneficiaries with heart failure and atrial fibrillation. JACC Heart Fail 2014;2:41–8.

132. Givertz MM. Heart allocation in the United States: intended and unintended consequences. Circ Heart Fail 2012;5:140–3.

Cost of Heart Failure

Containing the Cost of Heart Failure Management
A Focus on Reducing Readmissions

 CrossMark

Dwarakraj Soundarraj, MD[a], Vini Singh, MD[b],
Vaibhav Satija, MD[b], Ranjan K. Thakur, MD, MPH, MBA, FHRS[b],*

KEYWORDS

- Heart failure • Cost • Readmissions

KEY POINTS

- Heart failure (HF) consumes a large proportion of the total national health care budget. Incidence and prevalence of HF are increasing, and this may give rise to unsustainable increase in health care spending.
- Hospitalizations account for the vast majority of HF-related expenses, and 20% to 25% of patients discharged with a diagnosis of HF are readmitted within 60 days; thus, efforts to reduce HF readmissions are a reasonable target for reducing overall expenses.
- Readmission rates are influenced by factors inherent to the patient (severity of illness, determinants of social status, such as education and income and race) and community resources for social services as well as by the quality of care (effectiveness of in-patient care, quality of discharge instructions, accuracy of medication reconciliation, access to ambulatory care, and communication between providers).
- There is an emphasis in the US health care system on reducing readmission rates as a means to reduce the overall cost of care.
- Although the Centers for Medicare and Medicaid Services readmission measure is risk adjusted, it does not account for differences in social support and economic inequalities, which play a significant role in the ability of patients to adhere to treatment recommendations and may dampen cost reductions.

US health care expenses as a percentage of gross domestic product (GDP) have increased from 5% in 1960 to almost 18% in 2011.[1] The annual percentage increase in health care expenses far exceeded that of the increase in GDP over these years. A report by the Agency for Healthcare Research and Quality identified heart failure (HF) as the eighth most expensive condition treated in US hospitals in 2011, accounting for $10.5 billion in hospitalization expenses alone (2.7% of total national hospitalization expense).[2] Total annual medical care cost for HF, currently at $20.9 billion, is projected to increase to $53.1 billion in 2030 at the current health care inflation rates. These direct costs do not include lost productivity from HF morbidity and mortality. Increase in expenditures over the next 15 years is largely due to a projected increase in prevalence of HF from the current 2.4% to an estimated 3% of the population by 2030, coupled with population growth. The total number of patients with HF is projected to increase by 46% to greater than 8 million by 2030.[3] Such data have

[a] Liberty Cardiovascular Associates, Liberty Hospital, Liberty, MO, USA; [b] Thoracic and Cardiovascular Institute, Michigan State University, Lansing, MI, USA
* Corresponding author. Sparrow Thoracic and Cardiovascular Institute, Michigan State University, 1200 East Michigan Avenue, Suite 585, Lansing, MI 48912.
E-mail address: thakur@msu.edu

Card Electrophysiol Clin 7 (2015) 577–584
http://dx.doi.org/10.1016/j.ccep.2015.08.002

cardiacEP.theclinics.com

led to a general consensus that the current rate of increase in health care spending is not sustainable and effective measures must be taken immediately.

READMISSIONS

Hospitalizations are expensive and account for 31% of all health care expenses and for the vast majority of HF-related expenses. Anderson and Steinberg[4] first reported in 1984 that 22% of a random sample of more than 270,000 Medicare hospitalizations were readmitted within 60 days of discharge. HF is the most common diagnosis associated with readmissions.[5] It is disappointing, however, that 30 years of improved care, technology, and new additions to our pharmacologic armamentarium have not been enough to reduce readmission rates significantly. Bueno and colleagues[6] reported in 2010 that a decrease in length of stay was accompanied by an increase in readmission rates over a period extending from 1993 to 2006. They opined that incentives related to the prospective payment system and fee-for-service payment structure could have contributed to this trend. Of interest, there is a wide variation in regional rates of readmissions (45% more in the 5 states with highest readmissions compared with the 5 states with lowest readmissions).[5] Further analysis of this issue of regional variation showed that all-cause admission rates were the strongest predictors of regional variation in readmission rates, indicating that incentives favoring hospitalization (fee for service) may result in unnecessary reliance on hospitalizations.[7]

Section 3025 of the Affordable Care Act includes provisions that require Centers for Medicare and Medicaid Services (CMS) to reduce payments to hospitals with excess readmissions (after being admitted for certain diagnoses including HF) for discharges occurring on and after October 1, 2012. This reduction of payments has triggered a significant flurry of activity among hospitals to reduce their risk-adjusted readmission rates. As an increasing number of primary care physicians and cardiologists in the United States are now being employed by hospitals and as other physicians have entered into comanagement agreements with hospitals via accountable care organizations, physician interest is more aligned with hospital interests than it has been ever before.

CONTRIBUTORS TO EXCESSIVE READMISSIONS

Readmission rates are influenced by factors inherent to the patient, the community in which

the patient lives, as well as the quality of care. Patient factors include severity of illness, determinants of social status, such as education and income and race, whereas community factors include hospital resources and availability of social support institutions in the community.[8,9] However, even after adjustment for population factors, significant regional variation persists. Changes in readmission rates over time in the same population, without associated changes in population characteristics, point to the existence of modifiable factors. Quality-of-care factors include effectiveness of in-patient care, quality of discharge instructions, accuracy of medication reconciliation, access to ambulatory care, and communication between providers.

Most readmissions within 30 days after discharge for HF are for HF itself, indicating either incomplete treatment before discharge or lack of adequate discharge planning could have contributed to clinical worsening. Based on CMS data, the first physician contact for 52% of Medicare HF patients readmitted within 30 days was during the readmission itself. It is tempting to postulate that early outpatient intervention may prevent early readmissions for HF.

PREDICTING READMISSIONS

Predicting which patients are more likely to be readmitted has been challenging. Hence, resources targeting readmission reduction cannot be focused on high-risk patients alone. Multiple risk prediction models have been tested in populations ranging from a few hundred patients to greater than 2 million. The models were based on data extracted from either administrative sources or chart review. Kansagara and colleagues[10] reviewed 26 such models and generally found them to have poor predictive ability with c-statistics in the 0.6 range. A few models that incorporated social factors and functional status had improved predictive ability, with c-statistics improving to 0.72 to 0.83. Particularly, the model being used by CMS to define expected readmission rates for hospitals showed poor predictive ability (c-statistic of 0.61), leading the investigators to conclude that it is inappropriate to penalize hospitals for excessive readmissions based on this data.

STRATEGIES TO REDUCE READMISSION
Transitional Care Programs

Patient's health status continues to evolve after discharge from the hospital and effects of in-patient treatments continue to have an effect on their physiology. However, there tends to be an abrupt drop in the intensity of follow-up after discharge, allowing for unpredictable deterioration in health status and unnecessary readmissions. An observational study on patients participating in the OPTIMIZE-HF and GWTG-HF registries showed a wide variation among hospitals in the rate of early follow-up, which was defined as less than 7 days from discharge. Hospitals that had a higher rate of early follow-up had lower readmissions.[11] Early access to ambulatory care after hospitalization may offer a cost-effective way to reduce readmissions.

Care coordination for patients with coronary artery disease, HF, diabetes, and chronic pulmonary disease was evaluated by demonstration projects, funded by CMS at 15 sites across the country.[12] Only 1 of the 15 centers was able to demonstrate reduction in hospitalizations, and none demonstrated savings. Lack of a transitional care element was thought to be the reason for failure of these programs.

Rich and colleagues[13] demonstrated that a nurse-led program that focused on care transition, patient education, medication simplification, and close outpatient follow-up was effective in reducing costs and readmissions in elderly patients with HF. A recent meta-analysis reviewed 42 randomized controlled interventions intended to reduce 30-day readmissions. Each study intervention was rated on its ability to increase patient's capacity for self-care as well as affect workload positively or adversely. The study interventions were very diverse, ranging from telephone follow-up of high-risk patients only to out-patient clinic visits to home visits. Some of the studies used telehealth and home remote monitoring technology. Interventions that enhanced patient capacity for self-care were more effective than those that did not. Interestingly, interventions that relied on newer technology like telehealth and remote monitoring were not as effective as those interventions that relied solely on face-to-face patient contact. Interventions that used such technology were associated with significantly high patient workload and could have resulted in poor adherence.[11] Cumulative data from all 42 trials showed a net benefit of reduced readmissions from the interventions.

Evidence-based Interventions that Reduce Readmissions

Neurohormonal blockade
Well-studied disease-modifying agents like angiotensin-converting-enzyme (ACE) inhibitors, β-blockers, and aldosterone antagonists have been shown to reduce HF-related readmissions as well **(Table 1)**.[14–20] Although digoxin disappointed in the DIG trial, failing to show a mortality benefit, there was a 2.8% absolute reduction in the number of patients hospitalized for any reason among patients randomized to digoxin, over a mean follow-up period of 37 months.[21] It is important to recognize that these benefits are limited to patients with systolic HF. Ejection fraction cutoff for the above-mentioned studies varied from 25% in the COPERNICUS trial to 45% in the DIG trial.

Diastolic heart failure Although the dearth of data demonstrating mortality benefit in diastolic HF continues with the recently published TOPCAT trial, there was a statistically significant 1.5% absolute risk reduction (21.7% relative risk reduction) in HF hospitalizations among patients randomized to spironolactone.[22] However, post-hoc analysis of the TOPCAT trial has raised the possibility that low event rates in one geographic region (due to enrollment of low-risk patients) and the possibility of inadequate treatment in the active group in the same region as suggested by lower magnitude of study drug effects could have contributed to the negative results of the study.[23] Based on the

Table 1
Medical therapy for heart failure

Trial/Drug Class	Drug	Δ All-Cause Readmissions (%)	Δ HF Readmissions (%)
SOLVD/ACE inhibitor	Enalapril	−6.7	−16.7
VALHeFT/angiotensin receptor blocker	Valsartan	—	−24.2
CHARM-ALT, angiotension receptor blocker	Candesartan	—	−27.6
COPERNICUS, β-blocker	Carvedilol	−15.5	—
CIBIS-II/β-blocker	Bisoprolol	−15.4	—
RALES/aldosterone antagonist	Spironolactone	—	−20.8
EPHESUS/aldosterone antagonist	Eplerenone	—	−11.9
DIG/digoxin	Digoxin	−4.5	−22.8

results of the TOPCAT trial and the lack of other evidence-based therapies, spironolactone therapy should be considered in patients with diastolic HF, with careful monitoring of renal function and potassium.

Cardiac resynchronization therapy

Intraventricular conduction delay causes dyssynchronous ventricular contraction, reduced left ventricular systolic function, and an increase in systolic volumes. In addition, it can be associated with worsening mitral regurgitation. CRT eliminates the dyssynchrony, resulting in improved ejection fraction and cardiac output. The COMPANION trial demonstrated a statistically significant reduction in the combined secondary endpoint of death or hospitalization from cardiovascular causes or HF among systolic HF patients (New York Heart Association [NYHA] class III or IV, ejection fraction ≤35%, QRS duration ≥120 ms) treated with a CRT device with or without a defibrillator.[24] In a similar population, CARE-HF trial investigators showed a significant reduction in the primary endpoint of all-cause death or unplanned cardiovascular hospitalization among patients treated with CRT without a defibrillator. HF hospitalization was almost reduced in half among patients treated with CRT.[25] A cost-effectiveness analysis based on the COMPANION study population revealed estimates of $43,000 per quality-adjusted life-year for CRT with defibrillators and a more favorable $19,600 for CRT only.[26] Patients with a left bundle branch morphology and QRS duration ≥150 ms derive more benefit from CRT than patients without such findings, and it is likely that CRT will be more cost-effective in such a population.[27]

Cardiac rehabilitation and exercise training

Studies published in the 1990s addressed physiologic benefits that accrue with physical activity in patients with systolic HF. Aerobic exercise training was shown to increase cardiac output at submaximal and peak exercise and reduce systemic vascular resistance and sympathetic activity.[28] An increase in skeletal muscle mitochondrial density and the resultant increase in oxidative capacity are other benefits of physical training.[29] Subsequently, a relatively small Italian single-center study (99 patients) demonstrated the possibility of reducing mortality and HF hospitalizations with long-term moderate exercise training.[30] This and 8 other small European trials were the subject of a meta-analysis of 801 patients, which concluded that aerobic exercise training reduced mortality and hospitalizations.[31] Last, HF-ACTION, a large, multicenter randomized control trial of exercise training in systolic HF showed a significant reduction in all-cause mortality and hospitalization, after adjusting for 4 highly prognostic baseline variables.[32] Based on these results, CMS expanded coverage for cardiac rehabilitation services for patients with chronic systolic HF (left ventricular ejection fraction of 35% or less) and NYHA class II to IV symptoms despite being on optimal therapy for at least 6 weeks. To qualify for coverage, patients should not have had recent (≤6 weeks) or planned (≤6 months) major cardiovascular hospitalizations or procedures. Exercise training has been shown to be very cost-effective compared with other therapies.[33]

Palliative care

Palliative care is widely misunderstood to represent only end-of-life care. The current World Health Organization definition of palliative care calls for its implementation early in the course of an eventually life-threatening illness, along with other treatments that are intended to prolong life. In addition to symptom and pain relief, palliative care should also enable patients to live an active life and offer support to the involved families.[34] In 2011, HF contributed to 284,388 deaths, which is similar to the same figure from 2005.[35] Palliative care utilization in advanced HF remains low despite the fact that total deaths related to HF is higher than the combined deaths from breast, lung, and prostate cancers as well as human immunodeficiency virus.[36] Consulting with palliative care teams has been shown to result in considerable cost savings among hospitalized patients with serious illnesses.[37] Timely initiation of palliative care will ensure that symptoms usually not perceived to be due to cardiovascular illness (such as pain and depression, which are rather common in HF patients) are addressed, and eventually hospice care does not get delayed unnecessarily.

ALTERNATIVES TO HOSPITALIZATION

At many of the US hospitals, it is an exception when a patient presenting to an emergency room (ER) with HF exacerbation does not get admitted. Hospital admissions are expensive and may not be necessary in all patients with HF exacerbation. The difficulty in predicting a patient's clinical course and fear of an adverse outcome might be factors that influence the physician decision to admit all patients with HF exacerbation. Many patients present with milder exacerbation of chronic HF that may be related to temporary diet indiscretion or medication nonadherence and may not require admission to the hospital. Local treatment patterns and culture may also play a role as evident from a multinational study, which showed a higher rate of patients being discharged home from the ER in Western Europe compared with the United States.[38] Only a minority of patients admitted for HF exacerbation undergoes invasive procedures or has a need for intense monitoring that could only be performed in a hospital setting.[39] Alternative approaches to managing certain patients with HF exacerbation may be cost-effective.

Discharge from Emergency Room

Currently, 80% of patients presenting to the ER with HF are admitted.[40] Although studies from the late 1990s showed a high post-ER discharge event rate, it is not clear if intensive outpatient follow-up will reduce such events.[41] A 2-step ER risk stratification has been suggested to divert patients toward 1 of 3 treatment pathways: inpatient admission, observation, or ER discharge, depending on their condition at presentation, comorbidities, and response to initial therapy in the ER.[42]

Observation Units

Observation units have been used for various diagnoses ranging from chest pain to minor infections, with the aim of discharging certain patients within a short period of time, usually within 10 to 24 hours. The cost of care for the payer is lower in an observation unit, because it is considered outpatient treatment and reimbursed at lower rates. It is estimated that 50% of HF patients presenting to the ED are eligible for treatment in observation units, and of these patients, 75% can be discharged from the observation unit.[42] Small studies have indicated that this approach is safe and feasible, with results comparable to inpatient admissions.[43]

Outpatient Infusion Centers

Chronic HF patients, being followed serially by a hospital-based team that is familiar with them, can have episodes of milder HF exacerbations managed by outpatient titration of oral diuretic therapy with provisional intravenous loop diuretics in an outpatient setting.[44,45]

DETECTING PRECLINICAL HEART FAILURE EXACERBATION

Technological advances have made it feasible to obtain continuous direct (pressure sensor) and indirect measurements (via measurement of intrathoracic impedance) of intracardiac pressures. It has been shown that right ventricular pressures increase well in advance of symptom deterioration leading to hospitalization.[46] However, a randomized trial evaluating the utility of a right ventricular pressure monitoring device (Chronicle; Medtronic Inc, Minneapolis, MN, USA) in 274 patients failed to demonstrate a statistically significant reduction in the primary endpoint of HF-related events.[47] A left atrial pressure monitoring device (HeartPOD; St Jude Medical Inc, Minneapolis, MN, USA) has been shown to be feasible and safe in a small observational study of 40 patients, and publication of a larger randomized trial is awaited.[48] Measurement of impedance across the thoracic cavity, which is inversely related to the pulmonary fluid content, has been shown to predict HF exacerbations.[49]

Impedance measurement could be performed with currently available implantable defibrillators as well as biventricular pacemakers and has the advantage of not needing a separate device. Monthly review of varying types of data including duration of atrial fibrillation, rapidity of ventricular response during atrial fibrillation, low patient activity level, defibrillator shocks, and evidence for autonomic dysfunction (poor heart rate variability) in addition to transthoracic impedance in patients with systolic HF who have a biventricular pacemaker-defibrillator identifies patients at high risk for HF hospitalizations.[50] However, randomized trial evidence validating this observation is still lacking.

Recently, a completely wireless, memoryless, and batteryless device that can be inserted into a pulmonary arterial branch and which could transmit radiofrequency signals to an external monitor (CardioMEMS; St. Jude Medical) has obtained approval from the US Food and Drug Administration for clinical use. A randomized trial of 550 patients, all of whom received the device, with 270 patients assigned to the treatment group, demonstrated a 39% reduction in HF hospitalizations.[51]

There is not enough evidence that such advanced technology makes a difference in real world clinical practice, and more importantly, if such technology is cost-effective.

CONTROVERSIES REGARDING READMISSION REDUCTION

Everyone agrees that reducing unnecessary hospitalizations and health care expenditure is a priority for the US health care system. However, hospitals are being penalized for exceeding an arbitrary target readmission rate, which although risk-adjusted has not been validated in multiple populations independently.[52] If a center admits a lot of low-risk, mild HF exacerbations, it is conceivable that their readmission rates will be lower. On the other hand, a center that effectively avoids admitting its lower risk HF patients will naturally select for a higher risk pool of patients being admitted, and it is likely that these patients will have a higher rate of readmissions and further efforts to reduce readmissions may be fruitless. Furthermore, there are not any rewards for preventing a target number of readmissions, but penalties are rather heavy for excess readmissions. Although the CMS readmission measure is risk adjusted, it does not account for differences in social support and economic inequalities, which play a significant role in the ability of patients to adhere to treatment recommendations. It is to be seen if targeting readmission rates will lead to significant cost savings, and more importantly, lead to improved patient outcomes.

REFERENCES

1. Available at: http://www.cdc.gov/nchs/data/hus/hus13.pdf#112. Accessed January 11, 2015.
2. Available at: http://www.hcup-us.ahrq.gov/reports/statbriefs/sb160.jsp. Accessed January 11, 2015.
3. Heidenreich PA, Albert NM, Allen LA, et al, American Heart Association Advocacy Coordinating Committee, Council on Arteriosclerosis, Thrombosis and Vascular Biology, Council on Cardiovascular Radiology and Intervention, Council on Clinical Cardiology, Council on Epidemiology and Prevention, Stroke Council. Forecasting the impact of heart failure in the United States: a policy statement from the American Heart Association. Circ Heart Fail 2013; 6(3):606–19.
4. Anderson GF, Steinberg EP. Hospital readmissions in the Medicare population. N Engl J Med 1984; 311(21):1349–53.
5. Jencks SF, Williams MV, Coleman EA. Rehospitalizations among patients in the Medicare fee-for-service program. N Engl J Med 2009;360(14):1418–28.
6. Bueno H, Ross JS, Wang Y, et al. Trends in length of stay and short-term outcomes among Medicare patients hospitalized for heart failure, 1993-2006. JAMA 2010;303(21):2141–7.
7. Epstein AM, Jha AK, Orav EJ. The relationship between hospital admission rates and rehospitalizations. N Engl J Med 2011;365(24):2287–95.
8. Joynt KE, Orav EJ, Jha AK. Thirty-day readmission rates for Medicare beneficiaries by race and site of care. JAMA 2011;305(7):675–81.
9. Joynt KE, Jha AK. Who has higher readmission rates for heart failure, and why? Implications for efforts to improve care using financial incentives. Circ Cardiovasc Qual Outcomes 2011;4(1):53–9.
10. Kansagara D, Englander H, Salanitro A, et al. Risk prediction models for hospital readmission: a systematic review. JAMA 2011;306(15):1688–98.
11. Hernandez AF, Greiner MA, Fonarow GC, et al. Relationship between early physician follow-up and 30-day readmission among Medicare beneficiaries hospitalized for heart failure. JAMA 2010;303(17): 1716–22.
12. Peikes D, Chen A, Schore J, et al. Effects of care coordination on hospitalization, quality of care, and health care expenditures among Medicare beneficiaries: 15 randomized trials. JAMA 2009;301(6): 603–18.
13. Rich MW, Beckham V, Wittenberg C, et al. A multidisciplinary intervention to prevent the readmission of elderly patients with congestive heart failure. N Engl J Med 1995;333(18):1190–5.
14. Effect of enalapril on survival in patients with reduced left ventricular ejection fractions and congestive heart failure. The SOLVD investigators. N Engl J Med 1991;325(5):293–302.
15. Cohn JN, Tognoni G, Valsartan Heart Failure Trial Investigators. A randomized trial of the angiotensin-receptor blocker valsartan in chronic heart failure. N Engl J Med 2001;345(23):1667–75.
16. Granger CB, McMurray JJ, Yusuf S, et al, CHARM Investigators and Committees. Effects of candesartan in patients with chronic heart failure and reduced left-ventricular systolic function intolerant to angiotensin-converting-enzyme inhibitors: the CHARM-alternative trial. Lancet 2003;362(9386): 772–6.
17. Packer M, Coats AJ, Fowler MB, et al, Carvedilol Prospective Randomized Cumulative Survival Study Group. Effect of carvedilol on survival in severe chronic heart failure. N Engl J Med 2001;344(22): 1651–8.
18. The Cardiac Insufficiency Bisoprolol Study II (CIBIS-II): a randomised trial. Lancet 1999;353(9146):9–13.
19. Pitt B, Zannad F, Remme WJ, et al. The effect of spironolactone on morbidity and mortality in patients with severe heart failure. Randomized Aldactone Evaluation Study investigators. N Engl J Med 1999; 341(10):709–17.
20. Pitt B, Remme W, Zannad F, et al, Eplerenone Post-Acute Myocardial Infarction Heart Failure Efficacy and Survival Study Investigators. Eplerenone, a selective aldosterone blocker, in patients with left ventricular dysfunction after myocardial infarction [Erratum appears in N Engl J Med. 2003;348(22):2271]. N Engl J Med 2003;348(14): 1309–21.
21. Digitalis Investigation Group. The effect of digoxin on mortality and morbidity in patients with heart failure. N Engl J Med 1997;336(8):525–33.
22. Pitt B, Pfeffer MA, Assmann SF, et al, TOPCAT Investigators. Spironolactone for heart failure with

preserved ejection fraction. N Engl J Med 2014; 370(15):1383–92.

23. Pfeffer MA, Claggett B, Assmann SF, et al. Regional variation in patients and outcomes in the treatment of preserved cardiac function heart failure with an aldosterone antagonist (TOPCAT) trial. Circulation 2015;131(1):34–42.

24. Bristow MR, Saxon LA, Boehmer J, et al, Comparison of Medical Therapy, Pacing, and Defibrillation in Heart Failure (COMPANION) Investigators. Cardiac-resynchronization therapy with or without an implantable defibrillator in advanced chronic heart failure. N Engl J Med 2004;350(21):2140–50.

25. Cleland JG, Daubert JC, Erdmann E, et al, Cardiac Resynchronization-Heart Failure (CARE-HF) Study Investigators. The effect of cardiac resynchronization on morbidity and mortality in heart failure. N Engl J Med 2005;352(15):1539–49.

26. Feldman AM, de Lissovoy G, Bristow MR, et al. Cost effectiveness of cardiac resynchronization therapy in the comparison of medical therapy, pacing, and defibrillation in heart failure (COMPANION) trial. J Am Coll Cardiol 2005;46(12): 2311–21.

27. Peterson PN, Greiner MA, Qualls LG, et al. QRS duration, bundle-branch block morphology, and outcomes among older patients with heart failure receiving cardiac resynchronization therapy. JAMA 2013;310(6):617–26.

28. Coats AJ, Adamopoulos S, Radaelli A, et al. Controlled trial of physical training in chronic heart failure. Exercise performance, hemodynamics, ventilation, and autonomic function. Circulation 1992;85(6):2119–31.

29. Hambrecht R, Niebauer J, Fiehn E, et al. Physical training in patients with stable chronic heart failure: effects on cardiorespiratory fitness and ultrastructural abnormalities of leg muscles. J Am Coll Cardiol 1995;25(6):1239–49.

30. Belardinelli R, Georgiou D, Cianci G, et al. Randomized, controlled trial of long-term moderate exercise training in chronic heart failure: effects on functional capacity, quality of life, and clinical outcome. Circulation 1999;99(9):1173–82.

31. Piepoli MF, Davos C, Francis DP, et al, ExTraMATCH Collaborative. Exercise training meta-analysis of trials in patients with chronic heart failure (ExTraMATCH). BMJ 2004;328(7433):189.

32. O'Connor CM, Whellan DJ, Lee KL, et al, HF-ACTION Investigators. Efficacy and safety of exercise training in patients with chronic heart failure: HF-ACTION randomized controlled trial. JAMA 2009; 301(14):1439–50.

33. Georgiou D, Chen Y, Appadoo S, et al. Cost-effectiveness analysis of long-term moderate exercise training in chronic heart failure. Am J Cardiol 2001; 87(8):984–8.

34. World Health Organization's definition of palliative care. Available at: http://www.who.int/cancer/palliative/definition/en/. Accessed January 11, 2015.

35. Mozaffarian D, Benjamin EJ, Go AS, et al, American Heart Association Statistics Committee and Stroke Statistics Subcommittee. Executive summary: heart disease and stroke statistics—2015 update: a report from the American Heart Association. Circulation 2015;131(4):434–41.

36. Adler ED, Goldfinger JZ, Kalman J, et al. Palliative care in the treatment of advanced heart failure. Circulation 2009;120(25):2597–606.

37. Morrison RS, Penrod JD, Cassel JB, et al, Palliative Care Leadership Centers' Outcomes Group. Cost savings associated with US hospital palliative care consultation programs. Arch Intern Med 2008; 168(16):1783–90.

38. Collins SP, Pang PS, Lindsell CJ, et al. International variations in the clinical, diagnostic, and treatment characteristics of emergency department patients with acute heart failure syndromes. Eur J Heart Fail 2010;12(11):1253–60.

39. Adams KF Jr, Fonarow GC, Emerman CL, et al, ADHERE Scientific Advisory Committee and Investigators. Characteristics and outcomes of patients hospitalized for heart failure in the United States: rationale, design, and preliminary observations from the first 100,000 cases in the Acute Decompensated Heart Failure National Registry (ADHERE). Am Heart J 2005;149(2):209–16.

40. Weintraub NL, Collins SP, Pang PS, et al, American Heart Association Council on Clinical Cardiology and Council on Cardiopulmonary, Critical Care, Perioperative and Resuscitation. Acute heart failure syndromes: emergency department presentation, treatment, and disposition: current approaches and future aims: a scientific statement from the American Heart Association. Circulation 2010; 122(19):1975–96.

41. Rame JE, Sheffield MA, Dries DL, et al. Outcomes after emergency department discharge with a primary diagnosis of heart failure. Am Heart J 2001; 142(4):714–9.

42. Collins SP, Pang PS, Fonarow GC, et al. Is hospital admission for heart failure really necessary?: the role of the emergency department and observation unit in preventing hospitalization and rehospitalization. J Am Coll Cardiol 2013;61(2):121–6.

43. Storrow AB, Collins SP, Lyons MS, et al. Emergency department observation of heart failure: preliminary analysis of safety and cost. Congest Heart Fail 2005;11(2):68–72.

44. Ryder M, Murphy NF, McCaffrey D, et al. Outpatient intravenous diuretic therapy; potential for marked reduction in hospitalisations for acute decompensated heart failure. Eur J Heart Fail 2008;10(3): 267–72.

45. Lazkani M, Ota KS. The role of outpatient intravenous diuretic therapy in a transitional care program for patients with heart failure: a case series. J Clin Med Res 2012;4(6):434–8.

46. Adamson PB, Magalski A, Braunschweig F, et al. Ongoing right ventricular hemodynamics in heart failure: clinical value of measurements derived from an implantable monitoring system. J Am Coll Cardiol 2003;41(4):565–71.

47. Bourge RC, Abraham WT, Adamson PB, et al, COMPASS-HF Study Group. Randomized controlled trial of an implantable continuous hemodynamic monitor in patients with advanced heart failure: the COMPASS-HF study. J Am Coll Cardiol 2008; 51(11):1073–9.

48. Ritzema J, Troughton R, Melton I, et al, Hemodynamically Guided Home Self-Therapy in Severe Heart Failure Patients (HOMEOSTASIS) Study Group. Physician-directed patient self-management of left atrial pressure in advanced chronic heart failure. Circulation 2010;121(9):1086–95.

49. Catanzariti D, Lunati M, Landolina M, et al, Italian Clinical Service Optivol-CRT Group. Monitoring intrathoracic impedance with an implantable defibrillator reduces hospitalizations in patients with heart failure. Pacing Clin Electrophysiol 2009;32(3): 363–70.

50. Whellan DJ, Ousdigian KT, Al-Khatib SM, et al, PARTNERS Study Investigators. Combined heart failure device diagnostics identify patients at higher risk of subsequent heart failure hospitalizations: results from PARTNERS HF (Program to Access and Review Trending Information and Evaluate Correlation to Symptoms in Patients With Heart Failure) study. J Am Coll Cardiol 2010; 55(17):1803–10.

51. Abraham WT, Adamson PB, Bourge RC, et al, CHAMPION Trial Study Group. Wireless pulmonary artery haemodynamic monitoring in chronic heart failure: a randomised controlled trial. Lancet 2011; 377(9766):658–66.

52. Keenan PS, Normand SL, Lin Z, et al. An administrative claims measure suitable for profiling hospital performance on the basis of 30-day all-cause readmission rates among patients with heart failure. Circ Cardiovasc Qual Outcomes 2008;1(1):29–37.

Ventricular Dyssynchrony and Resynchronization: From Bench to Bedside

Cellular and Molecular Aspects of Dyssynchrony and Resynchronization

Jonathan A. Kirk, PhD*, David A. Kass, MD

KEYWORDS

- Dyssynchrony • Cardiac resynchronization therapy • Animal models • Myocyte • Myofilament

KEY POINTS

- In some instances, cardiac resynchronization therapy (CRT) does not simply reverse the damage done by dyssynchrony, but acts in novel ways to improve function.
- Progress has been made to understand the cellular and molecular mechanisms of cardiac dyssynchrony and resynchronization therapy and these insights are helping both understand the key pathways involved and establish better biomarkers for CRT responsiveness.
- It may be possible to extract a mechanism pertinent to a CRT benefit, and then apply this as its own therapy to patients who have synchronous HF and thus are not suitable for CRT.

INTRODUCTION: CARDIAC DYSSYNCHRONY AND RESYNCHRONIZATION THERAPY

Contraction of the left ventricle is precisely coordinated by the His-Purkinje system, which rapidly conducts electrical excitation to the myocardium. This system ensures that fiber shortening throughout the muscle wall occurs synchronously and by a similar magnitude to help optimize pump efficiency. Diseases of the conducting system, such as a left bundle branch block (LBBB), lead to a loss of synchrony, and occur in 30% to 50% of patients with dilated cardiomyopathy.[1,2] As a result, regions of the heart stimulated early contract sooner and at reduced load,[3] and, rather than generating sufficient pressure to open the aortic valve and eject blood, they impart energy to stretch the later-activated regions. The opposite happens in late systole, in which delayed-contracting regions can stretch regions stimulated earlier.[3] The net transfer of blood internally within the heart results in heterogeneity of myocardial work[4] and a reduction in mechanoenergetic performance.[5,6] In the failing heart, in which function is already reduced, dyssynchrony worsens both morbidity and mortality.[7]

Pioneering studies in the 1990s[8–10] showed that multisite artificial pacing improved left ventricular (LV) function, and this ultimately led to cardiac resynchronization therapy (CRT). CRT involves simultaneous biventricular preexcitation, and when applied to dyssynchronous hearts it improves function[10] and chamber efficiency,[11,12] while concomitantly reducing morbidity and mortality.[13,14] To date, CRT remains the singular therapy for heart failure (HF) that simultaneously improves both acute and chronic systolic function, increases cardiac work, and also prolongs survival.

CRT has traditionally been viewed as a mechanical tuning of the heart. Its simplicity and ease of

Disclosure: The authors have nothing to disclose.
Funding Sources: This work was supported by NIH grants P01-HL077180, HL-114910, HL-112586, Fondation Leducq and Peter Belfer Laboratory, Proteomic Initiative contract HHSN268201000032C, and Abraham and Virginia Weiss Professorship (D.A. Kass), and the American Heart Association (14SDG20380148 to J.A. Kirk).
Division of Cardiology, Department of Medicine, Johns Hopkins University School of Medicine, Ross Research Building, Room 858, 720 Rutland Avenue, Baltimore, MD 21205, USA
* Corresponding author. North Entrance, Building 102, 2160 S. First Avenue, Maywood, IL 60153.
E-mail address: jkirk2@luc.edu

entry into the clinic led to rapid development, testing, and approval; all performed in human subjects. There was little basic science on CRT reported before its clinical adaption. However, there have recently been efforts to reverse engineer CRT, exploring the cellular and molecular mechanisms that are involved. Dyssynchrony and resynchronization therapy induce a wide range of changes beyond the mechanical effects, many of which are unique to both the disease and the treatment.[15–19] In some instances, CRT does not simply reverse the damage done by dyssynchrony, it acts in novel ways to improve function. This article explores the extensive set of cellular and molecular mechanisms chronically and acutely induced by dyssynchrony and CRT.

BEYOND LEFT VENTRICULAR MECHANICS

Although there is little doubt that global cardiac mechanics is a major mechanism behind dysfunction of dyssynchrony and recovery with CRT, key issues indicate that there is more going on. The first is what is referred to as the nonresponder rate, and the second is the lack of relationship between apparent resynchronization and response.

Current guidelines identify CRT as a class I recommendation for patients with a QRS complex greater than 150 milliseconds (and ejection fraction <35%), and a class IIa recommendation for patients with a QRS complex between 120 and 150 milliseconds.[20,21] However, of the patients who receive CRT, approximately one-third show no clinical or morphometric response to the therapy.[22,23] This nonresponder rate has plagued the field, and despite significant efforts, has remained steady. One of these major efforts was the multicenter PROSPECT (Predictors of Response to CRT) trial, which used tissue-Doppler techniques to quantify regional wall motion to determine dyssynchrony and predict response to CRT. However, despite the rigorous study design, there was little predictive capability[24] and the nonresponder rate persisted. Although efforts continue in this area, alternative hypotheses have emerged to identify responders from other biomarkers. In this regard, understanding the cellular and molecular mechanisms of dyssynchrony and CRT may provide targets that could serve as such biomarkers.

Beyond the nonresponder rate, once a patient has been implanted with a CRT device and responds to the therapy, the relationship between the magnitude of resynchronization that occurs and magnitude of chronic improvement is weak at best. For example, in a cohort of patients with class I indications for CRT, there was a clear lower limit of resynchronization necessary to observe improvement (based on 10% or greater decline in end-systolic volume).[25] However, if the group of patients who did not resynchronize at all with CRT is removed, there is no correlation between the magnitude of resynchronized wall motion and long-term remodeling (**Fig. 1**). Other studies found similar results using different indices.[26] This finding suggests that there are other important aspects to both dyssynchrony and resynchronization.

MYOCYTE FUNCTION, CALCIUM HANDLING, AND β-ADRENERGIC SIGNALING

Experimental access to myocardial tissue in humans is limited to end-stage hearts at time of transplantation, limiting studies of CRT. Thus, most of the present understanding comes from animal models. Cardiac dyssynchrony can be induced either by right ventricular pacing or from ablation of the left bundle branch, recreating an LBBB. With dog and pigs, it is possible to use existing human pacemaker systems to introduce right ventricular pacing and CRT, superimposed over models of HF such as tachypacing,[27] pressure overload,[28] or volume overload.[29] It is also possible to study dyssynchrony without any underlying HF.[30]

Cardiomyocytes isolated from dyssynchronous failing canine hearts show severely reduced peak sarcomere shortening and slowed contractile kinetics.[31] Similarly, whole-cell calcium transients and their dynamics are reduced.[32–34] These cellular defects are observed globally,[31] rather than being

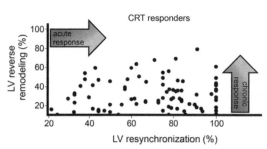

Fig. 1. Immediate LV resynchronization with CRT and change in LV end-systolic volume at 6-month follow-up. An acute response to CRT (>20% LV resynchronization) is necessary for a positive chronic response (>10% LV reverse remodeling), but among these responders there is almost no relationship between acute and chronic response. Therefore, acute hemodynamic response to CRT has little ability to predict long-term benefit. (*From* Bleeker GB, Mollema SA, Holman ER, et al. Left ventricular resynchronization is mandatory for response to cardiac resynchronization therapy: analysis in patients with echocardiographic evidence of left ventricular dyssynchrony at baseline. Circulation 2007;116:1444; with permission.)

specific to early-activated or late-activated territories. CRT significantly reverses most of these abnormalities[31–33] (**Fig. 2**A). HF without dyssynchrony also impairs calcium handling[35] and sarcomere shortening (see **Fig. 2**A), so these detriments and their reversal by CRT might be considered a function of HF rather than being specific to dyssynchrony. However, despite marked improvement in myocyte function in the canine model, global function is far less enhanced,[35] whereas dyssynchrony is resolved. The former occurs because the model involves tachycardia pacing that is present whether the heart is dyssynchronous or resynchronized, and prevents significant reversal of HF.

Mechanisms underlying calcium handling have been suggested (see **Fig. 2**B), although this remains incompletely understood. Biopsies from humans who responded to CRT showed increased messenger RNA (mRNA) expression of phospholamban (PLN),[36,37] sarcoplasmic reticular Ca^{2+}

ATPase 2A (Serca2A),[38] and sarcolemmal sodium calcium exchanger (NCX).[37] In a canine model of dyssynchronous HF, protein expression of PLN and Serca2A decreased[39] (NCX increased), but CRT did not improve their expression levels despite enhanced calcium transients.[33] Alternative mechanisms include structural changes to the T-tubules and sarcoplasmic reticulum, where the registration of the ryanodine receptor and membranes in which voltage-gated channels reside becomes disrupted.[34] This is partially reversed toward normal by CRT (see **Fig. 2**C). Another alternative is posttranslational protein modifications (such as phosphorylation or oxidation), although specific causes remain unresolved.

Cardiomyocytes were not just weaker with dyssynchronous HF and stronger with CRT, they also show differences in response to β-adrenergic stimulation.[35] Healthy cardiac myocytes significantly increase both intracellular calcium transients and

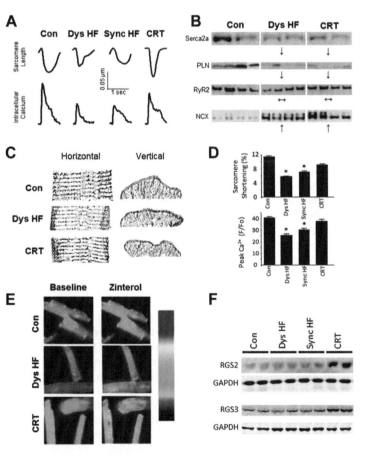

Fig. 2. Dyssynchrony reduced baseline cellular function, which is restored by CRT. (*A*) Myocyte sarcomere shortening and corresponding whole-cell calcium transients in myocytes taken from control (Con), dyssynchronous HF (Dys HF), synchronous HF (Sync HF), and CRT. (*B*) Western blots for calcium handling proteins. Arrows show the direction of change in Dys HF and CRT groups compared with control. (*C*) Three-dimensional reconstructions from confocal microscopic images showing t-tubule structure (*blue*) and ryanodine receptors (*red*). (*D*) In response to isoproterenol, Dys HF showed a much smaller augmentation in sarcomere shortening and calcium transient amplitude, which was reversed by CRT. * *P*<.01 versus all other groups. (*E*) Cell fluorescence ratio–encoded images from myocytes from Con, Dys HF, and CRT. The CRT myocytes showed increased cyclic AMP generation when stimulated with zinterol (β2-adrenergic receptor stimulation). (*F*) RGS2/3 can inhibit Gαi, and were significantly upregulated in CRT. RGS2, Regulator of G-Protein signaling 2. (*Adapted from* Chakir K, Depry C, Dimaano VL, et al. Galphas-biased beta2-adrenergic receptor signaling from restoring synchronous contraction in the failing heart. Sci Transl Med 2011;3:100ra88; with permission; [B] Aiba T, Hesketh GG, Barth AS, et al. Electrophysiological consequences of dyssynchronous heart failure and its restoration by resynchronization therapy. Circulation 2009;119:1220–30; and [C] Sachse FB, Torres NS, Savio-Galimberti E, et al. Subcellular structures and function of myocytes impaired during heart failure are restored by cardiac resynchronization therapy. Circ Res 2012;110:588–97.)

sarcomere shortening when stimulated with isoproterenol. However, myocytes from dyssynchronous HF showed little response to isoproterenol stimulation, whereas CRT restores this to almost normal/healthy levels (see **Fig. 2**D).[35] This finding mirrors changes observed in patients having CRT, who show enhanced responses to cardiac sympathetic stimulation,[40,41] although CRT acutely blunts sympathetic tone.[42]

The mechanism for restored β-adrenergic signaling shows that CRT is not just reestablishing electromechanical synchrony but engages subcellular mechanisms that improve reserve function. HF is characterized by a decline in β-adrenergic stimulation signaling, and this is observed in both synchronous or dyssynchronous forms. β1-Adrenergic receptor plasma membrane density increases with CRT in both humans and canines,[31,43] but CRT also has a novel impact on β2-adrenergic signaling, as shown by a greater increase in cyclic AMP after β2-adrenergic receptor stimulation (zinterol) in myocytes from CRT-treated hearts (see **Fig. 2**E). Inhibitory G protein Gαi couples to β2-adrenergic receptors, and its levels increase in dyssynchronous and synchronous human and canine HF.[44] In canine HF, augmented Gαi signaling reduced cyclic AMP levels and consequent protein kinase A activation at the sarcoplasmic reticulum (SR). Correspondingly, inhibiting Gαi with pertussis toxin (PTX) increased β2-adrenergic stimulation. However, in cells from CRT-treated dogs, the resting β2-adrenergic receptor stimulation response is near normal, and PTX has no further effect, indicating that CRT effectively decouples Gαi signaling. CRT achieved this by increasing expression of 2 negative regulators of this G protein, Regulator of G-Protein signaling 2 (RGS2) and RGS3.[35] This increase did not reverse depression of RGS2/RGS3 expression in dyssynchronous HF, but was a specific change observed in response to resynchronization. Human CRT responders also show increased cardiac LV mRNA levels for RGS2/RGS3, but this is lacking in nonresponders[35] (see **Fig. 2**F).

Another mechanism for altered β-adrenergic signaling involves a shift in parasympathetic modulation by muscarinic acetylcholine receptors (mAChRs). The M2-mAChR couples to Gαi,[45] whereas the M3-mAChR couples to Gq and exerts cardioprotective effects.[46] Dyssynchrony results in an increase in M2-mAChR, and CRT reverses this, while additionally increasing M3-mAChRs.[47]

ION CHANNELS

HF is often associated with prolonged action potential duration (APD)[48] caused by abnormalities of many membrane channels.[49–52] Dyssynchrony

introduces marked heterogeneity in APD, further lengthening APD in the late-activated lateral wall.[32,33] This heterogeneity can contribute to ventricular arrhythmias, a common cause of death from HF, and in human patients CRT reduces ventricular arrhythmias.[53–58] Even in dogs without LV dysfunction, dyssynchrony from left bundle branch ablation introduces regional APD heterogeneity.[30]

APD is determined by the magnitude and timing of inward and outward currents in the myocyte. Dyssynchronous HF reduces repolarizing potassium currents, including the inward rectifier K^+ current (I_{K1}), transient outward K^+ current (I_{to}), and delayed rectifier K^+ current (I_K),[33] concordant with less protein expression in corresponding channel proteins: Kir 2.1, Kv4.3 and KChIP2, and KvLQT1, respectively. CRT partially reverses changes in I_{K1}, and I_K (but not I_{to}) and their related proteins.[33,59]

One current whose increase is linked to prolongation of APD is the late sodium current, and this is augmented in HF.[60] Treating cells from dyssynchronous HF dogs with ranolazine, a relatively selective I_{Na-L} inhibitor, significantly reduces APD (**Fig. 3**), but has little impact on myocytes from nonfailing dogs or dogs having CRT.[61] It is known that Ca^{2+}/calmodulin protein kinase II (CaMKII) increases I_{Na-L},[62] and dyssynchrony is associated with an increase in CaMKII activity in the late-activated lateral wall, whereas CRT decreases this activity.[61,63]

MYOFILAMENT FUNCTION AND STRUCTURE

Length-dependent cardiac muscle tension is also an important contributor to CRT efficacy.[64] The dynamic properties of the myofilament are carefully controlled during a normal cardiac cycle, but introduction of systolic stretch, as occurs in dyssynchrony, perturbs this.[65] By precisely timing stretch in isolated mouse papillary muscles relative to their electrical stimulation, Tangney and colleagues[66] developed an in vitro model of acute dyssynchrony. Time-varying stiffness and force-velocity relationships played only a small role in explaining the tension that a dyssynchronous muscle generated. Instead, the dominant mechanism was transient deactivation,[66] in which stretching the activated muscle led to cross-bridge detachment.[67] Thus, acute electromechanical decoupling alters myofilament properties.

Chronic dyssynchrony further changes myofilament function, depressing the responsiveness of sarcomere force development to calcium stimulation (**Fig. 4**A).[68] This change is opposite that observed with synchronous HF, which increases

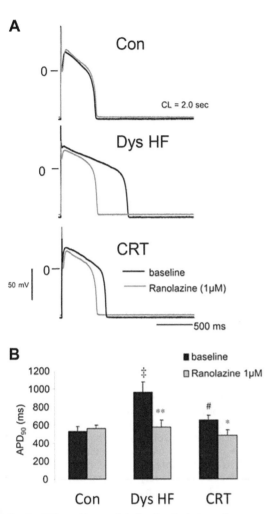

Fig. 3. APD and its modulation by the late sodium current. (A) Action potentials from myocytes isolated from the lateral wall in Con, Dys HF, and CRT, showing significantly longer APD in Dys HF, which is mostly reversed with CRT. Using ranolazine to block the late sodium current (I_{Na-L}) shortened APD in Dys HF, but had no affect on Con or CRT myocytes. CL, cycle length. (B) APD duration at 90% repolarization at baseline and after ranolazine. ‡ $P<0.01$ vs NF; # $P<0.01$ vs DHF by ANOVA with Bonferroni test; ** $P<0.01$; * $P<0.05$ vs baseline by paired t test. (Adapted from Aiba T, Barth AS, Hesketh GG, et al. Cardiac resynchronization therapy improves altered Na channel gating in canine model of dyssynchronous heart failure. Circ Arrhythm Electrophysiol 2013;6:551; with permission.)

calcium sensitivity in humans[69] and canines,[68,70] changes thought to be caused by a decline of protein kinase A (PKA)-phosphorylation of cardiac troponin I (TnI) at serines 22 and 23.[71] This oversensitization can result in diastolic dysfunction[72] and arrhythmias.[73] Because reduced TnI phosphorylation is also observed in dyssynchronous HF,

something else must explain the decline in sensitivity in this setting. To determine this mechanism, we first explored how CRT affects the myofilament and found that it fully recovers calcium sensitivity (see **Fig. 4**B) to normal/healthy levels.[74,75] The mechanism of improvement involved enhanced phosphorylation of myofilament proteins and, from proteomic analysis, a candidate kinase that could explain this was shown to be glycogen synthase kinase 3β[68] (GSK-3β; see **Fig. 4**A, B). This kinase acted on several proteins in the M band and Z disk, regions considered essential for structural scaffolding of the myofilament, which was a novel role for GSK-3β. Dyssynchrony specifically results in GSK-3β inactivation, and CRT reverses this. Treating normal or CRT-treated myocytes with activated GSK-3β had no effect on calcium sensitivity, but restored it in cells from dyssynchronous failing hearts.

In addition to the changes in calcium sensitivity, there is a significant reduction in maximal calcium activated force (F_{max}) with HF in both dyssynchronous and synchronous forms, and this too is restored by CRT[68] (see **Fig. 4**C, D). F_{max} is conventionally normalized to cellular cross-sectional area because it is assumed that a larger cell has more myofibers and thus can generate more force. Myocytes in dyssynchronous HF are enlarged and then return to normal size with CRT (see **Fig. 4**C, D). A similar reduction in myocyte size has been reported in humans after receiving CRT.[76] However, if F_{max} is not normalized to cell cross-sectional area, the forces produced in all 3 groups (healthy, dyssynchronous HF, CRT) are similar,[68] despite the middle group having much larger cells. This similarity could imply that, despite having more myofibers, these are in some way defective. Myocytes from dyssynchronous paced dog hearts show decreased regularity of α-actinin (an integral myofilament Z-disk protein) in both the transverse and longitudinal directions.[77] CRT improves sarcomeric organization, although it does not entirely restore it.

Myofilament structure and tethering are also maintained by the cytoskeleton. In myocytes a major intermediate filament that plays this role, co-localizing with the Z disk, is desmin. In dyssynchronous HF, desmin moves away from the Z disk.[78] Desmin's mechanisms reach beyond myofilament structure in this case, because desmin cleavage products also increase in dyssynchrony and have amyloidlike toxicity for the myocyte. CRT reverses both phenotypes, reducing desmin oligomers and reassociating desmin to the Z-disk.[78] Importantly, desmin cleavage is mediated by its phosphorylation by GSK-3β, the same kinase involved in regulated Z-disk myofilament calcium sensitivity.[68]

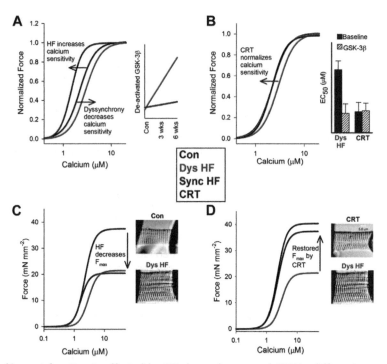

Fig. 4. Myofilament function is affected by HF, dyssynchrony, and CRT in different ways. (*A*) Compared with healthy myocytes (*black*) calcium sensitivity is increased in HF (Sync HF, *dark red*) and decreased in dyssynchronous HF (Dys HF, *red*). This difference is caused by deactivation of glycogen synthase kinase 3β (GSK-3β) in dyssynchronous HF, but not in synchronous HF (*inset*). (*B*) CRT (*blue*) restores calcium sensitivity to normal levels via reactivation of GSK-3β. If Dys HF myocytes are treated with active GSK-3β, the recovery with CRT is recapitulated. However, treating CRT myocytes with GSK-3β had no effect, because the myofilament is already resensitized via this mechanism (*inset*). (*C*) Both Dys HF and Sync HF see a decrease in maximal calcium activated force (F_{max}), and this is caused by an increase in myocyte size (*inset*). (*D*) CRT restores F_{max} by reversing the change in cell size (*inset*). (*Adapted from* Kirk JA, Holewinski RJ, Kooij V, et al. Cardiac resynchronization sensitizes the sarcomere to calcium by reactivating GSK-3beta. J Clin Invest 2014;124:132; with permission.)

MITOCHONDRIA, BIOENERGETICS, AND METABOLOMICS

Changes in energy consumption are a hallmark of HF,[79] and dyssynchronous HF also affects this, not only at the chamber level but also in isolated mitochondria. Molecular metabolic remodeling may be more severe in dyssynchronous HF compared with synchronous HF.[80] Regional disparities in glucose uptake, indicating altered metabolism, occur in the dyssynchronous failing human heart,[81,82] along with diminished substrate metabolism indicated by succinate/glutamate and citrate/glutamate ratios.[83] A pig model of dyssynchronous HF showed a global increase in glucose uptake,[84] but regional changes in hibernation, metabolic activity, and energy turnover.[85] CRT normalizes and harmonizes the metabolic fingerprint,[11,83,86] although it remains distinct from healthy controls.

These findings are further supported by an extensive analysis of the circulating glycoproteome

from the dog model of dyssynchrony. There were 32 glycosite-containing peptides in dyssynchronous HF, and these suggested altered cardiac metabolism; CRT fixed about one-third of these.[87] There remains ongoing debate as to whether a patient's metabolomic profile may also prove a useful biomarker to predict response to CRT.[88,89]

Corresponding with changes in global metabolism, dyssynchrony and CRT also affect mitochondrial function, with increased basal mitochondrial oxygen consumption with dyssynchronous HF compared with healthy controls or CRT-treated hearts.[90] Metabolites that feed into the Krebs cycle are increased in CRT, including pyruvate carboxylase and pyruvate dehydrogenase, and a proteomic analysis revealed 31 mitochondrial proteins altered by CRT, almost half of these involved in the respiratory chain.[90]

Cardiac dyssynchrony has also been associated with a decrease in ATPase activity, whereas CRT increased ATP synthetic capacity to healthy levels.[91] When exposed to reducing conditions, ATPase activity in dyssynchronous HF increased to levels similar to control and CRT myocardium, suggesting an increased oxidative environment in dyssynchronous HF. Cys294 was S-glutathionylated and CRT suppressed this while favoring S-nitrosylation at the same residue. S-nitrosylation of ATP synthase alpha occurs in ischemic precondioning and may be cardioprotective.[92] Thus, the S-nitrosylation/S-glutathionylation balance seems to be a regulatory mechanism for ATP-synthase that is targeted by CRT.

CIRCULATING INDICATORS OF DYSSYNCHRONY AND RESYNCHRONIZATION THERAPY

Several circulating biomarkers have also been explored for their potential to identify patient responsiveness to CRT.[93] For some this may reflect improved HF, whereas others are more specific to the restoration of synchrony. One example involves members of the extracellular matrix (ECM) regulating proteins, matrix metalloproteinases (MMPs), which degrade the ECM, and tissue inhibitors of matrix metalloproteinases (TIMPs), which inhibit MMPS. In a prospective study involving 42 patients who received CRT, baseline plasma TIMP-1 levels predicted CRT response (MMP-2 was borderline) at 12-month follow-up,[94] as well as long-term mortality.[95] Plasma levels of another ECM regulatory protein, galectin-3, predicted patients who benefited most from CRT, because the highest quartile of pre-CRT serum galectin-3 levels showed a disproportionately larger benefit from CRT.[96]

However, there is variability in these results. Other studies using serum found no baseline differences in MMP-1 or TIMP-1 between responders and nonresponders, but did find that MMP-1 and MMP-9 levels correlated with outcomes.[97–99] Another study showed a decrease in MMP-2 and an increase in TIMP-2 in 27 CRT responders, but had no nonresponders to compare them with.[100] Whether these enzymes will provide a useful biomarker to predict CRT response remains unclear, but the studies show that ECM remodeling is involved with both dyssynchrony and CRT.

Several other circulating biomarkers show promise as predictors of response before CRT. CRT responders showed lower baseline (pre-CRT) plasma levels of cardiotrophin-1, which induces a hypertrophic response, and tumor necrosis factor alpha, which can trigger apoptosis, compared with nonreponders.[101,102] Endothelial progenitor cells (EPCs) are stem cells that can mature into endothelial cells that contribute to neoangiogenesis. They are a heterogeneous population of cells, but 2 distinct types ($CD34^+CD133^+KDR^+$ and $CD45^{dim}CD34^+KDR^+CXCR4^+$) were at significantly higher levels at baseline in responders than in nonresponders.[103] CRT super-responders (patients who experience a near normalization of cardiac function with CRT[104]) showed still higher levels of both types of EPCs. Thus, it seems that CRT responders (and super-responders) have an increased capacity for vascular remodeling before CRT.

Recent evidence has shown that tiny noncoding RNAs (microRNAs [miRNAs]) are important regulators of cardiac function.[105] Using a small discovery cohort, and a validation cohort of 40 patients, circulating levels of miR-30d were predictors of beneficial remodeling 6 months post-CRT.[106] It was independent from and had better predictive capacity than any clinical variable. Mechanistically, miR-30d is expressed in myocytes, increased in response to cell stretch, and protects against apoptosis.[106] Another study examined 84 circulating miRNAs, and found that patients with dyssynchronous HF showed a decrease in 24, compared with healthy control patients.[107] Post-CRT, responders saw an increase in 19 circulating miRNAs, whereas nonresponders only saw an increase in 6, and even these 6 increased less than responders.[107] However, there were no baseline differences between responders and nonresponders, so these could not act as predictive biomarkers. However, these circulating miRNAs that were improved by CRT are known to regulate a variety of cellular functions that CRT has been shown to improve, including apoptosis, membrane ion currents, hypertrophic signaling, and fibrosis.[108]

There are other circulating markers that mirror the cellular and molecular mechanisms of CRT but fail to predict response to CRT. Annexin A5 levels decrease in CRT responders and are unchanged in nonresponders.[109] Annexin A5 is a proapoptotic protein,[110,111] and resynchronization has been shown to have antiapoptotic effects.[63,112] The neutrophil/lymphocyte ratio decreases in responders and increases in nonresponders, and although there were no baseline differences, there was a trend ($P = .20$) toward lower levels in responders.[113] Responses also correlated with changes in levels of G-coupled receptor ligand apelin[37,114] (increases with CRT) and various glycoproteins.[87]

FUTURE DIRECTIONS

Progress has been made in understanding the cellular and molecular mechanisms of cardiac dyssynchrony and CRT (**Fig. 5**) and these insights

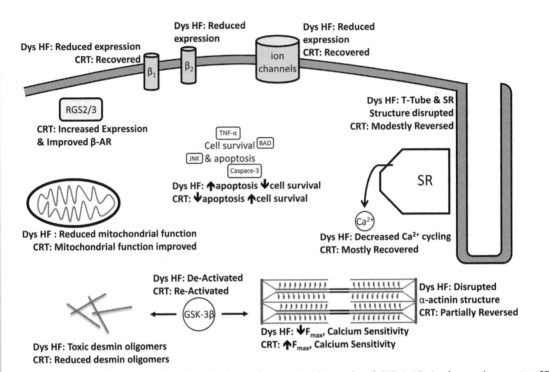

Fig. 5. Summary of molecular alterations in dyssynchronous HF (Dys HF) and CRT. β-AR, β-adrenergic receptor; SR, sarcoplasmic reticulum.

are helping both to understand the key pathways involved and to establish better biomarkers for CRT responsiveness. However, to date, no controlled studies have been performed to test these novel biomarkers. Another potential application of these insights is to extract a mechanism pertinent to a CRT benefit and then apply this as its own therapy to patients who have synchronous HF and thus are not suitable for CRT. At present, the benefits of CRT can only be applied to the subset of patients with HF with underlying dyssynchrony.[115] The large animal models used to date have yielded substantial insights, but they have their limitations, including cost and lack of genetic control. The only article to date reported results from an acute (7–10 days) mouse model of dyssynchrony,[116] and methodological development continues to establish robust chronic pacing in mice.[117] As these efforts begin to produce results, it should allow unprecedented exploration of the cellular and molecular aspects of regional mechanosignaling in the heart relevant to the mysteries of dyssynchrony and improvements from CRT.

REFERENCES

1. Ghio S, Constantin C, Klersy C, et al. Interventricular and intraventricular dyssynchrony are common in heart failure patients, regardless of QRS duration. Eur Heart J 2004;25:571–8.

2. Schuster I, Habib G, Jego C, et al. Diastolic asynchrony is more frequent than systolic asynchrony in dilated cardiomyopathy and is less improved by cardiac resynchronization therapy. J Am Coll Cardiol 2005;46:2250–7.

3. Prinzen FW, Hunter WC, Wyman BT, et al. Mapping of regional myocardial strain and work during ventricular pacing: experimental study using magnetic resonance imaging tagging. J Am Coll Cardiol 1999;33:1735–42.

4. Vernooy K, Verbeek XA, Peschar M, et al. Left bundle branch block induces ventricular remodelling and functional septal hypoperfusion. Eur Heart J 2005;26:91–8.

5. Burkhoff D, Oikawa RY, Sagawa K. Influence of pacing site on canine left ventricular contraction. Am J Physiol 1986;251:H428–35.

6. Park RC, Little WC, O'Rourke RA. Effect of alteration of left ventricular activation sequence on the left ventricular end-systolic pressure-volume relation in closed-chest dogs. Circ Res 1985;57:706–17.

7. Bader H, Garrigue S, Lafitte S, et al. Intra-left ventricular electromechanical asynchrony. A new independent predictor of severe cardiac events in heart failure patients. J Am Coll Cardiol 2004;43:248–56.

8. Cazeau S, Ritter P, Bakdach S, et al. Four chamber pacing in dilated cardiomyopathy. Pacing Clin Electrophysiol 1994;17:1974–9.

9. Auricchio A, Stellbrink C, Block M, et al. Effect of pacing chamber and atrioventricular delay on

acute systolic function of paced patients with congestive heart failure. The Pacing Therapies for Congestive Heart Failure Study Group. The Guidant Congestive Heart Failure Research Group. Circulation 1999;99:2993–3001.

10. Kass DA, Chen CH, Curry C, et al. Improved left ventricular mechanics from acute VDD pacing in patients with dilated cardiomyopathy and ventricular conduction delay. Circulation 1999;99:1567–73.

11. Nelson GS, Berger RD, Fetics BJ, et al. Left ventricular or biventricular pacing improves cardiac function at diminished energy cost in patients with dilated cardiomyopathy and left bundle-branch block. Circulation 2000;102:3053–9.

12. Ukkonen H, Beanlands RS, Burwash IG, et al. Effect of cardiac resynchronization on myocardial efficiency and regional oxidative metabolism. Circulation 2003;107:28–31.

13. Bristow MR, Saxon LA, Boehmer J, et al. Cardiac-resynchronization therapy with or without an implantable defibrillator in advanced chronic heart failure. N Engl J Med 2004;350:2140–50.

14. Cleland JG, Daubert JC, Erdmann E, et al. The effect of cardiac resynchronization on morbidity and mortality in heart failure. N Engl J Med 2005;352:1539–49.

15. Kirk JA, Kass DA. Electromechanical dyssynchrony and resynchronization of the failing heart. Circ Res 2013;113:765–76.

16. Chakir K, Kass DA. Rethinking resynch: exploring mechanisms of cardiac resynchronization beyond wall motion control. Drug Discov Today Dis Mech 2010;7:e103–7.

17. Helm RH, Spragg DD, Chakir K, et al. Pathobiology of left ventricular dyssynchrony and resynchronization. In: Pacing to support the failing heart. Wiley-Blackwell; 2009. p. 31–56.

18. Spragg DD, Kass DA. Pathobiology of left ventricular dyssynchrony and resynchronization. Prog Cardiovasc Dis 2006;49:26–41.

19. Kass DA. Pathobiology of cardiac dyssynchrony and resynchronization. Heart Rhythm 2009;6:1660–5.

20. Epstein AE, DiMarco JP, Ellenbogen KA, et al. ACC/AHA/HRS 2008 guidelines for device-based therapy of cardiac rhythm abnormalities: a report of the American College of Cardiology/American Heart Association Task Force on Practice Guidelines (Writing Committee to Revise the ACC/AHA/NASPE 2002 Guideline Update for Implantation of Cardiac Pacemakers and Antiarrhythmia Devices): developed in collaboration with the American Association for Thoracic Surgery and Society of Thoracic Surgeons. Circulation 2008;117:e350–408.

21. Tracy CM, Epstein AE, Darbar D, et al. 2012 ACCF/AHA/HRS focused update of the 2008 guidelines

for device-based therapy of cardiac rhythm abnormalities: a report of the American College of Cardiology Foundation/American Heart Association Task Force on Practice Guidelines. J Am Coll Cardiol 2012;60:1297–313.

22. Delgado V, Bax JJ. Assessment of systolic dyssynchrony for cardiac resynchronization therapy is clinically useful. Circulation 2011;123:640–55.

23. Sung RK, Foster E. Assessment of systolic dyssynchrony for cardiac resynchronization therapy is not clinically useful. Circulation 2011;123:656–62.

24. Chung ES, Leon AR, Tavazzi L, et al. Results of the predictors of response to CRT (PROSPECT) trial. Circulation 2008;117:2608–16.

25. Bleeker GB, Mollema SA, Holman ER, et al. Left ventricular resynchronization is mandatory for response to cardiac resynchronization therapy: analysis in patients with echocardiographic evidence of left ventricular dyssynchrony at baseline. Circulation 2007;116:1440–8.

26. Kydd AC, Khan FZ, O'Halloran D, et al. Radial strain delay based on segmental timing and strain amplitude predicts left ventricular reverse remodeling and survival after cardiac resynchronization therapy. Circ Cardiovasc Imaging 2013;6:177–84.

27. Wolff MR, de Tombe PP, Harasawa Y, et al. Alterations in left ventricular mechanics, energetics, and contractile reserve in experimental heart failure. Circ Res 1992;70:516–29.

28. van Oosterhout MF, Arts T, Muijtjens AM, et al. Remodeling by ventricular pacing in hypertrophying dog hearts. Cardiovasc Res 2001;49:771–8.

29. Peschar M, Vernooy K, Vanagt WY, et al. Absence of reverse electrical remodeling during regression of volume overload hypertrophy in canine ventricles. Cardiovasc Res 2003;58:510–7.

30. Spragg DD, Akar FG, Helm RH, et al. Abnormal conduction and repolarization in late-activated myocardium of dyssynchronously contracting hearts. Cardiovasc Res 2005;67:77–86.

31. Chakir K, Daya SK, Aiba T, et al. Mechanisms of enhanced beta-adrenergic reserve from cardiac resynchronization therapy. Circulation 2009;119:1231–40.

32. Nishijima Y, Sridhar A, Viatchenko-Karpinski S, et al. Chronic cardiac resynchronization therapy and reverse ventricular remodeling in a model of nonischemic cardiomyopathy. Life Sci 2007;81:1152–9.

33. Aiba T, Hesketh GG, Barth AS, et al. Electrophysiological consequences of dyssynchronous heart failure and its restoration by resynchronization therapy. Circulation 2009;119:1220–30.

34. Sachse FB, Torres NS, Savio-Galimberti E, et al. Subcellular structures and function of myocytes

impaired during heart failure are restored by cardiac resynchronization therapy. Circ Res 2012; 110:588–97.

35. Chakir K, Depry C, Dimaano VL, et al. Galphas-biased beta2-adrenergic receptor signaling from restoring synchronous contraction in the failing heart. Sci Transl Med 2011;3:100ra88.

36. Iyengar S, Haas G, Lamba S, et al. Effect of cardiac resynchronization therapy on myocardial gene expression in patients with nonischemic dilated cardiomyopathy. J Card Fail 2007;13: 304–11.

37. Mullens W, Bartunek J, Wilson Tang WH, et al. Early and late effects of cardiac resynchronization therapy on force-frequency relation and contractility regulating gene expression in heart failure patients. Heart Rhythm 2008;5:52–9.

38. Vanderheyden M, Mullens W, Delrue L, et al. Myocardial gene expression in heart failure patients treated with cardiac resynchronization therapy responders versus nonresponders. J Am Coll Cardiol 2008;51:129–36.

39. Spragg DD, Leclercq C, Loghmani M, et al. Regional alterations in protein expression in the dyssynchronous failing heart. Circulation 2003; 108:929–32.

40. Najem B, Unger P, Preumont N, et al. Sympathetic control after cardiac resynchronization therapy: responders versus nonresponders. Am J Physiol Heart Circ Physiol 2006;291:H2647–52.

41. Cha YM, Chareonthaitawee P, Dong YX, et al. Cardiac sympathetic reserve and response to cardiac resynchronization therapy. Circ Heart Fail 2011;4: 339–44.

42. Hamdan MH, Zagrodzky JD, Joglar JA, et al. Biventricular pacing decreases sympathetic activity compared with right ventricular pacing in patients with depressed ejection fraction. Circulation 2000; 102:1027–32.

43. Vanderheyden M, Mullens W, Delrue L, et al. Endomyocardial upregulation of beta1 adrenoreceptor gene expression and myocardial contractile reserve following cardiac resynchronization therapy. J Card Fail 2008;14:172–8.

44. Feldman AM, Cates AE, Veazey WB, et al. Increase of the 40,000-mol wt pertussis toxin substrate (G protein) in the failing human heart. J Clin Invest 1988;82:189–97.

45. Haga K, Haga T, Ichiyama A, et al. Functional reconstitution of purified muscarinic receptors and inhibitory guanine nucleotide regulatory protein. Nature 1985;316:731–3.

46. Hang P, Zhao J, Qi J, et al. Novel insights into the pervasive role of M(3) muscarinic receptor in cardiac diseases. Curr Drug Targets 2013;14:372–7.

47. DeMazumder D, Kass DA, O'Rourke B, et al. Cardiac resynchronization therapy restores sympathovagal balance in the failing heart by differential remodeling of cholinergic signaling. Circ Res 2015;116(10):1691–9.

48. Tomaselli GF, Marban E. Electrophysiological remodeling in hypertrophy and heart failure. Cardiovasc Res 1999;42:270–83.

49. Beuckelmann DJ, Nabauer M, Erdmann E. Alterations of K+ currents in isolated human ventricular myocytes from patients with terminal heart failure. Circ Res 1993;73:379–85.

50. Akar FG, Rosenbaum DS. Transmural electrophysiological heterogeneities underlying arrhythmogenesis in heart failure. Circ Res 2003;93:638–45.

51. Tsuji Y, Zicha S, Qi XY, et al. Potassium channel subunit remodeling in rabbits exposed to longterm bradycardia or tachycardia: discrete arrhythmogenic consequences related to differential delayed-rectifier changes. Circulation 2006;113: 345–55.

52. Nuss HB, Kääb S, Kass DA, et al. Cellular basis of ventricular arrhythmias and abnormal automaticity in heart failure. Am J Physiol 1999;277:H80–91.

53. Higgins SL, Yong P, Sheck D, et al. Biventricular pacing diminishes the need for implantable cardioverter defibrillator therapy. Ventak CHF Investigators. J Am Coll Cardiol 2000;36:824–7.

54. Kiès P, Bax JJ, Molhoek SG, et al. Effect of cardiac resynchronization therapy on inducibility of ventricular tachyarrhythmias in cardiac arrest survivors with either ischemic or idiopathic dilated cardiomyopathy. Am J Cardiol 2005;95:1111–4.

55. Cleland JG, Daubert JC, Erdmann E, et al. Longerterm effects of cardiac resynchronization therapy on mortality in heart failure [the CArdiac REsynchronization-Heart Failure (CARE-HF) trial extension phase]. Eur Heart J 2006;27:1928–32.

56. Markowitz SM, Lewen JM, Wiggenhorn CJ, et al. Relationship of reverse anatomical remodeling and ventricular arrhythmias after cardiac resynchronization. J Cardiovasc Electrophysiol 2009;20: 293–8.

57. Kutyifa V, Zareba W, McNitt S, et al. Left ventricular lead location and the risk of ventricular arrhythmias in the MADIT-CRT trial. Eur Heart J 2013;34: 184–90.

58. Ouellet G, Huang DT, Moss AJ, et al. Effect of cardiac resynchronization therapy on the risk of first and recurrent ventricular tachyarrhythmic events in MADIT-CRT. J Am Coll Cardiol 2012;60:1809–16.

59. Saba S, Mehdi H, Mathier MA, et al. Effect of right ventricular versus biventricular pacing on electrical remodeling in the normal heart. Circ Arrhythm Electrophysiol 2010;3:79–87.

60. Valdivia CR, Chu WW, Pu J, et al. Increased late sodium current in myocytes from a canine heart failure model and from failing human heart. J Mol Cell Cardiol 2005;38:475–83.

61. Aiba T, Barth AS, Hesketh GG, et al. Cardiac resynchronization therapy improves altered Na channel gating in canine model of dyssynchronous heart failure. Circ Arrhythm Electrophysiol 2013;6: 546–54.

62. Wagner S, Dybkova N, Rasenack EC, et al. Ca2+/calmodulin-dependent protein kinase II regulates cardiac Na+ channels. J Clin Invest 2006;116: 3127–38.

63. Chakir K, Daya SK, Tunin RS, et al. Reversal of global apoptosis and regional stress kinase activation by cardiac resynchronization. Circulation 2008; 117:1369–77.

64. Niederer SA, Plank G, Chinchapatnam P, et al. Length-dependent tension in the failing heart and the efficacy of cardiac resynchronization therapy. Cardiovasc Res 2011;89:336–43.

65. Pfeiffer ER, Tangney JR, Omens JH, et al. Biomechanics of cardiac electromechanical coupling and mechanoelectric feedback. J Biomech Eng 2014;136:021007.

66. Tangney JR, Campbell SG, McCulloch AD, et al. Timing and magnitude of systolic stretch affect myofilament activation and mechanical work. Am J Physiol Heart Circ Physiol 2014;307:H353–60.

67. Edman KA. Mechanical deactivation induced by active shortening in isolated muscle fibres of the frog. J Physiol 1975;246:255–75.

68. Kirk JA, Holewinski RJ, Kooij V, et al. Cardiac resynchronization sensitizes the sarcomere to calcium by reactivating GSK-3beta. J Clin Invest 2014;124:129–38.

69. Wolff MR, Buck SH, Stoker SW, et al. Myofibrillar calcium sensitivity of isometric tension is increased in human dilated cardiomyopathies: role of altered beta-adrenergically mediated protein phosphorylation. J Clin Invest 1996;98:167–76.

70. Wolff MR, Whitesell LF, Moss RL. Calcium sensitivity of isometric tension is increased in canine experimental heart failure. Circ Res 1995;76:781–9.

71. Zhang P, Kirk JA, Ji W, et al. Multiple reaction monitoring to identify site-specific troponin I phosphorylated residues in the failing human heart. Circulation 2012;126(15):1828–37.

72. Fraysse B, Weinberger F, Bardswell SC, et al. Increased myofilament Ca2+ sensitivity and diastolic dysfunction as early consequences of Mybpc3 mutation in heterozygous knock-in mice. J Mol Cell Cardiol 2012;52:1299–307.

73. Schober T, Huke S, Venkataraman R, et al. Myofilament Ca sensitization increases cytosolic Ca binding affinity, alters intracellular Ca homeostasis, and causes pause-dependent Ca-triggered arrhythmia. Circ Res 2012;111:170–9.

74. Neubauer S, Redwood C. New mechanisms and concepts for cardiac-resynchronization therapy. N Engl J Med 2014;370:1164–6.

75. Shah SR, Fatima K, Ansari M. Recovery of myofilament function through reactivation of glycogen synthase kinase 3beta (GSK-3beta): mechanism for cardiac resynchronization therapy. J Interv Card Electrophysiol 2014;41:193–4.

76. Orrego CM, Nasir N, Oliveira GH, et al. Cellular evidence of reverse cardiac remodeling induced by cardiac resynchronization therapy. Congest Heart Fail 2011;17:140–6.

77. Lichter JG, Carruth E, Mitchell C, et al. Remodeling of the sarcomeric cytoskeleton in cardiac ventricular myocytes during heart failure and after cardiac resynchronization therapy. J Mol Cell Cardiol 2014; 72:186–95.

78. Agnetti G, Halperin VL, Kirk JA, et al. Desmin modifications associate with amyloid oligomers deposition in heart failure. Cardiovasc Res 2014;102(1): 24–34.

79. Gupta A, Akki A, Wang Y, et al. Creatine kinase-mediated improvement of function in failing mouse hearts provides causal evidence the failing heart is energy starved. J Clin Invest 2012;122:291–302.

80. Shibayama J, Yuzyuk TN, Cox J, et al. Metabolic remodeling in moderate synchronous versus dyssynchronous pacing-induced heart failure: integrated metabolomics and proteomics study. PLoS One 2015;10:e0118974.

81. Altehoefer C, vom Dahl J, Buell U. Septal glucose metabolism in patients with coronary artery disease and left bundle-branch block. Coron Artery Dis 1993;4:569–72.

82. Zanco P, Desideri A, Mobilia G, et al. Effects of left bundle branch block on myocardial FDG PET in patients without significant coronary artery stenoses. J Nucl Med 2000;41:973–7.

83. Nemutlu E, Zhang S, Xu YZ, et al. Cardiac resynchronization therapy induces adaptive metabolic transitions in the metabolomic profile of heart failure. J Card Fail 2015;21(6):460–9.

84. Lionetti V, Guiducci L, Simioniuc A, et al. Mismatch between uniform increase in cardiac glucose uptake and regional contractile dysfunction in pacing-induced heart failure. Am J Physiol Heart Circ Physiol 2007;293:H2747–56.

85. Lionetti V, Aquaro GD, Simioniuc A, et al. Severe mechanical dyssynchrony causes regional hibernation-like changes in pigs with nonischemic heart failure. J Card Fail 2009;15:920–8.

86. Nowak B, Sinha AM, Schaefer WM, et al. Cardiac resynchronization therapy homogenizes myocardial glucose metabolism and perfusion in dilated cardiomyopathy and left bundle branch block. J Am Coll Cardiol 2003;41:1523–8.

87. Yang S, Chen L, Sun S, et al. Glycoproteins identified from heart failure and treatment models. Proteomics 2015;15:567–79.

88. Obrzut S, Tiongson J, Jamshidi N, et al. Assessment of metabolic phenotypes in patients with non-ischemic dilated cardiomyopathy undergoing cardiac resynchronization therapy. J Cardiovasc Transl Res 2010;3:643–51.

89. Padeletti L, Modesti PA, Cartei S, et al. Metabolomic does not predict response to cardiac resynchronization therapy in patients with heart failure. J Cardiovasc Med (Hagerstown) 2014;15:295–300.

90. Agnetti G, Kaludercic N, Kane LA, et al. Modulation of mitochondrial proteome and improved mitochondrial function by biventricular pacing of dyssynchronous failing hearts. Circ Cardiovasc Genet 2010;3:78–87.

91. Wang SB, Foster DB, Rucker J, et al. Redox regulation of mitochondrial ATP synthase: implications for cardiac resynchronization therapy. Circ Res 2011;109:750–7.

92. Sun J, Morgan M, Shen RF, et al. Preconditioning results in S-nitrosylation of proteins involved in regulation of mitochondrial energetics and calcium transport. Circ Res 2007;101:1155–63.

93. Bose A, Truong QA, Singh JP. Biomarkers in electrophysiology: role in arrhythmias and resynchronization therapy. J Interv Card Electrophysiol 2015; 43:31–44.

94. Tolosana JM, Mont L, Sitges M, et al. Plasma tissue inhibitor of matrix metalloproteinase-1 (TIMP-1): an independent predictor of poor response to cardiac resynchronization therapy. Eur J Heart Fail 2010; 12:492–8.

95. Trucco E, Tolosana JM, Castel MÁ, et al. Plasma tissue inhibitor of matrix metalloproteinase-1 a predictor of long-term mortality in patients treated with cardiac resynchronization therapy. Europace 2015. http://dx.doi.org/10.1093/europace/euv054.

96. Stolen CM, Adourian A, Meyer TE, et al. Plasma galectin-3 and heart failure outcomes in MADIT-CRT (Multicenter Automatic Defibrillator Implantation Trial with Cardiac Resynchronization Therapy). J Card Fail 2014;20:793–9.

97. Hessel MH, Bleeker GB, Bax JJ, et al. Reverse ventricular remodelling after cardiac resynchronization therapy is associated with a reduction in serum tenascin-C and plasma matrix metalloproteinase-9 levels. Eur J Heart Fail 2007;9:1058–63.

98. Lopez-Andrès N, Rossignol P, Iraqi W, et al. Association of galectin-3 and fibrosis markers with long-term cardiovascular outcomes in patients with heart failure, left ventricular dysfunction, and dyssynchrony: insights from the CARE-HF (Cardiac Resynchronization in Heart Failure) trial. Eur J Heart Fail 2012;14:74–81.

99. García-Bolao I, López B, Macías A, et al. Impact of collagen type I turnover on the long-term response to cardiac resynchronization therapy. Eur Heart J 2008;29:898–906.

100. Stanciu AE, Vatasescu RG, Stanciu MM, et al. Cardiac resynchronization therapy in patients with chronic heart failure is associated with anti-inflammatory and anti-remodeling effects. Clin Biochem 2013;46:230–4.

101. Rordorf R, Savastano S, Sanzo A, et al. Tumor necrosis factor-alpha predicts response to cardiac resynchronization therapy in patients with chronic heart failure. Circ J 2014;78:2232–9.

102. Limongelli G, Roselli T, Pacileo G, et al. Effect of cardiac resynchronization therapy on cardiotrophin-1 circulating levels in patients with heart failure. Intern Emerg Med 2014;9:43–50.

103. António N, Soares A, Carvalheiro T, et al. Circulating endothelial progenitor cells as a predictor of response to cardiac resynchronization therapy: the missing piece of the puzzle? Pacing Clin Electrophysiol 2014;37:731–9.

104. Castellant P, Fatemi M, Bertault-Valls V, et al. Cardiac resynchronization therapy: "nonresponders" and "hyperresponders". Heart Rhythm 2008;5:193–7.

105. Dorn GW 2nd. MicroRNAs in cardiac disease. Transl Res 2011;157:226–35.

106. Melman YF, et al. A novel functional and prognostic role for circulating microRNA- 30d after cardiac resynchronization therapy in advanced heart failure. Circulation 2015, in press.

107. Marfella R, Di Filippo C, Potenza N, et al. Circulating microRNA changes in heart failure patients treated with cardiac resynchronization therapy: responders vs. non-responders. Eur J Heart Fail 2013;15:1277–88.

108. Sardu C, Marfella R, Santulli G, et al. Functional role of miRNA in cardiac resynchronization therapy. Pharmacogenomics 2014;15:1159–68.

109. Ravassa S, García-Bolao I, Zudaire A, et al. Cardiac resynchronization therapy-induced left ventricular reverse remodelling is associated with reduced plasma annexin A5. Cardiovasc Res 2010;88:304–13.

110. Monceau V, Belikova Y, Kratassiouk G, et al. Externalization of endogenous annexin A5 participates in apoptosis of rat cardiomyocytes. Cardiovasc Res 2004;64:496–506.

111. Monceau V, Belikova Y, Kratassiouk G, et al. Myocyte apoptosis during acute myocardial infarction in rats is related to early sarcolemmal translocation of annexin A5 in border zone. Am J Physiol Heart Circ Physiol 2006;291:H965–71.

112. Klug D, Boule S, Wissocque L, et al. Right ventricular pacing with mechanical dyssynchrony causes apoptosis interruptus and calcium mishandling. Can J Cardiol 2012;29(4):510–8.

113. Agacdiken A, Celikyurt U, Sahin T, et al. Neutrophil-to-lymphocyte ratio predicts response to cardiac resynchronization therapy. Med Sci Monit 2013; 19:373–7.

114. Francia P, Salvati A, Balla C, et al. Cardiac resynch-ronization therapy increases plasma levels of the endogenous inotrope apelin. Eur J Heart Fail 2007;9:306–9.

115. Auger D, Bleeker GB, Bertini M, et al. Effect of car-diac resynchronization therapy in patients without left intraventricular dyssynchrony. Eur Heart J 2012;33:913–20.

116. Bilchick KC, Saha SK, Mikolajczyk E, et al. Differen-tial regional gene expression from cardiac dyssyn-chrony induced by chronic right ventricular free wall pacing in the mouse. Physiol Genomics 2006;26:109–15.

117. Laughner JI, Marrus SB, Zellmer ER, et al. A fully implantable pacemaker for the mouse: from battery to wireless power. PLoS One 2013;8:e76291.

Exploring the Electrophysiologic and Hemodynamic Effects of Cardiac Resynchronization Therapy
From Bench to Bedside and Vice Versa

Rick Schreurs, MD, Rob F. Wiegerinck, PhD,
Frits W. Prinzen, PhD*

KEYWORDS

- Left bundle branch block • Cardiac resynchronization therapy • Animal research
- Electrophysiology • Hemodynamics

KEY POINTS

- CRT reduces the dyssynchronous activation pattern caused by LBBB and improves the hemodynamic state. This results in reduced mortality and improved quality of life.
- For the best CRT response the LV lead should be positioned in a late activated area while avoiding sites with transmural myocardial infarction.
- The addition of more pacing sites further improves the hemodynamic state, but only if the first LV pacing site yielded a low hemodynamic response.
- An endocardial LV pacing site is superior to an epicardial LV pacing site with respect to CRT response.
- AV and VV optimization further increase the response to CRT by fusing intrinsic and paced electrical activation fronts.

INTRODUCTION

Patients with heart failure (HF) combined with left bundle branch block (LBBB) have broad QRS complexes and an impaired cardiac function. In these patients it is unclear whether HF leads to LBBB or vice versa. Animal models, however, have shown that induction of LBBB reduces cardiac contractility.[1] Similarly, inadvertent induction of LBBB during transcatheter aortic valve replacement worsens outcome.[2] In LBBB cardiac function is impaired because the left (LV) and right ventricle (RV) and various regions within the LV are not activated simultaneously, leading to dyssynchronous

Disclosure Statement: F.W. Prinzen received research grants from Medtronic, Boston Scientific, EBR Systems, St. Jude Medical, Biological Delivery System (Johnson and Johnson), MSD, and Proteus Medical. This research was performed within the framework of CTMM (Center for Translational Molecular Medicine), the Center for Translational Molecular Medicine (www.ctmm.nl), project COHFAR (COngestive Heart Failure and ARrhythmia; grant 01C-203), and supported by the Dutch Heart Foundation.
Department of Physiology, Cardiovascular Research Institute Maastricht, Maastricht University, Maastricht, The Netherlands
* Corresponding author. Department of Physiology, Maastricht University, PO Box 616, Maastricht 6200 MD, The Netherlands.
E-mail address: frits.prinzen@maastrichtuniversity.nl

Card Electrophysiol Clin 7 (2015) 599–608
http://dx.doi.org/10.1016/j.ccep.2015.08.012
1877-9182/15/$ – see front matter © 2015 Elsevier Inc. All rights reserved.

contraction and reduced cardiac pump function.[3] Animal studies have shown that isolated LBBB causes reduction in ejection time, slower rates of rise and fall of the LV pressure, and prolonged duration of isovolumic contraction and relaxation.[4]

Cardiac resynchronization therapy (CRT) aims to restore synchronous contraction of the heart by either LV free wall or biventricular (BiV) pacing. The first studies started during the late 1990s to evaluate the effect of CRT.[5–7] According to the current guidelines a CRT device is indicated for patients with HF and prolonged QRS duration, preferably with LBBB morphology on the electrocardiogram (ECG).[8] CRT reduces mortality and improves quality of life,[9] but additional research is needed to optimize this therapy. To this purpose investigations have also been performed in animal models of dyssynchrony.

Animals have long been used to study hemodynamics and electrophysiology in HF. As reviewed by Strik and colleagues[10] the canine seems to be the best species to study ventricular conduction abnormalities that occur during pacing and LBBB, because the anatomic structures of the bundle branches are comparable with those in human. Percutaneous radiofrequency ablation of the LBBB results in a model perfectly suited to study the effects of CRT.[1,4,11,12] This model enables the investigation of the role of LBBB and CRT in the absence of HF, but if needed, also in combination with HF (created by chronic tachypacing) or myocardial infarction.[10]

This article reviews the electrophysiologic and hemodynamic effects of CRT in animal models and patients with LBBB.

ELECTROMECHANICS OF DYSSYNCHRONY

In LBBB the normal activation pattern is disturbed because the LV is no longer activated via the left bundle branch and Purkinje fibers. Instead, the electrical activation spreads from the normally activated RV through the septum toward the LV. Because activation moving from myocyte to myocyte is much slower, the LV free wall, which is the site most remote from the RV, is activated latest. Several clinical[13,14] and preclinical[15] invasive electrocardiac mapping studies have shown that the activation in LBBB hearts follows a specific pattern. LV depolarization moves from the septum in a circumferential and longitudinal direction. However, because conduction often appears slow at the RV-LV junctions an important contribution of activation comes from the wavefront passing over the apex toward the LV lateral wall (referred to as U-shaped activation pattern). Another characteristic feature is the slow

transseptal conduction in LBBB, possibly caused by the vertical orientation of the laminar sheets of myocytes in the septum.[16,17] Epicardial activation maps generated with noninvasive electrocardiographic imaging show comparable electrical patterns, as illustrated by the *white arrow* in the upper left of **Fig. 1**.[18] The prolonged activation of the LV results in an increased total activation time (TAT) of both ventricles, which is characterized by a widened QRS complex on the surface ECG.[13] These findings are similar in dogs.[10]

Fig. 2 (*left*) describes how the dyssynchronous electrical activation of the LV causes the early activated septum to contract against a reduced load, which leads to prestretch of the LV lateral wall (ie, more positive strain; *middle, solid line*).[13] This prestretch increases contractile force of the LV free wall, which on its turn paradoxically stretches the septum later in systole (positive strain of the septum, *dashed line*). Both types of systolic stretching can be considered wasted work, which is the ratio of negative and positive work (*red and black lines*, respectively; *bottom*).[3,19]

In canine hearts, the maximum rates of rise and fall of the LV pressure (dP/dt_{max} and dP/dt_{min}) decrease immediately on creating LBBB and this decrease is still present after 8 weeks. Echocardiographic follow-up shows an increase of end-diastolic volume (EDV) and end-systolic volume (ESV) and decrease of ejection fraction (EF) with longer lasting LBBB.[3] These findings replicate the low EF, increased LV wall stress and ESV, and impaired myocardial relaxation as seen in patients with LBBB.[20]

ELECTROPHYSIOLOGIC EFFECTS OF CARDIAC RESYNCHRONIZATION THERAPY

The basic idea behind CRT is to resynchronize the late and more slowly activated LV by individually pacing both ventricles. **Fig. 1** shows that RV pacing alone results in an activation pattern that resembles the intrinsic activation pattern of LBBB and leads to a QRS duration of 250 milliseconds (ms) in this example. At a short atrioventricular (AV) delay LV pacing increases QRS duration, but with a completely reversed activation pattern compared with LBBB and RV pacing. With BiV pacing the left and right activation wavefronts fuse in the LV, which accelerates its activation, and consequently result in a shorter QRS duration of 150 ms.

In dogs simultaneous RV and LV pacing shortens TAT and QRS duration compared with the LBBB situation and immediately improves hemodynamics.[10] However, note that BiV pacing does not necessarily reduce QRS duration[6,7] or

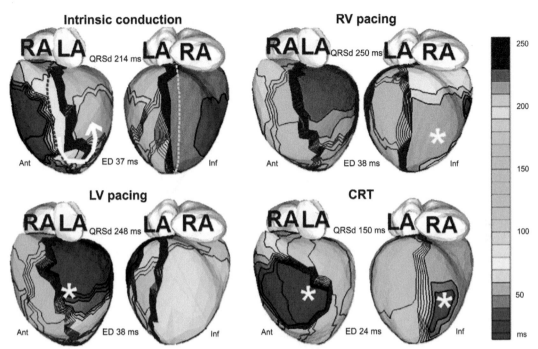

Fig. 1. Electrocardiographic images of an LBBB patient recorded during intrinsic conduction, RV pacing, LV pacing, and CRT. Each pair of images shows the anterior (Ant) and inferior (Inf) views. The black lines depict isochronal lines. Crowded isochronal lines indicate slow conduction. Thick black lines indicate conduction block. An asterisk indicates the pacing site. The *dotted lines* in the images of intrinsic conduction show the septal aspect of the epicardium. The QRS duration (QRSd) and the electrical dyssynchrony index (ED; calculated as the standard deviation of activation times at 500 sites in the LV) are indicated in the figure for each pacing modality. LA, left atrium; RA, right atrium. (*From* Ghosh S, Silva JN, Canham RM, et al. Electrophysiologic substrate and intraventricular left ventricular dyssynchrony in nonischemic heart failure patients undergoing cardiac resynchronization therapy. Heart Rhythm 2011;8(5):695; with permission.)

TAT,[14] which can be explained by prolonged activation of the RV that is not intrinsically activated anymore (ie, slower cell-to-cell conduction instead of activation through the Purkinje network; compare intrinsic conduction and RV pacing in **Fig. 1**). Moreover, in dogs it has been shown that hemodynamic improvement can even occur when the QRS duration has not shortened because of CRT.[1]

In responders CRT reduces LV dyssynchrony, measured as LV TAT or as the electrical dyssynchrony index (**Fig. 1**; lowest for BiV pacing).[18] CRT reduces the difference in the onset of electrical activation between LV and RV.[11] Ultimately, the intraventricular and interventricular (VV) resynchronization improve pump function.

ACUTE HEMODYNAMIC EFFECTS OF CARDIAC RESYNCHRONIZATION THERAPY

In dogs with LBBB acute BiV pacing raises dP/dt_{max} almost back to pre-LBBB levels, without affecting LV end-systolic or end-diastolic pressures. In canines with LBBB and tachypacing induced HF the relative increase in LV dP/dt_{max} is larger than in nonfailing LBBB hearts, but the absolute increase is comparable.[15] In patients the onset of BiV pacing immediately increases LV dP/dt_{max} compared with LBBB or RV pacing and this increase typically ranges from 10% to 30%.[6,7,21]

LV dP/dt_{max} has become an important variable for hemodynamic studies in CRT, but also pulse pressure and cardiac index increase during BiV stimulation.[6,21,22] Pressure-volume loop analysis in dogs with LBBB and HF shows an increase in stroke volume and stroke work (SW) in BiV pacing compared with baseline measurements.[7] It has been suggested that SW is a more reliable measure than increased LV dP/dt_{max}, because SW takes the complete systolic phase into account and comprises pressure and volume changes, whereas LV dP/dt_{max} only reflects the isovolumic contraction of cardiac systole.[23] However, the acute improvement in LV dP/dt_{max} may not be able to predict the clinical outcome on the long-term.[24]

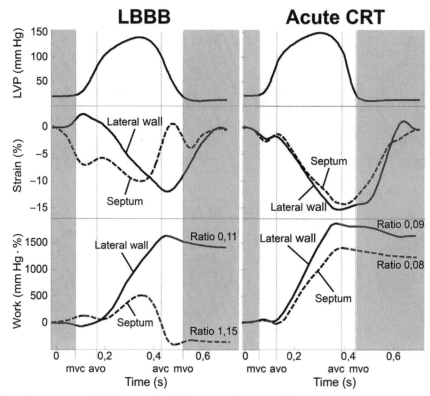

Fig. 2. Estimated LV pressure (*top*), strain (*middle*), and calculation of wasted work for the septum and lateral wall (*bottom*) in a representative patient with LBBB (*left*) and after treatment with CRT (*right*). Vertical lines indicate valvular events defined by echocardiography. Negative and positive work during systole is marked as red and black, respectively. Wasted work ratios were calculated using cumulated work between the closure and subsequent opening of the mitral valve (MVC and MVO, respectively). AVC, aortic valve closure; AVO, aortic valve opening. (*From* Russell K, Eriksen M, Aaberge L, et al. Assessment of wasted myocardial work: a novel method to quantify energy loss due to uncoordinated left ventricular contractions. Am J Physiol Heart Circ Physiol 2013;305(7):H998; with permission.)

LONG-TERM EFFECTS OF CARDIAC RESYNCHRONIZATION THERAPY

The favorable outcomes of CRT can be explained by reverse remodeling of the heart because of re-synchronization of the ventricles. Remodeling can be activated through neurohormonal activation, differences in mechanical load, and wall stress. Several studies in animal models of LBBB, sometimes in combination with tachypacing-induced HF, have shed led light on the cellular and molecular adaptations in asynchronous hearts. The expression of some genes and proteins is depressed uniformly, whereas others show regional differences in expression between early and late-activated areas. Changes occur related to myocyte function, calcium handling, β-adrenergic responsiveness, mitochondrial ATP synthase activity, cell survival signaling, and other functions. CRT reverses many of these alterations (discussed elsewhere in this issue).

These extensive reverse-remodelling processes may also explain the improvements in pressure-volume diagrams recorded after 6 months of CRT (**Fig. 3**). Note that after 6 months EDV and ESV show a leftward shift, whereas EF increases.[25] Moreover, whereas before CRT the loops decrease in size with increased heart rate, this was much less the case after 6 months of CRT, indicating better pump function. Other studies report higher EF and lower end-systolic ventricular dimensions after 1 year of follow-up.[23,26] A study in the LBBB canine model shows that acute CRT restores dP/dt_{max} almost back to pre-LBBB values and chronic CRT increases it slightly further, yet not completely back to pre-LBBB values.[12]

PACING LOCATION

The size of hemodynamic response to CRT depends on the location of the LV lead. Usually the

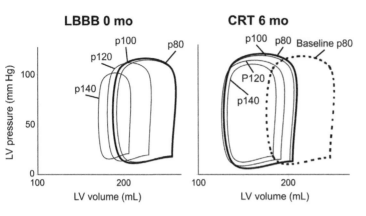

Fig. 3. Pressure-volume loops at baseline and after 6 months of CRT in a patient, measured at heart rates of 80, 100, 120, and 140 beats per minute. (*From* Steendijk P, Tulner SA, Bax JJ, et al. Hemodynamic effects of long-term cardiac resynchronization therapy: analysis by pressure-volume loops. Circulation 2006;113(10):1301; with permission.)

best location is in the latest activated region of the LV free wall.[27] Intriguingly, most studies fail to indicate an anatomic location that is clearly the best. A study in LBBB dogs showed that pacing in a rather large area of the LV free wall ($\pm$43%) yielded a dP/dt$_{max}$ larger than 70% of the maximal observed value.[28] This, coupled with the fact that anatomy limits the number of available pacing sites, may explain the lack of a clear anatomic defined location for pacing. Moreover, LV activation patterns vary considerably between patients. Therefore, it seems advisable to estimate the ideal LV pacing region in each individual patient.[27] To this purpose, the CardioInsight technique (see **Fig. 1**), other electroanatomic techniques,[29] and echocardiographic speckle tracking[30] may be used to determine the latest activated regions.

Currently, the site of latest activation is determined during intrinsic activation, but it is probably wiser to determine it during RV apex pacing because during CRT the RV is paced, which may shift the site of latest activation (see **Fig. 1**; compare intrinsic conduction and RV pacing).[31,32]

MYOCARDIAL SCARRING

Myocardial scarring plays a dual role in CRT response. First, the response to CRT is inversely related to the total amount of ventricular scar tissue.[33] Second, CRT response is poor, and potentially adverse if the LV lead is positioned in a region with extensive scar tissue.[33,34] This may be because scar tissue slows electrical conduction and may give rise to ventricular arrhythmias. However, a study in canines indicates that CRT should still be considered for patients with a myocardial scar.[35] In this study CRT reduces LV TAT and increases LV dP/dt$_{max}$ to similar values in LBBB dogs with and without infarction when pacing sites are selected outside of the infarcted region (**Fig. 4**).

MULTIPLE PACING SITES

Because BiV pacing leads to electrical resynchronization of the LV, it has been argued that increasing the number of LV pacing sites (multi-LV) will further improve resynchronization and cardiac function. The prospective TRIP-HF study shows that reverse remodelling is more pronounced after 3 months of triventricular pacing (two LV leads) compared with conventional BiV pacing, with higher EF and lower ESV in patients who did not respond to conventional BiV pacing.[36] Experiments using a strategy to maximally resynchronize the LV in the canine LBBB model show that additional pacing sites (up to seven) consistently decrease LV TAT, but only increase dP/dt$_{max}$ if the hemodynamic effect of pacing the initial single-site is small (**Fig. 5A**).[37] Similar findings were reported later for CRT patients (**Fig. 5B**).

Although multisite pacing often requires leads in multiple veins, the recently introduced quadripolar leads enable multipoint pacing at two LV sites in one cardiac vein. The first studies on multipoint pacing have shown a small but significant increase in dP/dt$_{max}$ and decrease in QRS duration compared with BiV pacing.[38,39] Although these results are promising, all studies so far relate to individual optimization using invasive hemodynamic measurements and no long-term benefits and clinical implications have yet been reported.

ENDOCARDIAL PACING

Previous paragraphs mostly discussed (multiple) LV epicardial pacing sites, because the conventional lead position in the coronary vein is epicardial. However, both animal and patient studies indicate that LV endocardial pacing is more promising (see **Fig. 5**).[39,40] Several other studies corroborated these findings.[41,42] The better resynchronization with endocardial CRT is explained

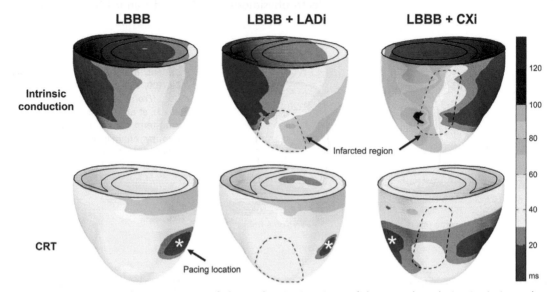

Fig. 4. Three-dimensional reconstruction of electrical activation times of the LV and RV during intrinsic conduction (LBBB, *top*) and CRT using midlateral LV wall pacing (*bottom*) in representative hearts with LBBB (*left*), and LBBB combined with an infarction of the left anterior ascending artery (LBBB + LADi, *middle*) or left circumflex artery (LBBB + LCXi, *right*). (*From* Rademakers LM, van Kerckhoven R, van Deursen CJ, et al. Myocardial infarction does not preclude electrical and hemodynamic benefits of cardiac resynchronization therapy in dyssynchronous canine hearts. Circ Arrhythm Electrophysiol 2010;3(4):363; with permission.)

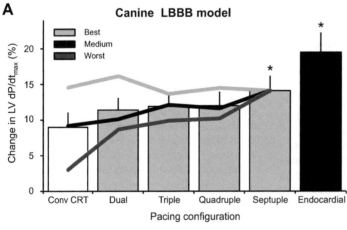

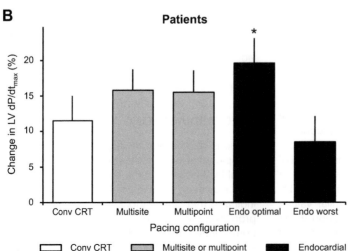

Fig. 5. Percentage change in LV dP/dt$_{max}$ versus baseline during conventional (Conv) CRT (*white bars*), multisite or multipoint (*gray bars*), and endocardial pacing (*black bars*) measured in a canine LBBB model (*A*) and in patients (*B*). The values in the bars are presented as mean + SEM. The three lines in *A* are the pooled data for the two "worst," the three "intermediate," and two "best" single LV pacing sites (*red, black,* and *green,* respectively). [a] $P \leq .05$ versus conventional CRT. (*Adapted from* Ploux S, Strik M, van Hunnik A, et al. Acute electrical and hemodynamic effects of multisite left ventricular pacing for cardiac resynchronization therapy in the dyssynchronous canine heart. Heart Rhythm 2014;11(1):123; and Shetty AK, Sohal M, Chen Z, et al. A comparison of left ventricular endocardial, multisite, and multipolar epicardial cardiac resynchronization: an acute haemodynamic and electroanatomical study. Europace 2014;16(6):875.)

by three factors: (1) a shorter path length for the depolarization wave to reach all regions of the ventricles, (2) more rapid impulse conduction in the endocardium than in the epicardium, and (3) a more rapid transmural conduction from endocardium to epicardium than in the opposite direction.[40,43] Unfortunately, practical implementation of endocardial CRT is still problematic, because currently leads placed in the LV cavity require anticoagulation and also show significant dislodgement.[44]

OPTIMIZATION OF TIMING OF PACING

All CRT devices have the option to adjust the AV and VV delay to the individual patient. **Fig. 6**A shows schematically how these different settings can influence the electrical activation of the LV. The VV intervals (y-axis) can be chosen such that either the RV or the LV is activated first or that both are activated simultaneously. This determines the relative contribution to the complete electrical activation of the LV by activation fronts initiated by the LV pacing site and the RV pacing site and/ or intrinsic activation from the RBB. AV delays (x-axis) shorter, equal to, or longer than the intrinsic

AV delay influence the relative contribution of the intrinsic and paced activation wavefronts to the complete activation of the LV (see **Fig. 6**A). These settings affect pump function primarily by optimizing the degree of resynchronization.[12,45] **Fig. 6**B shows the relative changes in LV dP/dt$_{max}$, SW, and electrical resynchronization in response to 100 different combinations of LV (x-axis) and RV (y-axis) AV delays. Note the similar leftward turn (*white arrows*) of the optimal values for all three parameters, occurring at an RV AV delay just shy of their respective intrinsic PQ duration.

Several parameters have been used to judge which AV and VV delays result in the best CRT response. These include diastolic filling time, aortic velocity time integral, arterial blood pressure, LV dP/dt$_{max}$, SW, and vectorcardiography.[46,47] However, a major problem seems to be that the increase in pump function is in the same order of magnitude as the biologic variability. According to basic rules for accurate measurements, reliable results are only observed if repeated measurements are performed.[48] That this has rarely been done may explain the variable results on the best way and clinical effect of AV and VV optimization. A possible solution to this problem is the

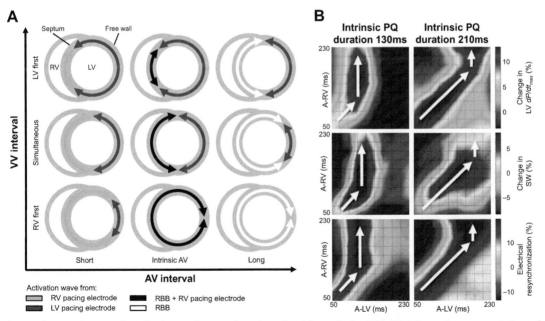

Fig. 6. Changes in resynchronization and pump function after biventricular CRT. (*A*) Schematic representation of interactions between activation wavefronts originating from the RV and LV pacing electrodes and from the right bundle branch (RBB). (*B*) Contour plots of percentage change in LV dP/dtmax (maximal rate of rise of left ventricular pressure; *top*), stroke work (SW) (*middle*), and electric resynchronization (*bottom*) in 100 different combinations of atrio-left ventricular (A-LV) and atrio-right ventricular (A-RV) intervals in two different experiments with an intrinsic PQ duration of 130 (*left*) and 210 ms (*right*). (*Adapted from* Strik M, van Middendorp LB, Houthuizen P, et al. Interplay of electrical wavefronts as determinant of the response to cardiac resynchronization therapy in dyssynchronous canine hearts. Circ Arrhythm Electrophysiol 2013;6(5):928; with permission.)

use of ECG or vectorcardiogram variables for optimization, which are both easy to acquire and have considerably lower variability.[49]

SUMMARY

CRT successfully improves cardiac function in HF patients with LBBB by resynchronizing the dyssynchronous contraction of the LV. Studies in patients and animals have indicated that the best electromechanical improvement is achieved by selecting the proper site for LV lead placement and by avoiding areas with transmural scarring. The acute effects of multiple pacing locations, endocardial pacing, and optimized timing of pacing are superior to conventional CRT, but further research on the long-term effects of these promising approaches is still needed.

REFERENCES

1. Verbeek XA, Vernooy K, Peschar M, et al. Quantification of interventricular asynchrony during LBBB and ventricular pacing. Am J Physiol Heart Circ Physiol 2002;283(4):H1370–8.
2. Houthuizen P, Van Garsse LA, Poels TT, et al. Left bundle-branch block induced by transcatheter aortic valve implantation increases risk of death. Circulation 2012;126(6):720–8.
3. Leclercq C, Kass DA. Retiming the failing heart: principles and current clinical status of cardiac resynchronization. J Am Coll Cardiol 2002;39(2):194–201.
4. Verbeek XA, Vernooy K, Peschar M, et al. Intra-ventricular resynchronization for optimal left ventricular function during pacing in experimental left bundle branch block. J Am Coll Cardiol 2003;42(3):558–67.
5. Daubert JC, Ritter P, Le Breton H, et al. Permanent left ventricular pacing with transvenous leads inserted into the coronary veins. Pacing Clin Electrophysiol 1998;21(1 Pt 2):239–45.
6. Leclercq C, Cazeau S, Le Breton H, et al. Acute hemodynamic effects of biventricular DDD pacing in patients with end-stage heart failure. J Am Coll Cardiol 1998;32(7):1825–31.
7. Kass DA, Chen CH, Curry C, et al. Improved left ventricular mechanics from acute VDD pacing in patients with dilated cardiomyopathy and ventricular conduction delay. Circulation 1999;99(12):1567–73.
8. Brignole M, Auricchio A, Baron-Esquivias G, et al. 2013 ESC guidelines on cardiac pacing and cardiac resynchronization therapy: the task force on cardiac pacing and resynchronization therapy of the European Society of Cardiology (ESC). Developed in collaboration with the European Heart Rhythm Association (EHRA). Europace 2013; 15(8):1070–118.
9. Abraham WT, Fisher WG, Smith AL, et al. Cardiac resynchronization in chronic heart failure. N Engl J Med 2002;346(24):1845–53.
10. Strik M, van Middendorp LB, Vernooy K. Animal models of dyssynchrony. J Cardiovasc Transl Res 2012;5(2):135–45.
11. Liu L, Tockman B, Girouard S, et al. Left ventricular resynchronization therapy in a canine model of left bundle branch block. Am J Physiol Heart Circ Physiol 2002;282(6):H2238–44.
12. Vernooy K, Cornelussen RN, Verbeek XA, et al. Cardiac resynchronization therapy cures dyssynchronopathy in canine left bundle-branch block hearts. Eur Heart J 2007;28(17):2148–55.
13. Auricchio A, Fantoni C, Regoli F, et al. Characterization of left ventricular activation in patients with heart failure and left bundle-branch block. Circulation 2004;109(9):1133–9.
14. Lambiase PD, Rinaldi A, Hauck J, et al. Non-contact left ventricular endocardial mapping in cardiac resynchronisation therapy. Heart 2004;90(1):44–51.
15. Strik M, Regoli F, Auricchio A, et al. Electrical and mechanical ventricular activation during left bundle branch block and resynchronization. J Cardiovasc Transl Res 2012;5(2):117–26.
16. Strik M, van Deursen CJ, van Middendorp LB, et al. Transseptal conduction as an important determinant for cardiac resynchronization therapy, as revealed by extensive electrical mapping in the dyssynchronous canine heart. Circ Arrhythm Electrophysiol 2013;6(4):682–9.
17. Helm PA, Younes L, Beg MF, et al. Evidence of structural remodeling in the dyssynchronous failing heart. Circ Res 2006;98(1):125–32.
18. Ghosh S, Silva JN, Canham RM, et al. Electrophysiologic substrate and intraventricular left ventricular dyssynchrony in nonischemic heart failure patients undergoing cardiac resynchronization therapy. Heart Rhythm 2011;8(5):692–9.
19. Russell K, Eriksen M, Aaberge L, et al. Assessment of wasted myocardial work: a novel method to quantify energy loss due to uncoordinated left ventricular contractions. Am J Physiol Heart Circ Physiol 2013; 305(7):H996–1003.
20. Leyva F, Nisam S, Auricchio A. 20 years of cardiac resynchronization therapy. J Am Coll Cardiol 2014; 64(10):1047–58.
21. Auricchio A, Stellbrink C, Block M, et al. Effect of pacing chamber and atrioventricular delay on acute systolic function of paced patients with congestive heart failure. The Pacing Therapies for Congestive Heart Failure Study Group. The Guidant Congestive Heart Failure Research Group. Circulation 1999; 99(23):2993–3001.
22. Gold MR, Auricchio A, Hummel JD, et al. Comparison of stimulation sites within left ventricular veins on the acute hemodynamic effects of cardiac

resynchronization therapy. Heart Rhythm 2005;2(4): 376–81.

23. de Roest GJ, Allaart CP, Kleijn SA, et al. Prediction of long-term outcome of cardiac resynchronization therapy by acute pressure-volume loop measurements. Eur J Heart Fail 2013;15(3):299–307.

24. Bogaard MD, Houthuizen P, Bracke FA, et al. Baseline left ventricular dP/dtmax rather than the acute improvement in dP/dtmax predicts clinical outcome in patients with cardiac resynchronization therapy. Eur J Heart Fail 2011;13(10):1126–32.

25. Steendijk P, Tulner SA, Bax JJ, et al. Hemodynamic effects of long-term cardiac resynchronization therapy: analysis by pressure-volume loops. Circulation 2006;113(10):1295–304.

26. Yu CM, Chau E, Sanderson JE, et al. Tissue Doppler echocardiographic evidence of reverse remodeling and improved synchronicity by simultaneously delaying regional contraction after biventricular pacing therapy in heart failure. Circulation 2002;105(4): 438–45.

27. Vernooy K, van Deursen CJ, Strik M, et al. Strategies to improve cardiac resynchronization therapy. Nat Rev Cardiol 2014;11(8):481–93.

28. Helm RH, Byrne M, Helm PA, et al. Three-dimensional mapping of optimal left ventricular pacing site for cardiac resynchronization. Circulation 2007; 115(8):953–61.

29. Rad MM, Blaauw Y, Dinh T, et al. Left ventricular lead placement in the latest activated region guided by coronary venous electroanatomic mapping. Europace 2015;17(1):84–93.

30. Khan FZ, Virdee MS, Palmer CR, et al. Targeted left ventricular lead placement to guide cardiac resynchronization therapy: the TARGET study: a randomized, controlled trial. J Am Coll Cardiol 2012; 59(17):1509–18.

31. Mafi Rad M, Blaauw Y, Dinh T, et al. Different regions of latest electrical activation during left bundle-branch block and right ventricular pacing in cardiac resynchronization therapy patients determined by coronary venous electro-anatomic mapping. Eur J Heart Fail 2014;16(11):1214–22.

32. Ludwig DR, Tanaka H, Friehling M, et al. Further deterioration of LV ejection fraction and mechanical synchrony during RV apical pacing in patients with heart failure and LBBB. J Cardiovasc Transl Res 2013;6(3):425–9.

33. Ypenburg C, Schalij MJ, Bleeker GB, et al. Impact of viability and scar tissue on response to cardiac resynchronization therapy in ischaemic heart failure patients. Eur Heart J 2007;28(1):33–41.

34. Bleeker GB, Kaandorp TA, Lamb HJ, et al. Effect of posterolateral scar tissue on clinical and echocardiographic improvement after cardiac resynchronization therapy. Circulation 2006; 113(7):969–76.

35. Rademakers LM, van Kerckhoven R, van Deursen CJ, et al. Myocardial infarction does not preclude electrical and hemodynamic benefits of cardiac resynchronization therapy in dyssynchronous canine hearts. Circ Arrhythm Electrophysiol 2010;3(4):361–8.

36. Leclercq C, Gadler F, Kranig W, et al. A randomized comparison of triple-site versus dual-site ventricular stimulation in patients with congestive heart failure. J Am Coll Cardiol 2008;51(15):1455–62.

37. Ploux S, Strik M, van Hunnik A, et al. Acute electrical and hemodynamic effects of multisite left ventricular pacing for cardiac resynchronization therapy in the dyssynchronous canine heart. Heart Rhythm 2014; 11(1):119–25.

38. Pappone C, Calovic Z, Vicedomini G, et al. Multipoint left ventricular pacing improves acute hemodynamic response assessed with pressure-volume loops in cardiac resynchronization therapy patients. Heart Rhythm 2014;11(3):394–401.

39. Shetty AK, Sohal M, Chen Z, et al. A comparison of left ventricular endocardial, multisite, and multipolar epicardial cardiac resynchronization: an acute haemodynamic and electroanatomical study. Europace 2014;16(6):873–9.

40. van Deursen C, van Geldorp IE, Rademakers LM, et al. Left ventricular endocardial pacing improves resynchronization therapy in canine left bundle-branch hearts. Circ Arrhythm Electrophysiol 2009; 2(5):580–7.

41. Garrigue S, Jais P, Espil G, et al. Comparison of chronic biventricular pacing between epicardial and endocardial left ventricular stimulation using Doppler tissue imaging in patients with heart failure. Am J Cardiol 2001;88(8):858–62.

42. Bordachar P, Grenz N, Jais P, et al. Left ventricular endocardial or triventricular pacing to optimize cardiac resynchronization therapy in a chronic canine model of ischemic heart failure. Am J Physiol Heart Circ Physiol 2012;303(2):H207–15.

43. Strik M, Rademakers LM, van Deursen CJ, et al. Endocardial left ventricular pacing improves cardiac resynchronization therapy in chronic asynchronous infarction and heart failure models. Circ Arrhythm Electrophysiol 2012;5(1):191–200.

44. Rademakers LM, van Gelder BM, Scheffer MG, et al. Mid-term follow up of thromboembolic complications in left ventricular endocardial cardiac resynchronization therapy. Heart Rhythm 2014;11(4): 609–13.

45. Strik M, van Middendorp LB, Houthuizen P, et al. Interplay of electrical wavefronts as determinant of the response to cardiac resynchronization therapy in dyssynchronous canine hearts. Circ Arrhythm Electrophysiol 2013;6(5):924–31.

46. International Working Group on Quantitative Optimization, Sohaib SM, Whinnett ZI, et al. Cardiac

resynchronisation therapy optimisation strategies: systematic classification, detailed analysis, minimum standards and a roadmap for development and testing. Int J Cardiol 2013;170(2):118–31.

47. van Deursen CJ, Strik M, Rademakers LM, et al. Vectorcardiography as a tool for easy optimization of cardiac resynchronization therapy in canine left bundle branch block hearts. Circ Arrhythm Electrophysiol 2012;5(3):544–52.

48. Whinnett ZI, Francis DP, Denis A, et al. Comparison of different invasive hemodynamic methods for AV delay optimization in patients with cardiac resynchronization therapy: implications for clinical trial design and clinical practice. Int J Cardiol 2013;168(3):2228–37.

49. van Deursen CJ, Wecke L, van Everdingen WM, et al. Vectorcardiography for optimization of stimulation intervals in cardiac resynchronization therapy. J Cardiovasc Transl Res 2015;8(2):128–37.

Assessment of Dyssynchrony

Newer Echocardiographic Techniques in Cardiac Resynchronization Therapy

John Gorcsan III, MD*, Bhupendar Tayal, MD

KEYWORDS

- Heart failure • Echocardiography • Cardiac resynchronization therapy • Ventricular function

KEY POINTS

- Left ventricular (LV) ejection fraction remains widely as the current accepted criterion for cardiac resynchronization therapy (CRT) selection, along with electrocardiographic (ECG) features, but ECG criteria are imperfect.
- Promising echocardiographic techniques may assist with identifying appropriate electromechanical substrate of CRT response, guide LV lead positioning, and identify risk for ventricular arrhythmias after CRT.
- New echocardiographic methods continue to evolve and future clinical experience and emerging evidence will determine eventual usage.

Echocardiographic imaging has played a major role in patient selection for cardiac resynchronization therapy (CRT) as the most commonly used clinical means to determine left ventricular (LV) ejection fraction (EF). A consistent selection criterion for CRT has been an LVEF of 35% or less.[1] Currently, nearly one-third of patients who undergo CRT do not benefit. CRT response relates to a complex interaction of the myocardial electromechanical substrate influenced by global and regional scar, irreversible myocardial dysfunction, and LV lead position, along with clinical and biological factors (**Fig. 1**). A major interest remains to apply advanced echocardiographic techniques beyond LVEF to improve patient selection and CRT delivery to influence patient outcomes favorably.[2,3] Applications of newer echocardiographic techniques to improve CRT response have included differentiating the electromechanical substrate responsive to CRT from nonelectrical substrates, mechanical mapping to guide LV lead, estimating location of regional scar to avoid, and determining profound myocardial dysfunction that is unresponsive to CRT. The large randomized clinical trials of CRT have included heart failure (HF) patients with electrocardiographic (ECG) QRS width of greater than 120 milliseconds[4,5] or of greater than 130 milliseconds,[6,7] subsequent substudies and metaanalyses showed that patients with left bundle branch block (LBBB) and a QRS duration of 150 milliseconds or greater derive most benefit with CRT.[8–12] Accordingly, current guidelines favor CRT implantation for patient with LBBB and QRS of 150 milliseconds or greater.[1] However, the ECG criteria are imperfect and nonresponse to CRT remains a clinical concern. There is less strong support for CRT in patients with LBBB with narrower QRS duration (120–149 ms), or non-LBBB morphology. A long-term follow-up study of the MADIT-CRT trial showed that CRT could lead to a 1.5-fold increased mortality in patients with

Disclosures: Dr J. Gorcsan receives research grant support from Medtronic, Biotronik, GE and Toshiba. There are no perceived conflicts of interest related to this work. Dr B. Tayal has nothing to disclose.
Heart and Vascular Institute, Division of Cardiology, University of Pittsburgh, Pittsburgh, PA, USA
* Corresponding author. University of Pittsburgh Medical Center, Scaife Hall, Suite S-564, 200 Lothrop Street, Pittsburgh, PA 15213.
E-mail address: gorcsanj@upmc.edu

Card Electrophysiol Clin 7 (2015) 609–618
http://dx.doi.org/10.1016/j.ccep.2015.08.013
1877-9182/15/$ – see front matter © 2015 Elsevier Inc. All rights reserved.

cardiacEP.theclinics.com

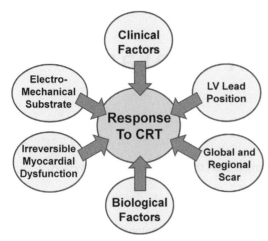

Fig. 1. Factors that alone or in combination have a potential impact on response to cardiac resynchronization therapy (CRT). Newer echocardiographic techniques may play a role in identifying the electromechanical substrate, quantifying irreversible myocardial dysfunction, estimating scar, and guiding left ventricular (LV) lead position to improve CRT response.

non-LBBB QRS morphology and the EchoCRT trial showed that CRT in patients with QRS less than 130 milliseconds and mechanical dyssynchrony may have increased mortality.[9] Therefore, there remains an interest in improvement in identifying CRT responders and also avoid possible harm by CRT. This discussion focuses on the application of newer echocardiographic methods to explore present and future means to improve patient selection for CRT, improve delivery of CRT by guiding LV lead placement and avoid scar, and identify patients who are at risk for poor outcomes and serious ventricular arrhythmias. Among the use of advances in echocardiographic methods in CRT, there is an additional opportunity currently to improve CRT delivery to the subgroup of patients in whom the ECG criteria alone are less clear.

EXPANDING UNDERSTANDING OF DYSSYNCHRONY

A discoordination of regional timing of LV contraction with the septum contracting earlier than the posteriorlateral free wall, usually termed mechanical dyssynchrony, has been an area of intense investigation to improve patient selection for CRT.[13] However, a multicenter observational study called PROSPECT showed that echocardiographic measures of dyssynchrony do not significantly improve patient selection for CRT convincingly beyond ECG criteria.[14] Accordingly,

although a large body of data demonstrates that patients with baseline mechanical dyssynchrony have a more favorable response after CRT than patients who lack dyssynchrony, the use of dyssynchrony measures have not gained widespread support for patient selection.[15–19] Echocardiographic dyssynchrony currently remains a prognostic marker for CRT response. It is reasonable to use measures of dyssynchrony as an adjunct to predict prognosis in patients undergoing CRT, but the guidelines currently do not support echocardiographic dyssynchrony to influence patient selection. Randomized clinical trials have shown that patients with narrow QRS width (<130 ms) with mechanical dyssynchrony do not benefit from CRT and may be harmed potentially with increased mortality.[20,21] Investigations continue to focus on expanding a newer understanding of mechanical dyssynchrony in patients undergoing CRT.

Mechanical dyssynchrony, or discoordination in timing of regional contraction, may occur from different mechanisms that were not previously appreciated. It seems that a minimum of electromechanical substrate, represented by QRS widening, is required for CRT response. In other words, it seems that patients may have mechanical delays in regional contraction from nonelectrical causes, such as differences in regional contractility or regional scar.[13,22] This is an important mechanistic explanation for why mechanical dyssynchrony may exist in a population of HF patients with narrow QRS duration. Recent work has shown that persistent or worsening dyssynchrony in HF patients with narrow QRS duration is associated with an increased incidence of HF hospitalizations, and may represent a new marker for disease severity.[23] Because the electromechanical substrate seems to be central to CRT response, efforts have focused on determining mechanical contraction patterns that reflect the substrate responsive to CRT.

Speckle Tracking Strain Imaging

The previous method of tissue Doppler echocardiography (TDI) can determine differences in timing of LV walls by longitudinal velocity as a measure of dyssynchrony and has been associated with CRT response in several studies. However, a limitation of TDI longitudinal velocity is that it cannot differentiate from passive motion, such as nonelectrical dyssynchrony caused by scar, and active contraction. Owing to this limitation, strain imaging is favored as a means to assess true regional mechanics. Strain methods seem to be more reflective of regional myocardial mechanics than TDI because of its angle independency and absence of the tethering effect. Among speckle tracking strain methods, dyssynchrony assessment by radial strain in the short axis is the most widely used method. A peak-to-peak radial strain cutoff of 130 milliseconds or greater between the anteroseptum and the posterior wall is defined as significant dyssynchrony and has been consistently associated with both response and survival after CRT (**Fig. 2**).[3,18,24,25] Comparative studies between different strain based peak-to-peak methods have also shown that radial strain dyssynchrony is associated most favorably with important patient outcomes after CRT.[3,25] The utility of radial dyssynchrony at baseline before CRT has been supported by its association with clinical outcomes in patients with non-LBBB QRS morphology.[26,27] Hara and colleagues[26] showed in a cohort of 121 non-LBBB patient that patients who lacked significant radial dyssynchrony had a 2.5 times increased risk of death, heart transplantation or LV device implantation after CRT (*P* = .002). Radial strain dyssynchrony was found to be associated independently with a poor prognosis in patients with interventricular conduction delay and right bundle branch block. A major limitation of speckle tracking echocardiography is that an adequate quality image is required and approximately 10% of patients need to be excluded from speckle tracking analysis owing to this. Furthermore, variability is a concern in speckle tracking dyssynchrony measures and proper training and experience is required to ensure high quality and reproducibility.[21]

Animal models and humans have shown that dyssynchrony resulting from an electrical delay, most commonly characterized by LBBB, shows a characteristic early septal contraction associated with lateral wall stretch followed by a delayed contraction of the lateral wall and septal stretch. This may be shown using speckle tracking radial strain from the midventricular level (see **Fig. 1**) or longitudinal strain using apical views (**Fig. 3**). This typical mechanical contraction pattern was described as early septal contraction, with free wall stretch followed by a delayed free wall contraction, represented the substrate for CRT response.[28,29] The absence of this typical baseline dyssynchronous contraction pattern was associated with 3-fold increase in mortality in a recently conducted study of 208 LBBB patients from 2 centers. Furthermore, this method seemed to identify the potential responders to CRT in LBBB morphology patients with QRS between 120 and 149 milliseconds, where the guidelines are still unclear.[29] One of the major advantages of this method was that the reported interobserver agreement was greater than 90%. However, these exciting new methods need to be tested in larger prospective trials to establish their validity and clinical utility.

Newer Tissue Doppler Echocardiography Methods

TDI measures of opposing wall longitudinal velocities were the first approach to demonstrate an association of baseline dyssynchrony before

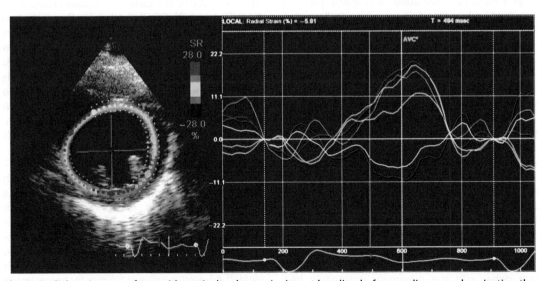

Fig. 2. Radial strain curves from midventricular short axis view at baseline before cardiac resynchronization therapy (CRT) in a 57-year-old woman with left bundle branch block and QRS duration of 164 milliseconds and nonischemic cardiomyopathy. This shows the appropriate electromechanical substrate that is associated with CRT response. This patient had a 55% favorable reduction in left ventricular end-systolic volume 6 months after CRT.

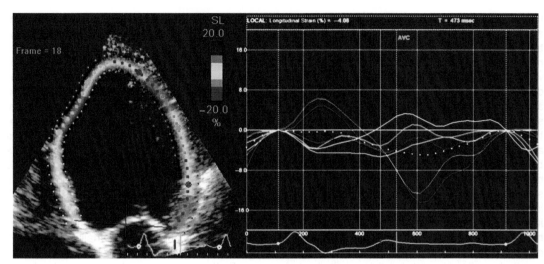

Fig. 3. Longitudinal strain curves at baseline before cardiac resynchronization therapy (CRT) in a 68-year-old man with left bundle branch block and QRS duration of 170 milliseconds. This shows the typical pattern of regional contraction and opposing wall stretch associated with CRT response. This patient had a 46% favorable reduction in left ventricular end-systolic volume 6 months after CRT.

CRT with favorable response. This finding was supported by the PROSPECT multicenter study that time difference between the peak velocities of septum and lateral wall during ejection phase in 4-chamber image was most favorably associated with LV reverse remodeling.[14] TDI measures also had a high yield in the EchoCRT study of a large sample of more than 600 patients with 99% TDI data available on follow-up study.[23] However, the 12-site standard deviation of TDI peak longitudinal velocities was not as successful in PROSPECT because of a lower yield of technically adequate studies and a smaller sample size.[14] Accordingly, TDI peak longitudinal velocity measures have been criticized and recent work has been focused on improving TDI methods. Cross-correlation analysis is a new echocardiographic technique using acceleration curves from the opposing walls and has less intraobserver and interobserver variability because it is largely automated and involves only manual timing of the end of systole.[30] Regions of interest are placed in the basal segments of opposing walls from 3 apical views (**Fig. 4**). Longitudinal velocity data are then converted to time differential acceleration curves. Acceleration curves from the opposing walls are correlated against each other by time shifting in either direction with a maximum of 15 frames. This time shifting results in determining the activation delay, which is the time delay with the maximum correlation between the opposing wall acceleration curves. A cut off of 35 milliseconds or greater in any of the 3 apical views would be used to characterize

as baseline dyssynchrony associated with favorable outcomes after CRT. Risum and colleagues[30] studied the cross-correlation of longitudinal velocities in 121 CRT patients with symptomatic HF, a LVEF of 35% or less, and a QRS duration of 120 milliseconds or greater. The patients with a cross-correlation maximum time delay of 35 milliseconds or greater had significantly more favorable clinical outcomes 4 years after CRT implantation with fewer deaths, heart transplants, or LV assist devices (14% vs 40%, P = .001). The patients' adjusted hazard ratio (HR) was 0.35 (95 CI, 0.16–0.76; P = .001). In a subgroup analysis of patients with QRS duration of 120 to 149 milliseconds, they reported that the absence of the cross correlation maximum time delay less than 35 milliseconds was associated with a 4 times increased risk of unfavorable events. Thus, this method could possibly play a role in patient selection for CRT implantation, including patients with intermediate QRS duration.

Another new TDI-based method used in CRT patients is to quantify the apical rocking with the calculation of apical transverse motion. It has suggested promising results in patients with LBBB.[31,32] Apical rocking is described as the passive transverse motion of the apex by the contraction of the opposing walls at different point of time. Apical transverse motion is calculated from TDI data.[31] A baseline value of 1.5 mm for apical transverse motion was associated with favorable reverse LV remodeling as well as improved survival after CRT.

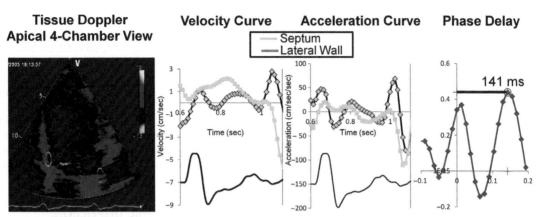

| Tissue Doppler Apical 4-Chamber View | Velocity Curve | Acceleration Curve | Phase Delay |

Fig. 4. Calculation of cross-correlation phase delay in a patient with significant baseline dyssynchrony before cardiac resynchronization therapy. (*Left panel*) Tissue Doppler image with regions of interest in basal 2 mitral annular regions. (*Middle panels*) Velocity and accelerations curves from septal and lateral walls. (*Right panel*) Calculation of a significant phase delay of 141 milliseconds.

Dyssynchrony by 3-Dimensional Echocardiography

Three-dimensional speckle tracking echocardiography is a new advancement to assess dyssynchrony in HF patients. Although the temporal resolution is lower than 2-dimensional methods, 3-dimensional (3D) methods may add information not appreciated by 2-dimensional imaging alone. Several approaches to assess dyssynchrony including standard deviation of time-to-peak of LV strain, 3D LV volume, LV area tracking have been described.[33–35] One of the most studied method is the standard deviation of the time to reach the minimum end-systolic volume of a 16-segment LV model. A metaanalysis of 73 studies reported a good accuracy of standard deviation of end-systolic volume to predict CRT response and a weighted mean of 9.8% was proposed as a cutoff to define dyssynchrony associated with CRT response.[36] In addition, intraobserver and interobserver reliability was reported to be favorable.[36] Another approach based on 3D strain described by Tanaka and colleagues[33] showed its ability to identify dyssynchrony and site of latest activation. This approach had the advantage of strain imaging, which measured wall thickening or thinning in 3 dimensions. An exciting advancement being developed is fusion imaging of the 3D echo images with fluoroscopy to facilitate the clinical usefulness in the electrophysiology laboratory (**Fig. 5**). Technical limitations of 3D imaging include inferior image resolution, lower frame rates, and the current lack of standardization between different software packages, which may result in variability in strain values.[37]

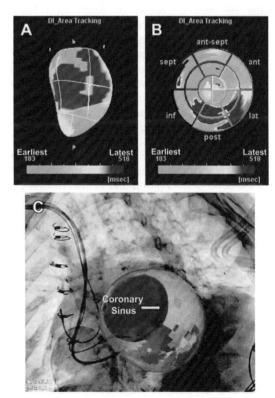

Fig. 5. Three-dimensional echocardiographic image (*A*) and polar map (*B*) with color-coded time to peak strain imaging showing site of late activation color coded as red. (*C*) Fusion of the echocardiographic image with the fluoroscopic image. ant, anterior; ant-sept, anteroseptum; inf, inferior; lat, lateral; post, posterior; sept, septum.

STRAIN IMAGING TO GUIDE PLACEMENT OF THE LEFT VENTRICULAR LEAD

Placement of the LV pacing lead at the optimal site could play an important role in the response after CRT. Echocardiographic strain imaging has been shown to map mechanical activation. Physiologic studies have suggested that LV pacing from the latest site of mechanical activation has the most efficient result from CRT. Two independent randomized trials named TARGET and STARTER showed improved patient outcomes after CRT with LV lead implantation guided by echocardiographic strain mapping to the site of latest activation. The TARGET trial enrolled 220 patients randomized in 1:1 fashion to echo-guided or routine LV lead implantation of CRT.[38] Echocardiographic guidance consisted of radial strain timing toward the latest activation and away from radial strain segments with less than 10% thickening, considered to be likely scar. There were 15% more patients with reverse LV remodeling in the echo-guided group (P = .03). As a secondary analysis, patients in the echo-guided group had less HF hospitalizations or death (Log Rank P = .03). Patients with LV lead placement concordant with the site of latest activation showed a 4-fold increase in their response rate. Similarly, LV lead placement remote from strain segments considered likely scar was associated with more favorable clinical outcomes. The TARGET investigators estimated that treatment by this in 6.6 patients will lead to a gain of an additional CRT responder.

The STARTER trial enrolled 187 patients, and with 3:2 randomization had 110 patients assigned to the echo-guided group and 77 had routine LV lead placement with coronary venography and fluoroscopy.[39] The total procedural time was similar between the 2 groups (134 vs 130 min). Site of latest mechanical activation was determined by speckle tracking radial strain from 12 segments including the basal and mid LV short axis views. Using an intention-to-treat analysis, patients randomized to the echo-guided strategy had a nearly 50% decrease in HF hospitalizations or death as the primary endpoint with a HR of 0.48 (95% CI, 0.28–0.82; P = .006) compared with the routine group. Interestingly, a substudy analysis revealed that benefit was particularly observed in patients with intermediate ECG criteria: QRS (120–149 ms) and non-LBBB QRS morphology.[40] Avoidance of LV positioning in a segment with likely scar was an important part of the STARTER analysis.[41] LV lead placement remote from scar estimated as segmental strain (<10%) was associated with a significantly lesser

risk of HF hospitalization or death after CRT compared with patients with LV leads concordant or adjacent to scar (HR, 0.46; 95% CI, 0.23–0.96; P = .04).[41] These 2 remarkable similar randomized clinical trials demonstrate improvements in patient outcomes with echo-guided LV lead placement for CRT. Future technical advancements, such as fusion of echocardiographic strain images showing site of latest activation and scar with the fluoroscopic images during CRT implantation, have promise to improve implementation.

ECHOCARDIOGRAPHIC DISPERSION, DYSSYNCHRONY, AND ARRHYTHMIAS

Newer echocardiographic approaches to characterize regional mechanics have played a role as a marker for ventricular arrhythmias after CRT. In a MADIT-CRT substudy, Kutyifa and colleagues[42] used the standard deviation of time-to-peak of the transverse strain from the 4-chamber and 2-chamber views. A total of 809 patients (CRT, n = 473; implantable cardioverter defibrillator, n = 336) had paired dyssynchrony analysis at baseline and 12-month follow-up. Patients with CRT were divided into 3 groups improved (15% decrease in baseline dyssynchrony after CRT; n = 281), worsened (15% decrease in baseline dyssynchrony; n = 96), and unchanged dyssynchrony (all others; n = 96). Baseline dyssynchrony was not associated with ventricular arrhythmias in the study. However, patients with improved dyssynchrony in the LBBB group had significantly fewer ventricular arrhythmias or deaths compared with groups of worsened dyssynchrony, unchanged dyssynchrony, or implantable cardioverter defibrillator control patients. LBBB patients with improved dyssynchrony had a reduced risk for ventricular arrhythmias with HR 0.30 (95% CI, 0.12–0.77; P = .01) in comparison with the implantable cardioverter defibrillator group. However, a similar association was not seen in the non-LBBB group of patients. One of the major limitations of the study was that they used transverse strain, which may have greater interobserver variability than other strain methods.

Haugaa and colleagues[43] recently studied the impact of change in dyssynchrony in a cohort of 266 HF patients undergoing CRT using radial strain peak-to-peak delay to identify dyssynchrony at baseline and 6 months after CRT. Patients were divided into 4 groups based on presence or absence of dyssynchrony before and after CRT. Patients with dyssynchrony after CRT had a nearly 4-fold increased risk of ventricular arrhythmias (antitachycardia pacing or appropriate shock) independent of all important baseline factors. The findings in this study were independent of QRS morphology. It also suggested that the onset of new radial strain dyssynchrony after CRT could be dangerous. Mechanical dispersion is a new echocardiographic measure of longitudinal strain introduced by Haugaa and colleagues[44] and these authors have showed it to be associated with ventricular arrhythmias in both ischemic and nonischemic cardiomyopathy groups.[45] Mechanical dispersion is defined by the standard deviation of the time to peak of the longitudinal segmental strain curves from the onset of QRS of the 18 segments in the apical views (**Fig. 6**). Hasselberg and colleagues[46] reported in 170 HF patients who had mechanical dispersion measured at baseline and at 6 months after CRT. Patients with serious ventricular arrhythmias had significantly greater mechanical dispersion 6 months after CRT (112 vs 80 ms; $P = .001$). Patients with improvement in mechanical dispersion had a significantly lesser risk of ventricular arrhythmias after CRT. Specifically, they reported that every 10-millisecond increase in mechanical dispersion at 6 months after CRT was associated with increased ventricular arrhythmias with a HR of 1.2 (95% CI, 1.06–1.35; $P = .005$).

A more recent study by Tayal and colleagues[47] used TDI cross-correlation to classify patients into 4 groups based on dyssynchrony before and 6 months after CRT. They studied 151 patients from 2 different centers who had CRT based on current guidelines. Patients with TDI cross-correlation maximum time delay of 35 milliseconds or greater[30] as a marker of dyssynchrony. Notably, the baseline characteristics of the study population were similar in all 4 groups. However, patients with TDI cross correlation maximum time delay of 35 milliseconds or greater that persisted after CRT or those with new-onset cross-correlation maximum phase delay after CRT had a significantly higher event rate of ventricular arrhythmia than patients with an improved cross-correlation maximum time delay. Specifically, they observed that patients had no significant cross-correlation delay at baseline but developed a new cross-correlation maximum time delay of 35 milliseconds or greater after CRT had a worse prognosis. This study further suggested that serial assessment TDI cross-correlation maximum time delay before and after CRT could have prognostic implication in patient receiving CRT regarding ventricular arrhythmias. These 4 studies combined together demonstrate that abnormal regional mechanical contraction assessed by newer echocardiographic methods after CRT are markers for increased risk of ventricular arrhythmias.

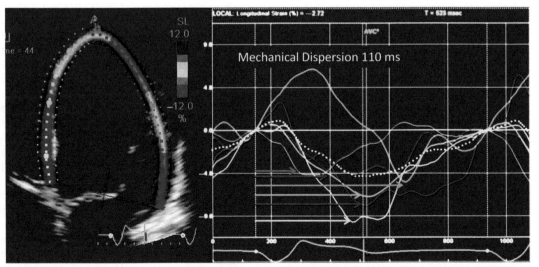

Fig. 6. Echocardiographic longitudinal velocity strain curves in a 69-year-old man with mechanical dispersion of time-to-peak longitudinal strain curves in each segment (*arrows*) after cardiac resynchronization therapy (CRT). The standard deviation in time-to-peak strain curves in the 4 chamber view was 110 milliseconds at 6 months after CRT. This patient experienced an episode of ventricular tachycardia with appropriate shock therapy approximately 1 year after CRT.

SUMMARY

LVEF remains widely as the currently accepted criterion for CRT selection, along with ECG features. Because ECG criteria are imperfect, several promising new echocardiographic techniques may assist with identification of the appropriate electromechanical substrate of CRT response, guide LV lead positioning toward latest site of mechanical activation and away from scar, and serve as a means to identify risk for ventricular arrhythmias after CRT. These new echocardiographic methods continue to evolve and future clinical experience and emerging evidence will determine their eventual usage.

REFERENCES

1. Tracy CM, Epstein AE, Darbar D, et al. 2012 ACCF/AHA/HRS focused update of the 2008 guidelines for device-based therapy of cardiac rhythm abnormalities: a report of the American College of Cardiology Foundation/American Heart Association Task Force on Practice Guidelines and the Heart Rhythm Society. [corrected]. Circulation 2012;126(14):1784–800.

2. Gorcsan J 3rd, Abraham T, Agler DA, et al. Echocardiography for cardiac resynchronization therapy: recommendations for performance and reporting–a report from the American Society of Echocardiography Dyssynchrony Writing Group endorsed by the Heart Rhythm Society. J Am Soc Echocardiogr 2008;21(3):191–213.

3. Gorcsan J 3rd, Oyenuga O, Habib PJ, et al. Relationship of echocardiographic dyssynchrony to long-term survival after cardiac resynchronization therapy. Circulation 2010;122(19):1910–8.

4. Bristow MR, Saxon LA, Boehmer J, et al. Cardiac-resynchronization therapy with or without an implantable defibrillator in advanced chronic heart failure. N Engl J Med 2004;350(21):2140–50.

5. Cleland JG, Daubert JC, Erdmann E, et al. The effect of cardiac resynchronization on morbidity and mortality in heart failure. N Engl J Med 2005;352(15):1539–49.

6. Abraham WT, Fisher WG, Smith AL, et al. Cardiac resynchronization in chronic heart failure. N Engl J Med 2002;346(24):1845–53.

7. Moss AJ, Hall WJ, Cannom DS, et al. Cardiac-resynchronization therapy for the prevention of heart-failure events. N Engl J Med 2009;361(14):1329–38.

8. Zareba W, Klein H, Cygankiewicz I, et al. Effectiveness of cardiac resynchronization therapy by QRS morphology in the Multicenter Automatic Defibrillator Implantation Trial-Cardiac Resynchronization Therapy (MADIT-CRT). Circulation 2011;123(10):1061–72.

9. Goldenberg I, Kutyifa V, Klein HU, et al. Survival with cardiac-resynchronization therapy in mild heart failure. N Engl J Med 2014;370(18):1694–701.

10. Gold MR, Thebault C, Linde C, et al. Effect of QRS duration and morphology on cardiac resynchronization therapy outcomes in mild heart failure: results from the Resynchronization Reverses Remodeling in Systolic Left Ventricular Dysfunction (REVERSE) study. Circulation 2012;126(7):822–9.

11. Sipahi I, Carrigan TP, Rowland DY, et al. Impact of QRS duration on clinical event reduction with cardiac resynchronization therapy: meta-analysis of randomized controlled trials. Arch Intern Med 2011;171(16):1454–62.

12. Sipahi I, Chou JC, Hyden M, et al. Effect of QRS morphology on clinical event reduction with cardiac resynchronization therapy: meta-analysis of randomized controlled trials. Am Heart J 2012;163(2):260–7.e3.

13. Lumens J, Leenders GE, Cramer MJ, et al. Mechanistic evaluation of echocardiographic dyssynchrony indices: patient data combined with multiscale computer simulations. Circ Cardiovasc Imaging 2012;5(4):491–9.

14. Chung ES, Leon AR, Tavazzi L, et al. Results of the Predictors of Response to CRT (PROSPECT) trial. Circulation 2008;117(20):2608–16.

15. Gorcsan J 3rd, Kanzaki H, Bazaz R, et al. Usefulness of echocardiographic tissue synchronization imaging to predict acute response to cardiac resynchronization therapy. Am J Cardiol 2004;93(9):1178–81.

16. Gorcsan J 3rd, Tanabe M, Bleeker GB, et al. Combined longitudinal and radial dyssynchrony predicts ventricular response after resynchronization therapy. J Am Coll Cardiol 2007;50(15):1476–83.

17. Sogaard P, Egeblad H, Kim WY, et al. Tissue Doppler imaging predicts improved systolic performance and reversed left ventricular remodeling during long-term cardiac resynchronization therapy. J Am Coll Cardiol 2002;40(4):723–30.

18. Suffoletto MS, Dohi K, Cannesson M, et al. Novel speckle-tracking radial strain from routine black-and white echocardiographic images to quantify dyssynchrony and predict response to cardiac resynchronization therapy. Circulation 2006;113(7):960–8.

19. Yu CM, Bax JJ, Gorcsan J 3rd. Critical appraisal of methods to assess mechanical dyssynchrony. Curr Opin Cardiol 2009;24(1):18–28.

20. Beshai JF, Grimm RA, Nagueh SF, et al. Cardiac-resynchronization therapy in heart failure with narrow QRS complexes. N Engl J Med 2007;357(24):2461–71.

21. Ruschitzka F, Abraham WT, Singh JP, et al. Cardiac-resynchronization therapy in heart failure with a narrow QRS complex. N Engl J Med 2013;369(15):1395–405.

22. Lumens J, Ploux S, Strik M, et al. Comparative electromechanical and hemodynamic effects of left ventricular and biventricular pacing in dyssynchronous heart failure: electrical resynchronization versus left-right ventricular interaction. J Am Coll Cardiol 2013;62(25):2395–403.

23. Gorcsan J, Sogaard P, Bax JJ, et al. Association of persistent or worsened echocardiographic dyssynchrony with unfavorable clinical outcomes in heart failure patients with narrow QRS width: a subgroup analysis of the EchoCRT trial. Eur Heart J 2015. [Epub ahead of print].

24. Tanaka H, Nesser HJ, Buck T, et al. Dyssynchrony by speckle-tracking echocardiography and response to cardiac resynchronization therapy: results of the Speckle Tracking and Resynchronization (STAR) study. Eur Heart J 2010;31(14):1690–700.

25. Delgado V, Ypenburg C, van Bommel RJ, et al. Assessment of left ventricular dyssynchrony by speckle tracking strain imaging comparison between longitudinal, circumferential, and radial strain in cardiac resynchronization therapy. J Am Coll Cardiol 2008;51(20):1944–52.

26. Hara H, Oyenuga OA, Tanaka H, et al. The relationship of QRS morphology and mechanical dyssynchrony to long-term outcome following cardiac resynchronization therapy. Eur Heart J 2012;33(21): 2680–91.

27. Bank AJ, Gage RM, Marek JJ, et al. Mechanical dyssynchrony is additive to ECG criteria and independently associated with reverse remodelling and clinical response to cardiac resynchronisation therapy in patients with advanced heart failure. Open Heart 2015;2(1):e000246.

28. Risum N, Strauss D, Sogaard P, et al. Left bundle-branch block: the relationship between electrocardiogram electrical activation and echocardiography mechanical contraction. Am Heart J 2013;166(2): 340–8.

29. Risum N, Tayal B, Fritz-Hansen T, et al. Identification of typical left bundle branch block contraction by strain echocardiography is additive to electrocardiography in prediction of long-term outcome after cardiac resynchronization therapy. J Am Coll Cardiol 2015;66(6):631–41.

30. Risum N, Williams ES, Khouri MG, et al. Mechanical dyssynchrony evaluated by tissue Doppler cross-correlation analysis is associated with long-term survival in patients after cardiac resynchronization therapy. Eur Heart J 2013;34(1):48–56.

31. Stankovic I, Aarones M, Smith HJ, et al. Dynamic relationship of left-ventricular dyssynchrony and contractile reserve in patients undergoing cardiac resynchronization therapy. Eur Heart J 2014;35(1): 48–55.

32. Szulik M, Tillekaerts M, Vangeel V, et al. Assessment of apical rocking: a new, integrative approach for selection of candidates for cardiac resynchronization therapy. Eur J Echocardiogr 2010;11(10):863–9.

33. Tanaka H, Hara H, Saba S, et al. Usefulness of three-dimensional speckle tracking strain to quantify dyssynchrony and the site of latest mechanical activation. Am J Cardiol 2010;105(2):235–42.

34. Kapetanakis S, Bhan A, Murgatroyd F, et al. Real-time 3D echo in patient selection for cardiac resynchronization therapy. JACC Cardiovasc Imaging 2011;4(1):16–26.

35. Thebault C, Donal E, Bernard A, et al. Real-time three-dimensional speckle tracking echocardiography: a novel technique to quantify global left ventricular mechanical dyssynchrony. Eur J Echocardiogr 2011;12(1):26–32.

36. Kleijn SA, Aly MF, Knol DL, et al. A meta-analysis of left ventricular dyssynchrony assessment and prediction of response to cardiac resynchronization therapy by three-dimensional echocardiography. Eur Heart J Cardiovasc Imaging 2012;13(9):763–75.

37. Aly MF, Kleijn SA, de Boer K, et al. Comparison of three-dimensional echocardiographic software packages for assessment of left ventricular mechanical dyssynchrony and prediction of response to cardiac resynchronization therapy. Eur Heart J Cardiovasc Imaging 2013;14(7):700–10.

38. Khan FZ, Virdee MS, Palmer CR, et al. Targeted left ventricular lead placement to guide cardiac resynchronization therapy: the TARGET study: a randomized, controlled trial. J Am Coll Cardiol 2012; 59(17):1509–18.

39. Saba S, Marek J, Schwartzman D, et al. Echocardiography-guided left ventricular lead placement for cardiac resynchronization therapy: results of the Speckle Tracking Assisted Resynchronization Therapy for Electrode Region trial. Circ Heart Fail 2013; 6(3):427–34.

40. Marek JJ, Saba S, Onishi T, et al. Usefulness of echocardiographically guided left ventricular lead placement for cardiac resynchronization therapy in patients with intermediate QRS width and non-left bundle branch block morphology. Am J Cardiol 2014;113(1):107–16.

41. Sade LE, Saba S, Marek JJ, et al. The association of left ventricular lead position related to regional scar by speckle-tracking echocardiography with clinical outcomes in patients receiving cardiac resynchronization therapy. J Am Soc Echocardiogr 2014;27(6): 648–56.

42. Kutyifa V, Pouleur AC, Knappe D, et al. Dyssynchrony and the risk of ventricular arrhythmias. JACC Cardiovasc Imaging 2013;6(4):432–44.

43. Haugaa KH, Marek JJ, Ahmed M, et al. Mechanical dyssynchrony after cardiac resynchronization therapy for severely symptomatic heart failure is associated with risk for ventricular arrhythmias. J Am Soc Echocardiogr 2014;27(8):872–9.

44. Haugaa KH, Goebel B, Dahlslett T, et al. Risk assessment of ventricular arrhythmias in patients with nonischemic dilated cardiomyopathy by strain echocardiography. J Am Soc Echocardiogr 2012; 25(6):667–73.

45. Haugaa KH, Smedsrud MK, Steen T, et al. Mechanical dispersion assessed by myocardial strain in patients after myocardial infarction for risk prediction of ventricular arrhythmia. JACC Cardiovasc Imaging 2010;3(3):247–56.

46. Hasselberg NE, Haugaa KH, Bernard A, et al. Left ventricular markers of mortality and ventricular arrhythmias in heart failure patients with cardiac resynchronization therapy. Eur Heart J Cardiovasc Imaging 2015. [Epub ahead of print].

47. Tayal B, Gorcsan Iii J 3rd, Delgado-Montero A, et al. Mechanical dyssynchrony by tissue Doppler cross correlation is associated with risk for complex ventricular arrhythmias after cardiac resynchronization therapy. J Am Soc Echocardiogr 2015. [Epub ahead of print].

The Role of Cardiovascular Magnetic Resonance in Cardiac Resynchronization Therapy

Francisco Leyva, MD, FRCP[a,b,*]

KEYWORDS

- Cardiac resynchronization therapy • Cardiovascular magnetic resonance • Heart failure

KEY POINTS

- Imaging in cardiac resynchronization therapy (CRT) patients is particularly important before implantation.
- Cardiovascular magnetic resonance (CMR) is the gold standard for the assessment of myocardial structure and function and its ability to image myocardial scar is unique.
- With the advent of CMR-compatible (conditional or safe) devices, CMR is likely to prove useful in the investigation of CRT nonresponders.

INTRODUCTION

Cardiac resynchronization therapy (CRT) is an established treatment for patients with heart failure with impaired left ventricular (LV) systolic function and a wide QRS complex. Early studies confirmed a benefit from CRT in patients with advanced heart failure (New York Heart Association [NYHA] class III and IV). More recently, emerging evidence supports the extension of CRT to patients mild heart failure (NYHA class I and II).

Cardiovascular magnetic resonance (CMR) is a radiation-free imaging modality that provides unparalleled spatial resolution. As well as providing measurements of global and segmental cardiac function, CMR also permits localization and quantification of myocardial perfusion and scars. These measures provide important information on the

cause and prognosis of patients with heart failure and may also be helpful in guiding LV lead deployment. This review explores the role of CMR in the preimplant workup for patients undergoing CRT.

CARDIAC FUNCTION AND CAUSE OF CARDIOMYOPATHY

Echocardiography is, and is likely to remain, the initial imaging modality in patients with heart failure. Although CMR is not a replacement for echocardiography, it provides complementary diagnostic information on cardiac structure, function, and myocardial viability in a single scan. For this reason, CMR is becoming a routine investigation in patients with cardiomyopathy and heart failure. A typical CMR scanning protocol is described in **Fig. 1.**

Conflicts of Interest: F. Leyva is a consultant for and has received research support from Medtronic, St. Jude Medical, Sorin, and Boston Scientific.
[a] Aston Medical Research Institute, Aston Medical School, Aston University, Aston Triangle, Birmingham, B4 7ET, UK; [b] Department of Cardiology, University Hospital Birmingham Queen Elizabeth, Mindelsohn Way, Edgbaston, Birmingham, B15 2WB, UK
* Aston Medical Research Institute, Aston Medical School, Aston University, Aston Triangle, Birmingham, B4 7ET, UK.
E-mail address: cardiologists@hotmail.com

Card Electrophysiol Clin 7 (2015) 619–633
http://dx.doi.org/10.1016/j.ccep.2015.08.003

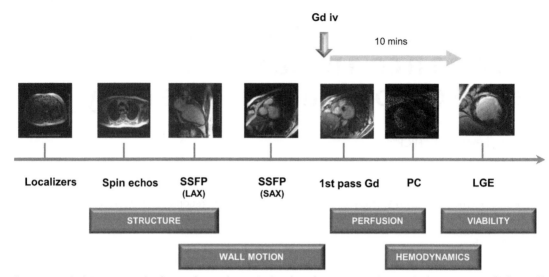

Fig. 1. A typical CMR scan. The figure shows the typical order of acquisitions in a typical CMR scan, which usually takes approximately 45 minutes to perform. From left to right, these consist of (1) Localizers: low-quality scans used to frame the region of interest; (2) Spin-echoes: these are black-blood scans that provide excellent anatomic border delineation, ideal for the assessment of cardiac structure; SSFP imaging in the long axes; (3) LAX (long-axis) and short axis (SAX); (4) SAX; (5) First-pass imaging immediately after administration of contrast (gadolinium chelate [Gd]); (6) Phase-contrast imaging, for the assessment of velocity and flow in the aorta and pulmonary arteries, ideal for the assessment of cardiac output, valvular stenosis, and regurgitation. It can be undertaken while waiting 10 minutes for the LGE acquisition; (7) LGE acquisition, for the assessment of myocardial scar. This basic protocol can be extended to include further sequences on the same sitting, such as tagging and T1 mapping.

Left Ventricular Function

The "work-horse," white-blood CMR sequence, steady-state free precession (SSFP), provides excellent spatial resolution and endocardial border delineation of cardiac chambers. Using 2- or 3-dimensional acquisitions, SSFP can be used for LV volumes with high precision.[1,2] Importantly, the interstudy variability of CMR for calculation of LV volumes and left ventricular ejection fraction (LVEF) is much lower than with echocardiography.[3]

Cause of Heart Failure

Establishing the cause of heart failure is pivotal in clinical management. Traditionally, the diagnosis of ischemic cardiomyopathy has been made on the basis of a history of a myocardial infarction,[4] and finding electrocardiogram (ECG) abnormalities, coronary artery stenoses on coronary angiography, and of regional wall motion abnormalities on echocardiography. Conversely, absence of these features has been used to support the diagnosis of nonischemic cardiomyopathy. Importantly, however, myocardial infarction can be silent in approximately 30% of patients, coronary arteries may appear unobstructed after a myocardial infarction, ECG abnormalities may not be present after a

myocardial infarction,[5] and regional wall motion abnormalities may also be found in patients with nonischemic cardiomyopathy.

Late gadolinium enhancement CMR (LGE-CMR) is the gold standard for the quantification and localization of myocardial scarring in vivo.[6] Characterization of the pattern of LGE is a key factor to the elucidation of cause (**Fig. 2**). A subendocardial or transmural distribution of scar along arterial territories is typical of a myocardial infarction. In contrast, the association of dilated ventricular cavities, impaired ventricular function, and no myocardial scarring, or LV midwall enhancement, indicates idiopathic dilated cardiomyopathy.[6,7] A more patchy, piecemeal, distribution of LGE is found in myocarditis, sarcoidosis, and arrhythmogenic right ventricular (RV) cardiomyopathy. Diffuse, subendocardial LGE is characteristic of amyloidosis, whereas as a basal inferior, LV distribution of LGE is typical of Anderson-Fabry disease. In the author's experience, nonischemic cardiomyopathy on the basis of a traditional definition may be reclassified as ischemic cardiomyopathy on CMR (see **Fig. 2**) in approximately 20% of cases (unpublished data, Leyva F, 2015). Importantly, LGE-CMR is superior to nuclear imaging in detecting scar, particularly in a subendocardial distribution (**Fig. 3**).[8]

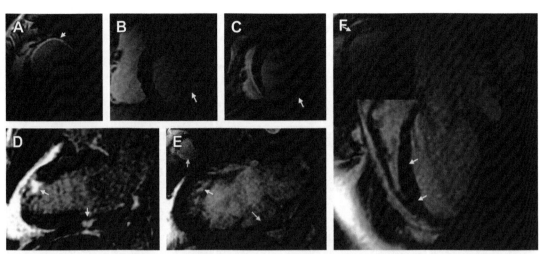

Fig. 2. CMR in the diagnosis of cardiomyopathy. All the CMR images pertain to patients who were initially diagnosed with nonischemic, dilated cardiomyopathy. Yellow arrows indicate areas of LGE. This diagnosis was reclassified on the basis of subsequent CMR scans, as shown. (*A*) LGE-CMR short-axis slice showing a subendocardial myocardial infarction in the territory of the left anterior descending artery, extending from a 9-o'clock to a 2-o'clock position; (*B*) LGE-CMR short-axis slice showing a transmural myocardial infarction the territory of the circumflex artery, extending from a 3-o'clock to a 7-o'clock position; (*C*) LGE-CMR showing a transmural myocardial infarction in the territory of the right coronary artery, extending from a 3-o'clock to a 7-o'clock position. This is associated with marked myocardial thinning; (*D*) Patchy LGE characteristic of myocarditis; (*E*) Mixed cardiomyopathy: LV noncompaction cardiomyopathy and ischemic cardiomyopathy. Note the transmural inferior myocardial infarction (see insert for LGE-CMR), which has led to myocardial thinning; (*F*) Four-chamber and short-axis LGE-CMR images showing midwall LGE, denoting fibrosis, in idiopathic dilated cardiomyopathy. (*From* Leyva F. Cardiac resynchronization therapy guided by cardiovascular magnetic resonance. J Cardiovasc Magn Reson 2010;12:17; with permission.)

CARDIOVASCULAR MAGNETIC RESONANCE IN RISK STRATIFICATION

Current guidelines require the physician to decide between CRT-pacing (CRT-P) or CRT-defibrillation (CRT-D), but no recommendations are made as to how to choose between these therapies. This choice depends on the expected benefits of these therapies as well as potential risks.

Risks of Implantable Cardioverter Defibrillator Therapy

The COMPANION (Comparison of Medical Therapy, Pacing, and Defibrillation in Heart Failure) study showed that CRT-D was superior to CRT-P in prolonging survival.[9] Currently, CRT-D accounts for 70% to 80% of all CRT therapies delivered worldwide. Importantly, however, only 35% of implantable cardioverter defibrillator (ICD) patients receive therapy for ventricular arrhythmia during the first 3 years following implantation.[10] In addition, ICD therapy is not without risks. Within 4 years of implantaton, more than 30% ICD patients suffer a complication.[11] These complications may include inappropriate shocks and their associated harm.[12] Generally, complications are higher for CRT-D than for CRT-P.[13]

An assessment of arrhythmic risk is therefore important in choosing between CRT-P, which will only prevent pump failure, and CRT-D, which will also prevent sudden cardiac death (SCD). Unfortunately, conventional measures, such as the presence of premature ventricular complexes, nonsustained ventricular tachycardia, and programmed ventricular stimulation, have proven to be of little value in assessing arrhythmic risk in primary prevention.[14]

Scar Burden

Increasing myocardial scar burden relates to a poor outcome from treatments such as revascularization[15–18] and pharmacologic therapy.[19] Similar findings have emerged in the context of CRT. In a study of 28 patients, White and colleagues[20] found a higher scar burden in nonresponders than in responders (median 24.7% vs 1.0% in responders, *P* = .0022). The author also showed that a clinical composite score, defined as survival for 1 year following implantation free of hospitalizations plus an improvement by greater than or equal to 1 NYHA classes or by greater than or equal to 25% in 6-minute walking distance was 2.3 times higher in patients with scar greater than or equal to 33%

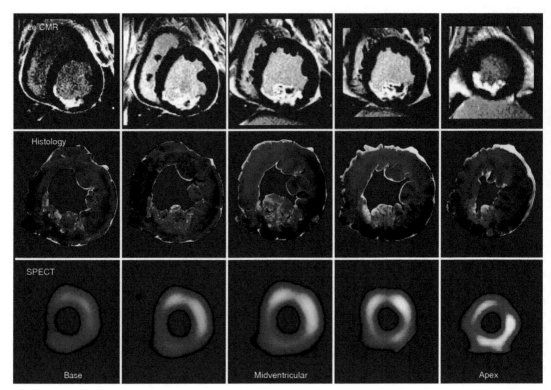

Fig. 3. Comparison of LGE-CMR and nuclear imaging for the detection of myocardial scar. Contrast-enhanced CMR (*upper row*) in which subendocardial scar appears white; histology (*middle row*) in which scar also appears white; and, single-photon emission computed tomography (SPECT; *lower row*), in which the same scar is not evident. Note the nearly perfect match between necrosis defined by histology and CMR. Although CMR allows the exact assessment of the transmural extent of infarction, SPECT defines segments as either viable or nonviable. In this study, CMR systematically detects subendocardial infarcts that were missed by SPECT. (*From* Wagner A, Mahrholdt H, Holly TA, et al. Contrast-enhanced MRI and routine single photon emission computed tomography (SPECT) perfusion imaging for detection of subendocardial myocardial infarcts: an imaging study. Lancet 2003;361:376; with permission.)

than in patients with scar less than 33%.[21] Although the notion that increasing scar burden should predict a poor outcome from CRT, a cutoff of scar burden above which CRT becomes ineffective has not been validated, internally or externally. Moreover, studies on the effects of scar burden in CRT recipients have not included a control group. Therefore, no conclusions can be made regarding the benefits of CRT according to scar burden. Accordingly, scar burden should not be used in selecting patients for CRT.

Scar Patterns

Midwall scar (fibrosis) (see **Fig. 2**), which is found in approximately one-third of patients with idiopathic dilated cardiomyopathy, has been linked to a poor outcome. In a study of 472 patients with dilated cardiomyopathy, Gulati and colleagues[22] showed that midwall fibrosis was independently associated with total mortality (hazard ratio [HR], 2.43; 95% confidence interval [CI],

1.50–3.92), cardiovascular mortality or cardiac transplantation (HR, 3.22; 95% CI, 1.95–5.31), and sudden cardiac death (HR, 4.61; 95% CI, 2.75–7.74). In patients undergoing CRT-P, Leyva and colleagues[23] found that midwall fibrosis was associated with an 18.5-fold risk of death from cardiovascular causes (**Fig. 4**). Although no patient of 77 without midwall fibrosis died suddenly, 15% of patients with midwall fibrosis died suddenly over a follow-up period of 8.7 years. These findings suggest that patients with nonischemic cardiomyopathy and midwall fibrosis are at a particularly high risk of cardiovascular events, including arrhythmic events. Conversely, patients with dilated cardiomyopathy and no myocardial scar are at a comparatively low risk of SCD.

Scar and Arrhythmias

Considerable attention has focused on myocardial scar as a possible predictor of arrhythmic events. Early studies showed that scar burden is a more

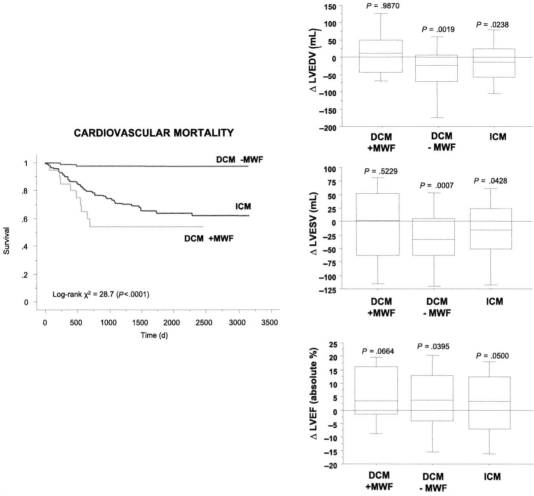

Fig. 4. Effects of midwall fibrosis after CRT. The left panel shows Kaplan-Meier survival curves for cardiovascular mortality in patients with dilated cardiomyopathy (DCM) with (+) and without (−) midwall fibrosis (MWF), and patients with ischemic cardiomyopathy (ICM). The right panel shows changes from baseline in box-and-whisker plots, in which the 5 horizontal lines represent the 10th, 25th, 50th, 75th, and 90th percentiles, from bottom to top. For left ventricular end-diastolic (LVEDV) and end-systolic (LVESV) volumes, the change is shown as the percentage change in relation to baseline volumes. For LVEF, changes are shown in terms of the absolute percentage change. (*Adapted from* Leyva F, Taylor RJ, Foley PW, et al. Left ventricular midwall fibrosis as a predictor of mortality and morbidity after cardiac resynchronization therapy in patients with nonischemic cardiomyopathy. J Am Coll Cardiol 2012;60:1664–5; with permission.)

powerful predictor of SCD than LVEF. In the MADIT-II (Multicentre Automatic Defibrillator Implantation Trial II) trial, the extent of fixed perfusion defects on nuclear imaging was a strong predictor of lethal arrhythmias over a follow-up of 30 months.[24] Using an LGE-CMR study of 65 patients with nonischemic cardiomyopathy undergoing ICD therapy, Wu and colleagues[25] found that SCD or appropriate ICD shock occurred in 22% patients with scar versus 8% of patients without scar (**Fig. 5**).

A relationship between patterns of myocardial scar and arrhythmogenesis is also apparent in nonischemic cardiomyopathy. In a study of 26 patients with nonischemic cardiomyopathy undergoing LGE-CMR and electrophysiological studies, Nazarian and colleagues[26] found that scar with a transmurality of 26% to 75% was predictive of inducible ventricular tachycardia (odds ratio, 9.125; $P = .020$), independent of LVEF. Scar heterogeneity has also been linked to arrhythmic risk.[27]

Current evidence is certainly supportive of a pathophysiologic link between scar, assessed using LGE-CMR, and arrhythmic events. There is, however, a considerable step from proof causality

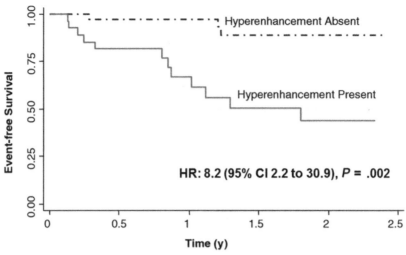

Fig. 5. Myocardial scar and survival in ICD patients. The figure shows survival from death, heart failure hospitalizations, or appropriate ICD shown in 65 patients with nonischemic cardiomyopathy, stratified according to the presence or absence of scar, assessed using LGE-CMR. After adjustment for LV volume index and functional class, patients with LGE had an 8-fold higher risk of experiencing the primary outcome (HR 8.2, 95% CI 2.2–30.9; $P = .002$). (*Adapted from* Wu KC, Weiss RG, Thiemann DR, et al. Late gadolinium enhancement by cardiovascular magnetic resonance heralds an adverse prognosis in nonischemic cardiomyopathy. J Am Coll Cardiol 2008;51:2418; with permission.)

between a biomarker and a clinical event and proof of a biomarker as a reliable predictor of outcome or benefit from ICD therapy. So far, no scar measure, or cutoff thereof, has been externally validated as a predictor of SCD, or benefit from defibrillation.

Global Dyssynchrony

Intuitively, the extent of mechanical dyssynchrony should correlate with the outcome of CRT. This question has been addressed by myriad echocardiographic studies over the past decade. The simplest measure is the septal-to-posterior wall motion delay,[28] which is the absolute time difference between peak septal and peak posterior LV wall motion displacement. Among the most sophisticated is the standard deviation of the time-to-peak systolic wall motion from multiple myocardial segments, derived using tissue Doppler imaging.[29] These and many other echocardiographic measures of mechanical dyssynchrony once held promise as predictors of response to and outcome of CRT in single-center studies.[28,30,31] Importantly, however, such measures did not predict LV reverse remodeling or clinical response to CRT in a multicenter study.[32] Mounting evidence from other groups[33–35] has led to the abandonment of dyssynchrony assessment in patient selection.

The gold-standard CMR technique for assessment of myocardial motion and deformation is

CMR tagging.[36] This technique involves tagging the myocardium with physical markers that, tracked through the cardiac cycle, can provide measures of myocardial displacement as well as strain. Although acquisition of tagged images can easily be incorporated into a routine CMR, postprocessing is laborious and not applicable to clinical practice. Similar obstacles apply to velocity-encoded CMR,[37,38] and strain-encoded CMR.[39] Importantly, these techniques have not been studied in relation to CRT.

The author used readily available SSFP short-axis imaging to quantify radial wall motion and to derive a global measure of dyssynchrony.[40] It was found that global LV mechanical dyssynchrony is present in almost all patients with heart failure[41] and that it also predicted the long-term clinical outcome of CRT.[40] Similar findings subsequently emerged from other groups.[42–44] Invariably, however, these studies have not involved randomization to CRT or usual care. As with echocardiography, CMR measures of global dyssynchrony should not be used in patient selection.

CARDIOVASCULAR MAGNETIC RESONANCE FOR GUIDING CARDIAC RESYNCHRONIZATION THERAPY IMPLANTATION

By the time a patient reaches CRT device implantation, the severity and cause of heart failure, as well as optimization of pharmacologic therapy, would have been addressed. Several aspects of CMR are relevant to implantation.

Right Ventricular Lead Position

Over the past 20 years, questions have arisen as to which site is best for RV pacing. In effect, RV pacing gives rise to similar hemodynamic effects to an intrinsic left bundle branch block.[45] These observations are in keeping with findings of a high prevalence of heart failure in patients with conventional pacemakers (mainly RV apical pacing).[46–48]

It has long been hypothesized that pacing the RV from the mid- or high-interventricular septum leads to a more physiologic mechanical activation and a better outcome. This question was addressed by the SEPTAL-CRT study, in which pacing the RV midseptum rather than the apex was not associated with a better outcome from CRT.[49] A recent CMR study, however, has suggested that scar in the vicinity of RV lead during CRT may be associated with suboptimal LV reverse remodeling.[50] Although the findings of SEPTAL-CRT may have been influenced by scar, there is no compelling evidence to position the RV lead anywhere else but the apex.

Coronary Venography

Retrograde cardiac venography via the coronary sinus, undertaken at the time of implantation, is the gold-standard approach to imaging the coronary veins. Some would argue that there is a clinical need for coronary vein imaging before CRT device implantation. In this respect, coronary venography is possible with both CMR[51] (Fig. 6) and computed tomography (CT). In the author's experience, however, retrograde venography and selective coronary vein intubation are superior to noninvasive imaging. Veins that are beyond the spatial resolution of CMR[52] and CT[51] may be suitable for implantation using advanced techniques, such as buddy-wiring or venoplasty. In addition, neither CMR nor CT provides adequate imaging of Thebesian and Viussen valves, or stenoses. For these reasons, implanters are unlikely to use noninvasive imaging routinely in planning implantation. It may, however, be useful that coronary vein abnormalities are expected, such as in congenital heart disease.

Scar and Left Ventricular Lead Position

The response to CRT can be suboptimal even when the LV lead is deployed in fluoroscopically optimal LV pacing positions[53–56]; this is perhaps not surprising, because fluoroscopy is opaque to properties of the myocardium that could influence the response to CRT.

Scar in the vicinity of the LV pacing stimulus can interfere with LV resynchronization and cause fragmentation and prolongation of the QRS complex.[57–60] As shown by animal studies, however, CRT can be effective in the presence of myocardial scar, provided lead position and timing of LV stimulation are optimized.[61] These findings are consistent with an acute pressure-volume loop study of patients undergoing CRT, in which stimulating scarred myocardium in a posterolateral segment actually resulted a reduction in stroke

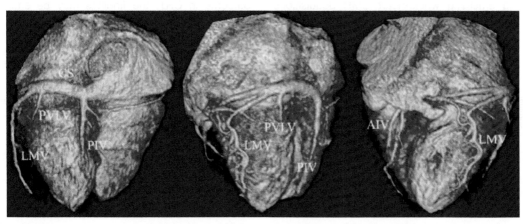

Fig. 6. CMR coronary sinus venography. These volume-rendered images show the posterior interventricular vein (PIV), posterior vein of the left ventricle (PVLV), left marginal vein (LMV), and anterior interventricular vein (AIV), obtained using contrast-enhanced whole-heart coronary magnetic resonance angiography. (*From* Ma H, Tang Q, Yang Q, et al. Contrast-enhanced whole-heart coronary MRA at 3.0T for the evaluation of cardiac venous anatomy. Int J Cardiovasc Imaging 2011;27:1005; with permission.)

work ($-17\% \pm 17\%$, $P = .018$), whereas pacing viable myocardium in the same segment led to an increase ($+62\% \pm 51\%$, $P<.001$).[62]

Long-term clinical studies of patients undergoing CRT are consistent with animal and acute human studies. Chalil and colleagues[21] showed that pacing over scar was associated with a higher risk of cardiac mortality or heart failure hospitalizations compared with pacing viable myocardium. Moreover, pacing a transmural scar was associated with a worse outcome than pacing a subendocardial scar (**Fig. 7**).[21] In a further study of 559 patients undergoing CRT, Leyva and colleagues[63] found that LV lead positions over scar was associated with a higher risk of cardiovascular death (HR 6.34) or hospitalizations for heart failure (HR 5.57) (both $P<.0001$), compared with LV lead positions over viable myocardium (**Fig. 8**). An intermediate risk of meeting these endpoints was observed for LV lead implantations, which were not guided by LGE-CMR. An LV lead position over scar was also associated with a higher risk of SCD (HR 4.40; $P = .0218$).

Importantly, the strategy avoiding myocardial scar in LV lead implantation has not been scrutinized by multicenter, randomized, controlled trials. It is, however, unlikely that further studies on this subject could include a control group not treated with CRT. It follows, therefore, that the true benefit of avoiding an LV scar may never be explored in a randomized, controlled trial. Demonstration of a better outcome from a CMR-guided approach versus the conventional fluoroscopic approach on an intention-to-treat basis would be feasible, but has not been undertaken. As it stands, the evidence for targeting the LV lead position away from scar seems compelling. Advanced fusion methods using emerging whole-heart CMR acquisitions

(**Fig. 9**)[64] are likely to make this type of imaging more accessible to implanters.

Late Mechanical Activation and Left Ventricular Lead Position

Intuitively, deploying the LV lead over late electrical or mechanical-activated segments is likely to maximize the effects of CRT.[65,66] Using CMR tagging in an animal model, Helm and colleagues[67] showed that LV sites yielding 70% or more of the maximum LV pressure derivative (dP/dt_{max}) increase after LV pacing covered approximately 43% of the LV free wall. The size and distribution of these pacing sites correlated with areas of dyssynchrony, assessed using CMR-tagging (**Fig. 10**).

In humans, the site of late activation is very variable between individuals.[65] Consequently, further studies have targeted sites of late mechanical activation in individual patients. Many early, small echocardiographic studies using tissue Doppler imaging,[68] tissue synchronization imaging,[69] 3-dimensional echocardiography,[70] and speckle-tracking echocardiography showed an intraindividual correlation between deployment of the LV lead in areas of late mechanical activation and response to CRT.

Recently, the Speckle Tracking Assisted Resynchronization Therapy for Electrode Region (STARTER)[71] (**Fig. 11**) and Targeted Left Ventricular Lead Placement to Guide Cardiac Resynchronization Therapy (TARGET)[72] studies set out to determine whether targeting late mechanically activated LV segments leads to a better response to CRT. Although the outcome of both studies has been regarded as supporting the hypothesis that targeting late activated segments improves outcome in CRT, the findings may be entirely

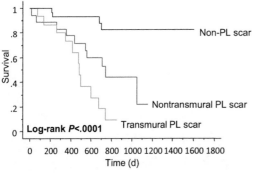
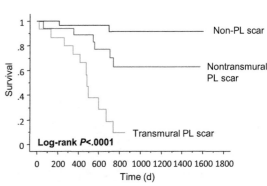

Fig. 7. LV lead position, transmurality of scar, and outcome after CRT. Survival from cardiovascular death or hospitalization for major adverse cardiovascular events (MACE) as well as cardiovascular death and hospitalization for heart failure (HF) after CRT, according to transmurality of posterolateral (PL) scar in the paced LV segment. (*Adapted from* Chalil S, Stegemann B, Muhyaldeen S, et al. Effect of posterolateral left ventricular scar on mortality and morbidity following cardiac resynchronization therapy. Pacing Clin Electrophysiol 2007;30:1204; with permission.)

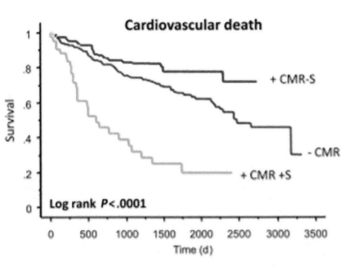

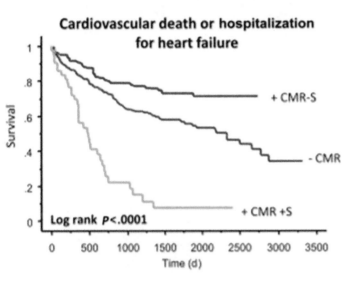

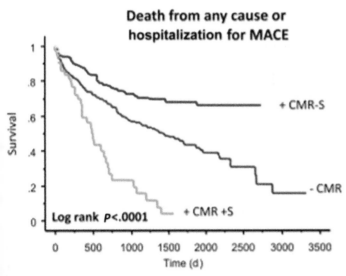

Fig. 8. Using LGE-CMR to target LV pacing sites. The clinical outcome of CRT according to implantation strategy. +CMR − S, group with CMR showing no scar at the LV pacing position; +CMR + S, group with CMR showing scar at the LV pacing position; −CMR, non-CMR-guided group; MACE, major adverse cardiovascular events. (*From* Leyva F, Foley P, Chalil S, et al. Cardiac resynchronization therapy guided by late gadolinium-enhancement cardiovascular magnetic resonance. J Cardiovasc Magn Reson 2011;13:32; with permission.)

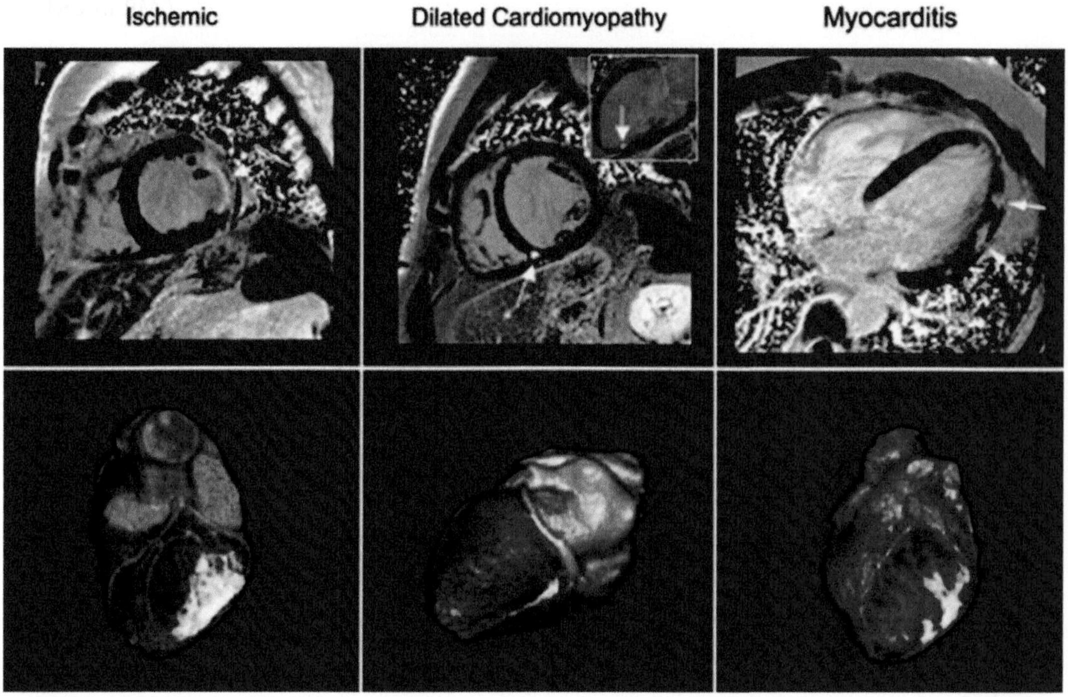

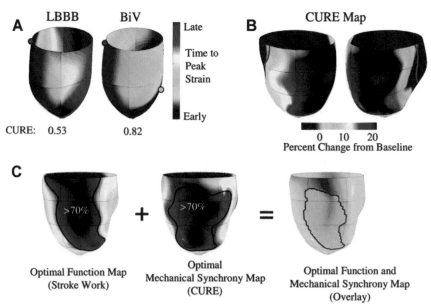

Fig. 9. Scar imaging using whole-heart imaging. The figure shows conventional 2-dimensional LGE images (*top row*) and fused, high-resolution 3-dimensional scar and coronary artery imaging (*bottom row*). Ischemic: lateral wall myocardial infarction due to ostial occlusion of ramus intermedius. Dilated cardiomyopathy: midwall scar in patient with nonischemic dilated cardiomyopathy. The inset shows small embolic infarction in apical segment of the inferior wall. Myocarditis: epicardial LGE, consistent with prior myocarditis. Note the coronary sinus in the middle panel, lower row. (*From* White JA, Fine N, Gula LJ, et al. Fused whole-heart coronary and myocardial scar imaging using 3-T CMR. Implications for planning of cardiac resynchronization therapy and coronary revascularization. JACC Cardiovasc Imaging 2010;3:925; with permission.)

Fig. 10. LV dyssynchrony and hemodynamic response to CRT. (*A*) Three-dimensional plot of relative mechanical activation time (time from QRS to peak circumferential strain) in a dog model of a dyssynchronous failing heart (with left bundle-branch block, LBBB) and during CRT (biventricular pacing, BiV). The green dot shows the LV stimulation site. (*B*) Synchrony indexed by the circumferential uniformity ratio estimate (CURE) was calculated as a function of varying LV pacing site and plotted on 3-dimensional maps, in which the color red denotes optimal mechanical resynchronization. (*C*) Combined maps derived for ventricular stroke work and synchrony (CURE) were determined in 4 failing hearts, and the territories producing optimal responses (70% maximal) for both were calculated and are displayed in green (*far right*). (*Adapted from* Helm RH, Byrne M, Helm PA, et al. Three-dimensional mapping of optimal left ventricular pacing site for cardiac resynchronization. Circulation 2007;115:956; with permission.)

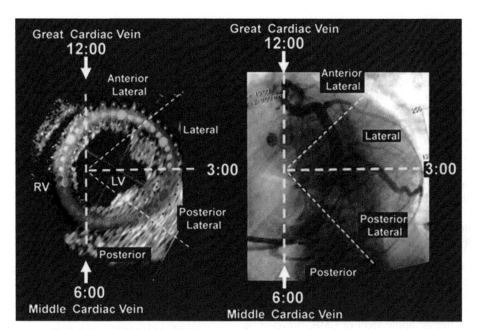

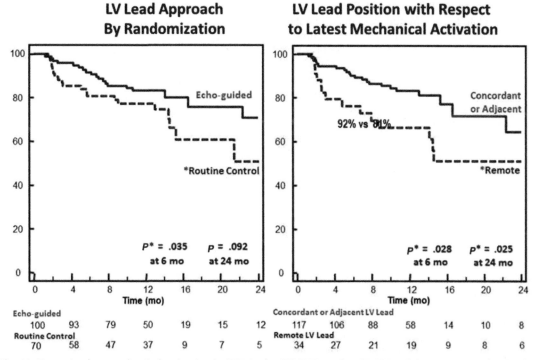

Fig. 11. Targeting late mechanical activation in CRT. In the STARTER study, 187 CRT recipients were randomized to echocardiographically guided (echo-guided) or non-echo-guided LV lead deployment. Concordance of LV lead position with segments with late mechanical activation (time-to-peak systolic radial strain) was associated with a more favorable event-free survival at 2 years than those with remote LV leads (*P* = .025). HF, heart failure; LVAD, left ventricular assist device. (*Adapted from* Saba S, Marek J, Schwartzman D, et al. Echocardiography-guided left ventricular lead placement for cardiac resynchronization therapy: results of the Speckle Tracking Assisted Resynchronization Therapy for Electrode Region trial. Circ Heart Fail 2013;6:429–32; with permission.)

attributable to the avoidance of scar. In STARTER,[71] myocardial scar was not formally assessed, but segments with low-amplitude strain curves were handled as missing data, and therefore, not available to implanters as a possible target at implantation. By virtue of study design, therefore, implanters were likely to avoid scar. In the TARGET study,[72,73] which included a prospective evaluation of scar (defined as <10% radial strain), the difference in outcome could be explained by scar alone. On this basis, neither STARTER nor TARGET provided support for targeting late mechanically activation but rather, nonscarred segments.

CARDIOVASCULAR MAGNETIC RESONANCE AFTER DEVICE IMPLANTATION

The most critical point for imaging in the CRT patient is before implantation. As noted earlier, CMR has a crucial role in determining the cause of heart failure and in planning LV lead deployment. A further application of CMR, however, is in identifying lead positions after implantation, particularly in nonresponders.

Concerns about the safety of CMR in device patients relate to radiofrequency-induced heating of the pacing leads[74] and the induction of currents by radiofrequency and magnetic gradients, which may interfere with detection and pacing and induce arrhythmias. Several groups, however, have reported on the safety of CMR in patients with conventional pacemakers. Sheldon and colleagues[75] found no adverse events from noncardiac magnetic resonance scans (1.5 T) in 40 non-pacemaker-dependent patients with non-MRI conditional CRT systems.

SUMMARY

Imaging in CRT patients is particularly important before implantation. CMR is the gold standard for the assessment of myocardial structure and function, and its ability to image myocardial scar is unique. These aspects of CMR are important in the identification of the cause of heart failure and in guiding LV lead deployment away from myocardial scar. With the advent of CMR-compatible (conditional or safe) devices, CMR is also likely to be proven useful in the investigation of CRT nonresponders.

REFERENCES

1. Kuhl HP, Spuentrup E, Wall A, et al. Assessment of myocardial function with interactive non-breath-hold real-time MR imaging: comparison with echocardiography and breath-hold Cine MR imaging. Radiology 2004;231:198–207.

2. Bellenger NG, Davies LC, Francis JM, et al. Reduction in sample size for studies of remodeling in heart failure by the use of cardiovascular magnetic resonance. J Cardiovasc Magn Reson 2000;2:271–8.

3. Grothues F, Smith GC, Moon JC, et al. Comparison of interstudy reproducibility of cardiovascular magnetic resonance with two-dimensional echocardiography in normal subjects and in patients with heart failure or left ventricular hypertrophy. Am J Cardiol 2002;90:29–34.

4. Alpert JS, Thygesen K, Antman E, et al. Myocardial infarction redefined–a consensus document of the Joint European Society of Cardiology/American College of Cardiology Committee for the redefinition of myocardial infarction. J Am Coll Cardiol 2000;36:959–69.

5. Schelbert EB, Cao JJ, Sigurdsson S, et al. Prevalence and prognosis of unrecognized myocardial infarction determined by cardiac magnetic resonance in older adults. JAMA 2012;308:890–6.

6. McCrohon JA, Moon JCC, Prasad SK, et al. Differentiation of heart failure related to dilated cardiomyopathy and coronary artery disease using gadolinium-enhanced cardiovascular magnetic resonance. Circulation 2003;108:54–9.

7. Assomull RG, Prasad SK, Lyne J, et al. Cardiovascular magnetic resonance, fibrosis, and prognosis in dilated cardiomyopathy. J Am Coll Cardiol 2006;48:1977–85.

8. Wagner A, Mahrholdt H, Holly TA, et al. Contrast-enhanced MRI and routine single photon emission computed tomography (SPECT) perfusion imaging for detection of subendocardial myocardial infarcts: an imaging study. Lancet 2003;361:374–9.

9. Bristow MR, Saxon LA, Boehmer J, et al, for the Comparison of Medical Therapy, Pacing and Defibrillation in Heart Failure (COMPANION) Investigators. Cardiac resynchronization therapy with or without an implantable defibrillator in advanced heart failure. N Engl J Med 2004;350:2140–50.

10. Moss AJ, Schuger C, Beck CA, et al. Reduction in inappropriate therapy and mortality through ICD programming. N Engl J Med 2012;367:2275–83.

11. Alter P, Waldhans S, Plachta E, et al. Complications of implantable cardioverter defibrillator therapy in 440 consecutive patients. Pacing Clin Electrophysiol 2005;28:926–32.

12. Poole JE, Johnson GW, Hellkamp AS, et al. Prognostic importance of defibrillator shocks in patients with heart failure. N Engl J Med 2008;359:1009–17.

13. Schuchert A, Muto C, Maounis T, et al. Lead complications, device infections, and clinical outcomes in the first year after implantation of cardiac resynchronization therapy-defibrillator and cardiac resynchronization therapy-pacemaker. Europace 2013;15:71–6.

14. Goldberger JJ, Cain ME, Hohnloser SH, et al. American Heart Association/American College of Cardiology Foundation/Heart Rhythm Society Scientific Statement on Noninvasive Risk Stratification Techniques for identifying patients at risk for sudden cardiac death. A scientific statement from the American Heart Association Council on Clinical Cardiology Committee on Electrocardiography and Arrhythmias and Council on Epidemiology and Prevention. J Am Coll Cardiol 2008;52:1179–99.

15. Allman KC, Shaw LJ, Hachamovitch R, et al. Myocardial viability testing and impact of revascularization on prognosis in patients with coronary artery disease and left ventricular dysfunction: a meta-analysis. J Am Coll Cardiol 2002;39:1151–8.

16. Wu E, Judd RM, Vargas JD, et al. Visualisation of presence, location and transmural extent of healed Q-wave and non-Q-wave myocardial infarction. Lancet 2001;357:21–8.

17. Kim RJ, Wu E, Rafael A, et al. The use of contrast-enhanced magnetic resonance imaging to identify reversible myocardial dysfunction. N Engl J Med 2000;343:1445–53.

18. Bellenger NG, Yousef Z, Kajappan K, et al. Infarct viability influences ventricular remodelling after late recanalisation of an occluded infarct related artery. Heart 2005;91:478–83.

19. Bello D, Shah DJ, Farah GM, et al. Gadolinium cardiovascular magnetic resonance predicts myocardial dysfunction and remodelling in patients with heart failure undergoing beta-blocker therapy. Circulation 2003;108:1945–53.

20. White JA, Yee R, Yuan X, et al. Delayed enhancement magnetic resonance imaging predicts response to cardiac resynchronization therapy in patients with intraventricular dyssynchrony. J Am Coll Cardiol 2006;48:1953–60.

21. Chalil S, Stegemann B, Muhyaldeen SA, et al. Effect of posterolateral left ventricular scar on mortality and morbidity following cardiac resynchronization therapy. Pacing Clin Electrophysiol 2007;30(10):1201–9.

22. Gulati A, Jabbour A, Ismail TF, et al. Association of fibrosis with mortality and sudden cardiac death in patients with nonischemic dilated cardiomyopathy. JAMA 2013;309:896–908.

23. Leyva F, Taylor RJ, Foley PW, et al. Left ventricular midwall fibrosis as a predictor of mortality and morbidity after cardiac resynchronization therapy in patients with nonischemic cardiomyopathy. J Am Coll Cardiol 2012;60:1659–67.

24. Morishima I, Sone T, Tsuboi H, et al. Risk stratification of patients with prior myocardial infarction and advanced left ventricular dysfunction by gated myocardial perfusion SPECT imaging. J Nucl Cardiol 2008;15:631–7.

25. Wu KC, Weiss RG, Thiemann DR, et al. Late gadolinium enhancement by cardiovascular magnetic resonance heralds an adverse prognosis in nonischemic cardiomyopathy. J Am Coll Cardiol 2008;51:2414–21.

26. Nazarian S, Bluemke DA, Lardo AC, et al. Magnetic resonance assessment of the substrate for inducible ventricular tachycardia in nonischemic cardiomyopathy. Circulation 2005;112:2821–5.

27. Roes SD, Borleffs CJ, van der Geest RJ, et al. Infarct tissue heterogeneity assessed with contrast-enhanced MRI predicts spontaneous ventricular arrhythmia in patients with ischemic cardiomyopathy and implantable cardioverter-defibrillator. Circ Cardiovasc Imaging 2009;2:183–90.

28. Pitzalis MV, Iacoviello M, Romito R, et al. Cardiac resynchronization therapy tailored by echocardiographic evaluation of ventricular asynchrony. J Am Coll Cardiol 2002;40:1615–22.

29. Yu CM, Zhang Q, Chan YS, et al. Tissue Doppler velocity is superior to displacement and strain mapping in predicting left ventricular reverse remodelling response after cardiac resynchronisation therapy. Heart 2006;92:1452–6.

30. Yu CM, Fung WH, Lin H, et al. Predictors of left ventricular reverse remodeling after cardiac resynchronization therapy for heart failure secondary to idiopathic dilated or ischemic cardiomyopathy. Am J Cardiol 2003;91:684–8.

31. Bax JJ, Bleeker GB, Marwick TH, et al. Left ventricular dyssynchrony predicts response and prognosis after cardiac resynchronization therapy. J Am Coll Cardiol 2004;44:1834–40.

32. Chung E, Leon A, Tavazzi L, et al. Results of the predictors of response to CRT (PROSPECT) Trial. Circulation 2008;117:2608–16.

33. Hawkins NM, Petrie MC, Burgess MI, et al. Selecting patients for cardiac resynchronization therapy: the fallacy of echocardiographic dyssynchrony. J Am Coll Cardiol 2009;53:1944–59.

34. Marwick T. Hype and hope in the use of echocardiography for selection for cardiac resynchronization therapy: the tower of Babel revisited. Circulation 2008;117:2573–6.

35. Fornwalt BK, Sprague WW, BeDell P, et al. Agreement is poor among current criteria used to define response to cardiac resynchronization therapy. Circulation 2010;121:1985–91.

36. Axel L, Dougherty L. MR imaging of motion with spatial modulation of magnetization. Radiology 1989;171:841–5.

37. Marsan NA, Bleeker GB, van Bommel RJ, et al. Comparison of time course of response to cardiac resynchronization therapy in patients with ischemic versus nonischemic cardiomyopathy. Am J Cardiol 2009;103:690–4.

38. Westenberg JJM, Lamb H, van der Geest RJ, et al. Assessment of left ventricular dyssynchrony in

patients with conduction delay and idiopathic dilated cardiomyopathy. J Am Coll Cardiol 2006; 47:2042–8.

39. Osman NF, Sampath S, Atalar E, et al. Imaging longitudinal cardiac strain on short-axis images using strain-encoded MRI. Magn Reson Med 2001;46: 324–34.

40. Chalil S, Stegemann B, Muhyaldeen S, et al. Intraventricular dyssynchrony predicts mortality and morbidity following cardiac resynchronization therapy: a study using cardiovascular magnetic resonance tissue synchronization imaging. J Am Coll Cardiol 2007;50:243–52.

41. Foley PW, Khadjooi K, Ward JA, et al. Radial dyssynchrony assessed by cardiovascular magnetic resonance in relation to left ventricular function, myocardial scarring and QRS duration in patients with heart failure. J Cardiovasc Magn Reson 2009; 11:50.

42. Delgado V, van Bommel R, Bertini M, et al. Relative merits of left ventricular dyssynchrony, left ventricular lead position, and myocardial scar to predict long-term survival of ischemic heart failure patients undergoing cardiac resynchronization therapy. Circulation 2011;123:70–8.

43. Petryka J, Misko J, Przybylski A, et al. Magnetic resonance imaging assessment of intraventricular dyssynchrony and delayed enhancement as predictors of response to cardiac resynchronization therapy in patients with heart failure of ischaemic and non-ischaemic etiologies. Eur J Radiol 2012;81: 2639–47.

44. Sohal M, Duckett SG, Zhuang X, et al. A prospective evaluation of cardiovascular magnetic resonance measures of dyssynchrony in the prediction of response to cardiac resynchronization therapy. J Cardiovasc Magn Reson 2014;16:58.

45. Prinzen FW, Hunter WC, Wyman BT, et al. Mapping of regional myocardial strain and work during ventricular pacing: experimental study using magnetic resonance imaging tagging. J Am Coll Cardiol 1999;33:1735–42.

46. Wilkoff BL, Cook JR, Epstein AE, et al. Dual-chamber pacing or ventricular back-up pacing in patients with an implantable defibrillator: the Dual Chamber and VVI Implantable Defibrillator (DAVID) Trial. JAMA 2002;288:3115–23.

47. Hayes JJ, Sharma AD, Love JC, et al. Abnormal conduction increases risk of adverse outcomes from right ventricular pacing. J Am Coll Cardiol 2006;48:1628–33.

48. Sweeney MO, Hellkamp AS, Ellenbogen KA, et al. Adverse effect of ventricular pacing on heart failure and atrial fibrillation among patients with normal baseline QRS duration in a clinical trial of pacemaker therapy for sinus node dysfunction. Circulation 2003;107:2932–7.

49. Leclercq C, Sadoul N, Mont L, et al. Comparison of right ventricular septal pacing and right ventricular apical pacing in patients receiving cardiac resynchronization therapy defibrillators: the SEPTAL CRT Study. Eur Heart J 2015. [Epub ahead of print].

50. Wong JA, Yee R, Stirrat J, et al. Influence of pacing site characteristics on response to cardiac resynchronization therapy. Circulation 2013;6:542–50.

51. Younger JF, Plein S, Crean A, et al. Visualization of coronary venous anatomy by cardiovascular magnetic resonance. J Cardiovasc Magn Reson 2009; 11:26.

52. Knackstedt C, Muhlenbruch G, Mischke K, et al. Imaging of the coronary venous system in patients with congestive heart failure: comparison of 16 slice MSCT and retrograde coronary sinus venography: comparative imaging of coronary venous system. Int J Cardiovasc Imaging 2008;24:783–91.

53. Foley P, Chalil S, Ratib K, et al. Fluoroscopic left ventricular lead position and the long-term clinical outcome of cardiac resynchronization therapy. Pacing Clin Electrophysiol 2011;34:785–97.

54. Gasparini M, Mantica M, Galimberti P, et al. Is the left ventricular lateral wall the best lead implantation site for cardiac resynchronization therapy? Pacing Clin Electrophysiol 2003;26:162–8.

55. Rossillo A, Verma A, Saad EB, et al. Impact of coronary sinus lead position on biventricular pacing: mortality and echocardiographic evaluation during long-term follow-up. J Cardiovasc Electrophysiol 2004;15:1120–5.

56. Kronborg MB, Albertsen AE, Nielsen JC, et al. Long-term clinical outcome and left ventricular lead position in cardiac resynchronization therapy. Europace 2009;11:1177–82.

57. Schwartzman D, Chang I, Michele JJ, et al. Electrical impedance properties of normal and chronically infarcted ventricular myocardium. J Interv Card Electrophysiol 1999;3:213–24.

58. Reddy VY, Wrobleski D, Houghtaling C, et al. Combined epicardial and endocardial electroanatomic mapping in a porcine model of healed myocardial infarction. Circulation 2003;107:3236–42.

59. Tedrow U, Maisel W, Epstein L, et al. Feasibility of adjusting paced left ventricular activation by manipulating stimulus strength. J Am Coll Cardiol 2004;44: 2249–51.

60. Breithardt OA, Stellbrink C, Kramer AP, et al. Echocardiographic quantification of left ventricular asynchrony predicts an acute hemodynamic benefit of cardiac resynchronization therapy. J Am Coll Cardiol 2002;40:536–45.

61. Rademakers LM, van Kerckhoven R, van Deursen CJ, et al. Myocardial infarction does not preclude electrical and hemodynamic benefits of cardiac resynchronization therapy in dyssynchronous canine hearts. Circ Arrhythm Electrophysiol 2010;3:361–8.

62. de Roest GJ, Wu L, de Cock CC, et al. Scar tissue-guided left ventricular lead placement for cardiac resynchronization therapy in patients with ischemic cardiomyopathy: an acute pressure-volume loop study. Am Heart J 2014;167:537–45.

63. Leyva F, Foley P, Chalil S, et al. Cardiac resynchronization therapy guided by late gadolinium-enhancement cardiovascular magnetic resonance. J Cardiovasc Magn Reson 2011;13:29–35.

64. White JA, Fine N, Gula LJ, et al. Fused whole-heart coronary and myocardial scar imaging using 3-T CMR. Implications for planning of cardiac resynchronization therapy and coronary revascularization. JACC Cardiovasc Imaging 2010;3:921–30.

65. Becker M, Franke A, Breithardt OA, et al. Impact of left ventricular lead position on the efficacy of cardiac re-synchronisation therapy: a two-dimensional strain echocardiography study. Heart 2007;93:1197–203.

66. Bedi M, Suffoletto M, Tanabe M, et al. Effect of concordance between sites of left ventricular pacing and dyssynchrony on acute electrocardiographic and echocardiographic parameters in patients with heart failure undergoing cardiac resynchronization therapy. Clin Cardiol 2006;29:498–502.

67. Helm RH, Byrne M, Helm PA, et al. Three-dimensional mapping of optimal left ventricular pacing site for cardiac resynchronization. Circulation 2007; 115:953–61.

68. Ansalone G, Giannantoni P, Ricci R, et al. Doppler myocardial imaging in patients with heart failure receiving biventricular pacing treatment. Am Heart J 2001;142:881–96.

69. Murphy RT, Sigurdsson G, Mulamalla S, et al. Tissue synchronization imaging and optimal left ventricular pacing site in cardiac resynchronization therapy. Am J Cardiol 2006;97:1615–21.

70. Becker M, Hoffmann R, Schmitz F, et al. Relation of optimal lead positioning as defined by three-dimensional echocardiography to long-term benefit of cardiac resynchronization. Am J Cardiol 2007; 100:1671–6.

71. Saba S, Marek J, Schwartzman D, et al. Echocardiography-guided left ventricular lead placement for cardiac resynchronization therapy: results of the Speckle Tracking Assisted Resynchronization Therapy for Electrode Region trial. Circ Heart Fail 2013; 6:427–34.

72. Khan FZ, Virdee MS, Palmer CR, et al. Targeted left ventricular lead placement to guide cardiac re-synchronization therapy: the TARGET study: a randomized, controlled trial. J Am Coll Cardiol 2012; 59:1509–18.

73. Kydd AC, Khan FZ, Watson WD, et al. Prognostic benefit of optimum left ventricular lead position in cardiac resynchronization therapy: follow-up of the TARGET Study Cohort (Targeted Left Ventricular Lead Placement to Guide Cardiac Resynchronization Therapy). JACC Heart Fail 2014; 2:205–12.

74. Achenbach S, Moshage W, Diem B, et al. Effects of magnetic resonance imaging on cardiac pacemakers and electrodes. Am Heart J 1997;134: 467–73.

75. Sheldon SH, Bunch TJ, Cogert GA, et al. Multicenter study of the safety and effects of magnetic resonance imaging in patients with coronary sinus left ventricular pacing leads. Heart Rhythm 2015;12: 345–9.

Implantation and Extraction Technique

Coronary Sinus Lead Positioning

Attila Roka, MD, PhD, Rasmus Borgquist, MD, PhD, Jagmeet Singh, MD, DPhil*

KEYWORDS

- Cardiac resynchronization therapy • Heart failure • Pacing • Targeted lead placement
- Coronary sinus

KEY POINTS

- Transvenous implantation of the left ventricular (LV) lead is still the most challenging part of cardiac resynchronization therapy (CRT); it can be hindered by suboptimal coronary sinus (CS) anatomy, phrenic nerve (PN) capture, lead instability, or unfavorable electrical properties at the pacing site.
- Optimal lead placement is of utmost importance to achieve electrical and mechanical resynchronization.
- Alternative techniques such as surgical lead placement or endocardial LV stimulation may be attempted when implantation of a transvenous CS lead is not feasible.
- Targeted LV lead placement may address individual patient factors and improve clinical outcomes. Several modalities are under investigation, evaluating anatomic, electrical, mechanical, and hemodynamic characteristics.

INTRODUCTION

The most frequent intraventricular conduction abnormality in heart failure is left bundle branch block (LBBB), occurring in 25% to 30% of patients. Regionally delayed electrical activation leads to dyssynchronous mechanical activity, affecting both systolic and diastolic function.[1,2] Even with similar QRS morphology, variations in ventricular activation pattern and mechanical dyssynchrony may be observed because factors such as scar affect electrical activation and electromechanical coupling.[3–5] Patients with non-LBBB morphology (IVCD [interventricular conduction delay], RBBB, left anterior fascicular block) are even more heterogeneous, and CRT is less effective in this population, emphasizing the need for an individualized approach in finding the lead locations to deliver effective CRT.[6]

Optimal placement of the LV lead remains the cornerstone of CRT. Despite advances in transvenous lead technology, the implantation is still challenging and a significant number of patients are nonresponders. Alternative lead implant strategies and individually targeted lead placement are methods of great interest and subjects of several ongoing trials.

Assessment of Coronary Sinus Anatomy

The CS runs between the left atrium and the LV, in the posterior coronary groove. The ostium is usually 5 to 15 mm in size, located in the posteroseptal right atrium (RA), close to the tricuspid annulus. The Thebesian valve is present in around 60% and may interfere with cannulation during implant.[7] In some instances, the CS entrance is in a more superior position, making it harder to slide a guiding catheter into the vein.[8] The ligament or vein of Marshall is located near the distal CS and may be an issue during cannulation because

Disclosure Statement: Consulting and research grants from Biotronik, Boston Scientific, Medtronic, St. Jude Medical, and Sorin Group; consulting for Respicardia & CardioInsight (J. Singh). None (A. Roka and R. Borgquist).
Cardiology Division, Cardiac Arrhythmia Service, Massachusetts General Hospital, 55 Fruit Street, Boston, MA 02114, USA
* Corresponding author.
E-mail address: jsingh@mgh.harvard.edu

inadvertent introduction of the balloon catheter or lead in this small vein may cause dissection or perforation. The valve of Vieussens is present in around 8% in this region, making access to the branches of distal CS difficult.[9]

The anatomy of the CS branches is highly variable,[10] and a median of 6 veins drain from the LV into the CS. The middle cardiac vein (MCV, posterior vein) is almost always present and may originate from the immediate proximity of the CS ostium or with a separate ostium. Inadvertent cannulation of the MCV may lead to misinterpretation of the true CS anatomy during angiogram. This vein is usually quite straight and large in caliber, not well suited for a stable LV lead position. Another prominent branch is the anterior interventricular vein (AIV), which is the continuation of the CS in the anterior interventricular groove. Although its course and size often allow stable lead placement, this area usually does not have enough electrical delay to allow effective CRT in typical LBBB. The size and number of posterolateral, lateral, and anterolateral branches, originating from the CS body between the MCV and AIV, is highly variable (usually 1–4), but presence of a vein does not guarantee that LV capture from a given spot will be possible. Anatomy is assessed during implant by occlusion retrograde venography (**Fig. 1**), and the area typically targeted for LV lead implantation (midlateral) is usually accessible from more than one CS branch: posterolateral, lateral, or a side-branch of the AIV. Occasionally, the MCV may also have a suitable sidebranch.[11]

Clues for difficult implant are enlarged or very small RA, severe tricuspid regurgitation (TR), or presence of a left-sided persistent superior vena cava. In these cases, preoperative evaluation of the CS anatomy can be helpful (**Box 1**), and depending on the results, alternative LV lead placement may be preferred.

Coronary angiography may visualize the CS ostium by using prolonged exposure to cover the contrast washout in the coronary venous phase (**Fig. 2**). A study compared preprocedural 3-dimensional (3D) rotational angiography (images of venous phase of the coronary angiogram) with conventional intraprocedural occlusive venogram: contrast use, time for CS lead placement after guiding catheter intubation (8.9 ± 5.5 vs 14.7 ± 7.4 min), total fluoroscopy, and procedure time were significantly lower in the 3D group. Occlusive venography was necessary only in 14% of the 3D group.[12]

Cardiac computed tomographic (CT) venography provides a detailed view of coronary venous anatomy (**Fig. 3**). The CS, posterior veins, and lateral veins were identified in 100%, 76%, and 91%, respectively, in a study of 51 patients.[11] Rotational CT angiography (CTA) may be superior to conventional CTA: in a retrospective study of 47 patients, the CS branch selected for lead placement was initially identified in 100% of patients using the rotational CTA, but only in 74% with conventional CTA.[13] Contemporary low-radiation-dose protocols with prospective electrocardiography-triggered CT acquisition may make preprocedural CT attractive as a standard evaluation before CRT implant.

Cardiac MRI can also be used to assess the coronary veins, scar burden and location (using late gadolinium enhancement), and mechanical dyssynchrony.[14–16] Limitations include low temporal resolution, less-detailed visualization of the coronary veins, and lack of availability outside large centers.

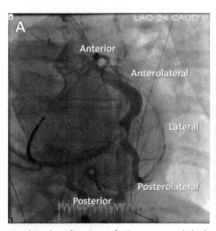
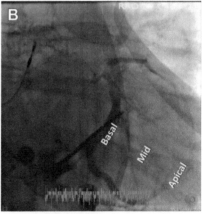

Fig. 1. Angiographic classification of CS anatomy. (*A*) The left anterior oblique (LAO) projection enables segmentation of the LV along the short axis, defining anterior, anterolateral, lateral, posterior, and posterior segments of the CS and its veins. (*B*) The right anterior oblique (RAO) projection shows the LV along the long axis, defining basal, mid, and apical segments.

Box 1
Methods to assess CS anatomy before CRT implant

- Coronary angiogram (venous phase)
- Cardiac CT angiogram
- Cardiac MR angiogram
- Echocardiography (gross chamber anatomy, TR, persistent left SVC)

Abbreviations: MR, magnetic resonance; SVC, superior vena cava.

Transvenous Coronary Sinus Lead Implant

Guidelines summarize the recommended approach for preoperative evaluation, implant technique, and follow-up.[17] It is recommended to place the RV lead first because it is less likely to dislodge during manipulation of other leads,

provides information about the position of the tricuspid valve and RA size, and can be used for backup pacing if the right bundle suffers mechanical trauma during CS cannulation, which can lead to atrioventricular block in patients with preexisting LBBB. A wide array of specialized tools have been developed to facilitate LV lead implantation (**Table 1**).

The implantation success rate for transvenous CS leads was around 90% in major CRT trials[18,19] but is likely to be higher with today's more refined delivery tools and also increases with individual operator experience. The challenging anatomy of the CS is the most common reason for implant failure, and LV lead dislodgement incidence has also been relatively high, up to 5.7% in the large clinical trials.[20] The use of quadripolar leads has led to a significant improvement in this respect.

Cannulation of the CS ostium is usually attempted with a guidewire (0.032 or similar size), a nonsteerable catheter, or a steerable electrophysiology

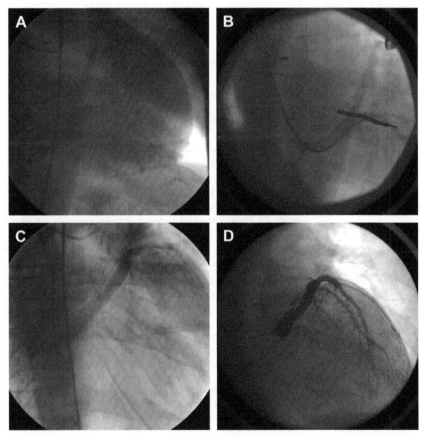

Fig. 2. Assessment of CS anatomy on the venous phase of left coronary angiogram. The CS body and ostium are visualized on delayed images (*A*), which correlated well with nonselective venogram during implant (*B*). The CS body and the proximal main branches are visualized in another patient (*C*), correlating with the image obtained with occlusive venogram during implant (*D*). The delayed-phase image from coronary venogram may be used to assess the location of the CS ostium and location of main branches, when planning for a transvenous implant.

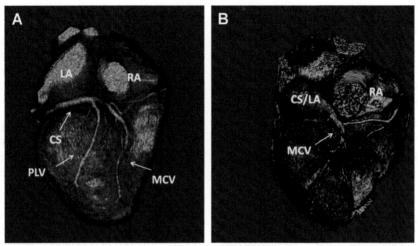

Fig. 3. CT coronary vein angiogram. (*A*) Normal CS anatomy. (*B*) Unroofed CS with direct communication with LA. There was no CS-RA communication in this patient, making transvenous LV lead implantation unfeasible. LA, left atrium; PLV, posterolateral vein.

catheter. Delivery catheters are available in multiple prefabricated shapes, allowing CS cannulation from left or right subclavian approach and accommodating for various RA sizes. If initial attempts to cannulate the CS ostium are not successful, a left coronary angiogram may be performed and the venous phase assessed to localize the ostium.

After successful CS cannulation, a balloon-tipped angiography catheter is advanced and an occlusion venogram is performed. CS dissection or perforation may occur if the balloon is inflated in a sidebranch or the tip is pressed against the wall—a small nonselective injection is recommended before balloon inflation. At least 2 projections

Table 1
Tools facilitating transvenous CS LV lead implantation

Tool	Description
Splittable guide catheter	• Serves as a preformed sheath to cannulate CS and provide support • Multiple shapes, allowing to accommodate variable RA sizes and positions of the CS ostium
Splittable subselector guide	• May be used if the origin of the vein is at a very acute angle from the main CS body, provides support for the lead during implant • Multiple shapes
Balloon-tipped angiography catheter	• Used to perform occlusive CS venography to identify branches
Soft (angioplasty) guidewire	• Over-the-wire lead implantation: advancing the wire into the distal part of the vein provides support for lead implant
LV (CS) lead	• Commercially available in unipolar, bipolar, and quadripolar configurations • Leads with less poles are thinner, although the size difference is minimal and maneuverability of the newest-generation multipolar leads is comparable to that of the older-generator leads with less poles • Quadripolar leads allow testing for sites with optimal electrical delay, avoid PN capture, and can be implanted distally in a stable position while still allowing paced stimulation from the mid or distal part of the LV
Steerable electrophysiology catheter	• Facilitates CS cannulation, especially in the case of a Thebesian valve, which needs to be penetrated (sometimes impossible using guidewire or guide catheter alone). Intracardiac signals can be helpful to determine when CS is engaged

of the occlusive venogram are recommended (right anterior oblique and left anterior oblique) to visualize both the long- and short-axes courses of the veins (see **Fig. 1**). The angiography catheter is then removed. If the guide cannot be advanced into the CS because of tortuosity, a stiffer guide-wire, a diagnostic coronary catheter, or the occlusive balloon catheter may be used as support.[21]

Most LV leads can be implanted using over-the-wire technique, using a soft coronary guidewire. The wire is atraumatic and unlikely to cause dissection or perforation, even if it is advanced until it is wedged. The leads also come with conventional stylets, which may be used to stiffen them, if a guidewire is not used. Preshaped telescopic sheaths with appropriate angulation of the tip can be used to engage the vein of interest and to advance the lead directly, a strategy that may be particularly useful for veins with a very acute takeoff angle from the main CS. In a nonrandomized study of 437 patients comparing the telescoping sheath versus the over-the-wire technique, the incidence of failed LV lead implantation was lower (1.9% vs 8.1%) and optimal lead positioning was achieved more often (87% vs 75%).[22]

Most current LV leads are bipolar or quadripolar with a low profile (5 Fr or less), thin, and flexible enough to be advanced at least into the midportion of a coronary vein. Quadripolar leads allow multiple pacing configurations, providing options to avoid PN stimulation or sites with high threshold, and have a stable distal lead tip position even while allowing pacing of the basal or mid-LV segments. Quadripolar leads in the More Options Available with a Quadripolar LV Lead Provide In-Clinic Solutions to CRT Challenges (MORE-CRT) trial had significantly less intraoperative and postoperative LV lead-related complications (14.0% vs 23.1% with bipolar leads), driven mainly by reduction of PN stimulation or lead instability (6.0% vs 13.7%). A multicenter study of 721 patients even showed a mortality benefit in patients who had quadripolar leads compared with those who had bipolar leads during 5 years of follow-up: 13.2% versus 22.5%.[23] PN stimulation was eliminated in the quadripolar group by switching pacing vectors in all cases, compared with in only 60% in the bipolar group. LV lead displacement (1.7% vs 4.6%) and repositioning (2.0% vs 5.2%) occurred significantly less often. Although patient demographics were similar in terms of most parameters, the quadripolar group did have a significantly lower proportion of ischemic heart disease (62.6% vs 54.1%). Quadripolar leads may also enable multipoint LV pacing with a compatible pulse generator, a strategy that is currently being tested in the multi point pacing (MPP) (NCT01786993) and the MORE-CRT MPP (NCT02006069) studies.

Familiarity with less-frequently used tools and techniques may facilitate the implant (**Table 2**). Stenosis or dissection may limit advancement of the guidewire or the lead. If the narrowing can be negotiated with an angioplasty guidewire, venoplasty may be attempted.[24] The risk of perforation and tamponade is low, although rupture has been reported.[25] Dilatation of the collateral veins may also be attempted to facilitate placement in the target vein.[26] The implantation success rate may be as high as 99% with access to angioplasty: a retrospective single-center analysis showed that 3.5% of patients required venoplasty (77% coronary vein, 13% subclavian vein, 10% valvular

Table 2
Techniques and tools for difficult transvenous CS lead implantation

Techniques and Tools	Role
Venous phase of coronary angiogram	• Visualize CS ostium—can be done during implant • With preoperative 3D angiogram, can decrease procedure time and contrast use during implant
Venoplasty	• Overcome venous stenosis or dissection • High-pressure inflation may be needed, low risk of perforation with short 3-mm balloon
Buddy wire	• Straighten the vein using a second angioplasty wire, placed parallel to the first one • The wire used for lead insertion can be anchored against the vein with an angioplasty balloon
Active fixation CS lead • Built-in lobes • Stent implantation	• Stabilization of lead tip location in proximal position to avoid PN pacing or high threshold • May become an issue if extraction is needed • With quadripolar leads, this is no longer recommended because this lead allows distal placement and provide the ability to pace proximally

structures within the CS or Marshall vein). The required inflation pressures for ringlike structures were high (16 ± 3 atm), but complications were rare. Mostly, short balloons with 3 mm diameter were used.[27] A coronary balloon can also be used to assist lead advancement through a tortuous branch by advancing a second wire into the vein and then inflating the balloon to anchor the second wire against the wall in a distal position in the branch. Back traction is then applied on the non-balloon wire, and the LV lead is advanced over it.

If support with wire is an issue in a tortuous vein, an angioplasty guidewire may be advanced distally and then back into the main CS via a collateral, if feasible. A gooseneck snare can be used to grab the free tip, and then traction is applied to support over-the-wire lead insertion in the antero-grade direction.[21] A long guidewire (300 cm) is best suited for this approach.

Before the availability of quadripolar leads, pacing the basal or mid-LV was not always feasible because the lead position was not stable. A single-center study of 312 patients used coronary stent implantation besides the LV lead into the vein to stabilize the lead tip position.[28] Active fixation CS leads were also available (Starfix, Medtronic, Minneapolis, MN, USA). With the advent of quadripolar leads and availability of multiple pacing vectors, active fixation is no longer recommended because it may interfere if lead removal is needed.[29] Stabilizing the lead position with retained guidewire or stylet is not recommended because of the risk of lead failure.[30]

Alternative LV lead implant methods are usually reserved for cases in which transvenous implant fails or does not seem to be feasible based on pre-procedural evaluation (**Table 3**).

TARGETING LEFT VENTRICULAR LEAD PLACEMENT
Targeting Maximal Anatomic Distance

The most commonly used strategy involves the placement of the LV lead in an anatomically favorable position (**Table 4**). The anatomic position of the LV lead can be described among the long and short axes of the LV, which can be readily assessed with fluoroscopy (see **Fig. 1**). The basal to midlateral or posterolateral areas are usually targeted for LV lead implant because these have the most delayed onset of activation in patients with typical LBBB.

Data from the large clinical trials have not been entirely consistent as to whether anatomic LV lead position can affect long-term outcome. There is general agreement that an apical lead position is less favorable,[31] as was shown in the Multicenter Automatic Defibrillator Implantation Trial-Cardiac Resynchronization Therapy (MADIT-CRT).[32] However, in both Comparison of Medical Therapy, Pacing, and Defibrillation in Heart Failure (COM-PANION) trial and MADIT-CRT, the anterior, lateral, and posterior lead locations all had comparable CRT outcome,[33] whereas the REVERSE HF (REsynchronization reVErses Remodeling in Systolic Left vEntricular Dysfunction) trial showed

Table 3
LV lead implantation methods

LV Lead Implant Method	Description
Transvenous, CS	• Standard method, success rate >90% • Well tolerated, low complication rate • Targeted placement limited by CS anatomy
Surgical epicardial • Thoracotomy • Video assisted thoracic surgery • Robotic	• Requires general anesthesia • Longer recovery time • Higher lead failure rate • Difficult to achieve posterolateral lead position
Transvenous, endocardial • Transseptal with conventional PM lead • Transseptal, leadless	• Need for anticoagulation • Electrically targeted placement possible • Limited data from small studies
Surgical, transapical endocardial	• Need for anticoagulation • May be an option if transvenous implantation fails and pericardial adhesions limit conventional surgical epicardial lead placement • Limited data from small studies
Multiple leads	• Allows for multipoint pacing • Limited data from small studies • May become obsolete if trials using multipoint pacing from a single quadripolar lead show similar results

Table 4
Methods for targeted LV lead implantation

	Method	Description
Anatomic		Based on observations from activation in LBBB
		Does not require specialized tools
		Relatively high rate of nonresponders
Electrical	3D contact mapping	High accuracy, map superimposed on true geometry
		Invasive
		Slow, requires serial acquisition of points
		Endocardial or epicardial map (from CS)
	3D noncontact mapping	Fast
		Invasive
		Endocardial map
	Body surface mapping	Noninvasive
		Allows quick repeated measurements: assess dyssynchrony before implant, targeted lead placement during implant, device optimization after implant
		Not widely available
	Q-LV	Measures epicardial activation
		Simple to measure during implant
		No consensus as for cutoff values
Mechanical	Echocardiography (Tissue doppler imaging, speckle tracking)	Lead placement that is concordant with latest activation improves outcome
		Requires significant echo expertise
		High interindividual and intraindividual variability
	Cardiac MRI	Requires significant expertise in image acquisition
		Limited time resolution
		Limited availability
		Expensive, not possible for patients with any cardiac device in situ
Hemodynamic	Invasive LV pressures, dp/dt, p/V (pressure/ volume) loop	Invasive
		Most accurate representation of hemodynamic changes
		Limited transformation of results to long-term prognosis

better outcome (combined end point of death and heart failure hospitalization) with lateral lead placement.[34]

One of the first attempts to improve CRT responder rate was to aim for an LV lead position with the greatest RV-LV lead separation.[35] In a study of 51 patients, acute hemodynamic changes (change in dP/dT by echo Doppler) correlated significantly with the magnitude of separation between the LV and RV lead tips on the lateral radiograph (r = 0.43) and the lateral distance in the horizontal plane (r = 0.58), but not in the vertical plane (r = −0.28).

Targeting Maximal Electrical Delay

Several algorithms based on intracardiac electrograms have been investigated to guide LV lead positioning. Measurement of the LV lead electrical delay (LVLED) (Q-LV and LVLED: Q-LV/QRS duration ratio) quantifies the delay in a given location (**Fig. 4**). By moving the LV lead within the coronary

veins, places suitable for implant can be mapped and the optimal one targeted (**Figs. 5** and **6**). LVLED overall correlated weakly with delta dP/dt in a study of 48 patients (r = 0.311), but strongly in the nonischemic subgroup (r = 0.48). LVLED was significantly longer in acute responders (70 ± 24% vs 32% ± 12%) among patients with nonischemic cardiomyopathy. A reduced LVLED (<50%) was associated with worse clinical outcome within the entire cohort (hazard ratio, 2.7).[36] The ongoing multicenter randomized ENHANCE CRT trial will compare targeted LV lead placement (based on Q-LV) with conventional implant in patients with non-LBBB QRS of 120 ms or greater duration, New York Heart Association class III, or ambulatory class IV, assessing a composite clinical end point at 12 months of follow-up.

A retrospective study using a combination of anatomic, hemodynamic, and electrical data (dorsoventral LV/RV interleaved distance >10 cm, LVLED ≥50%, baseline maximum + dP/dt <600 mm Hg/s, maximum time difference >100 ms, using a scale

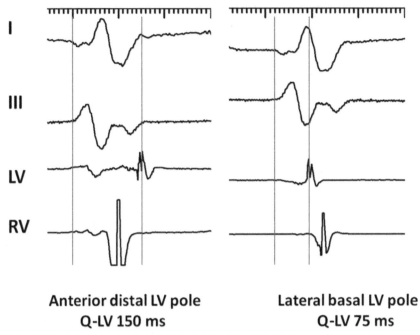

Anterior distal LV pole
Q-LV 150 ms

Lateral basal LV pole
Q-LV 75 ms

Fig. 4. Optimizing LV lead placement using electrical delay. The delay between the initiation of the QRS and the sensed LV signal (Q-LV) can be measured during lead positioning. The Q-LV/QRS duration ratio (LVLED) was shown to correlate with clinical outcome during CRT. In this patient with anterior scar, RBBB, and left anterior fascicular block, the Q-LV at the distal anterior site was longer than at the basal lateral segment.

up to 4 points) was able to accurately predict 12-month event-free survival.[37]

Both contact and noncontact electroanatomical methods can be used to create 3D maps of electrical activation of the LV and identify the area of latest activation.[38,39] Routine use of this technique during CRT implant is, however, limited by expense and practical considerations. An impedance-based 3D mapping system (NavX, St. Jude Medical, St Paul, MN, USA), has also been used for periprocedural electrical mapping. Although data correlated to mechanical delay, the use adds considerable expense and time to the standard CRT implant.[40]

Body surface electrical mapping is noninvasive and enables quick repeated measurements.[41,42] Potential uses include preprocedural assessment of dyssynchrony, intraprocedural use for targeted lead placement, and use for CRT optimization during follow-up, but so far limited data are available on its role in CRT.

Targeting Maximal Mechanical Delay

Targeting areas with maximum mechanical delay can also be used to guide CRT. The randomized Targeted Left Ventricular Lead Placement to Guide Cardiac Resynchronization Therapy (TARGET) study assessed the impact of targeted LV lead

placement in 220 patients. All patients had baseline echocardiographic speckle-tracking 2-dimensional radial strain imaging and were then randomized into 2 groups. In the TARGET group, the LV lead was positioned at the latest site of peak contraction with an amplitude of 10% or greater to signify freedom from scar. In the control group, patients underwent standard CRT. Patients were classified by the relationship of the LV lead to the optimal site as concordant (at optimal site), adjacent (within 1 segment), or remote (≥2 segments away). In the TARGET group, there was a greater proportion of responders at 6 months (70% vs 55%). Compared with controls, TARGET patients had a higher clinical response (83% vs 65%) and lower rates of the combined clinical end point.[43]

The STARTER study (Speckle Tracking Assisted Resynchronization Therapy for Electrode Region) used the same strategy with time to maximal radial strain for assessment of latest mechanical activation, but a qualitative evaluation of whether or not a specific segment had transmural scar (excluded scarred segments did not qualify as targets, regardless of timing). All 187 patients had baseline dyssynchrony studies and were randomized to echo-guided or routine strategies. The echo-guided strategy had better event-free survival (hazard ratio 0.48). Exact or adjacent concordance of LV lead with latest site could be achieved in 85%

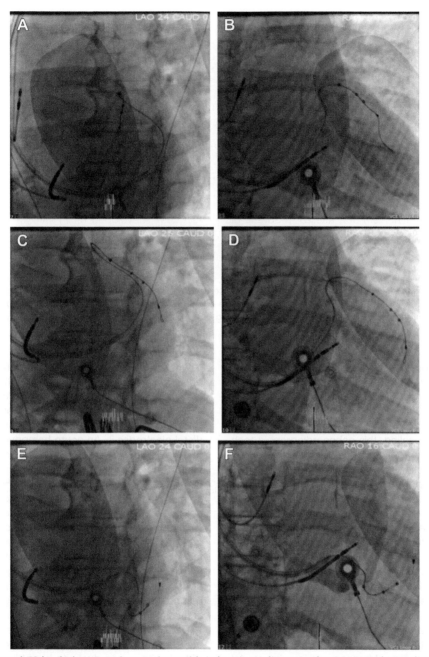

Fig. 5. Targeted CS lead placement in a patient with ischemic cardiomyopathy, RBBB, and LAD disease. The CS lead was placed into the anterior vein (*A, B*), anterolateral vein (*C, D*), and lateral vein (*E, F*) to measure the delay between the QRS and local LV activation on each electrode in each configuration. See **Fig. 6** for electrical data. LAO, left anterior oblique; RAO, right anterior oblique.

of the targeted group (occurred incidentally in 66%, significantly less in controls). Concordance was associated with an improvement in event-free survival (hazard ratio 0.40).[44] Cardiac MRI can assess scar burden besides dyssynchrony, which is a predictor of lack of response to CRT.[45,46]

The gold standard for selection of the optimal LV pacing segment has yet to be established. Although there is consensus to avoid apical segments and segments with transmural scar (>50%), there is no consensus on which exact segment to choose. Q-LV measurements are

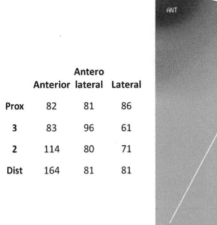
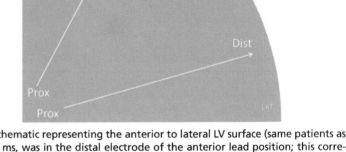

	Anterior	Antero lateral	Lateral
Prox	82	81	86
3	83	96	61
2	114	80	71
Dist	164	81	81

Fig. 6. The local Q-LVs are plotted in a schematic representing the anterior to lateral LV surface (same patients as in **Figs. 4** and **5**). The longest delay, 164 ms, was in the distal electrode of the anterior lead position; this corresponds to a midanterior location in this patient (see **Fig. 5B**). Ant, anterior; antlat, anterolateral; dist, distal; lat, lateral; prox, proximal.

promising but do not take electromechanical uncoupling into account, vary greatly depending on the underlying QRS width, and so far lack prospectively validated cutoff values for a good LV position. Although the late mechanical activation theory is appealing, this echocardiographic technique is prone to high intraindividual and interindividual variability and also depends on an exact virtual transformation of the cardiac segment localization from the echo machine to the mindset of the implanting physician. Several device manufacturers have developed proprietary optimization algorithms based on baseline or continuous electrical or mechanical input from the implanted CRT device.[47–49] Nevertheless, no optimization algorithm will be able to overcome the obstacle of a poorly placed LV lead far from the areas that need to be resynchronized, and these algorithms can at best be used as adjuncts to an optimal targeted LV lead implant. Determination of the optimal pacing site depends on input from several imaging modalities, and various image fusion strategies are currently being evaluated in the CRT setting.

MULTISITE AND MULTIPOINT PACING

Pacing from more than one LV site simultaneously during CRT may provide more effective resynchronization. Triple-site pacing showed promise (improved reverse remodeling and heart failure symptoms over a follow-up of 1 year), but implantation was difficult and the complication rate was higher.[50,51]

Quadripolar leads renewed the interest in multipolar pacing. Improved resynchronization (increase in acute systolic function, dP/dt) could be achieved through individualization of multipoint pacing, by pacing from the most proximal and distal electrodes.[52] An acute hemodynamic study of 44 patients showed improved systolic and diastolic parameters with multipoint pacing, compared with biventricular pacing.[53] In a direct comparison between multisite epicardial and endocardial LV pacing, the optimal pacing method was found to be individually specific, and on a group level, only endocardial pacing was superior to conventional CRT (improved acute hemodynamic response).[54] Multipoint pacing may be an option for nonresponders to conventional CRT, particularly for patients with heterogeneous LV activation due to underlying myocardial scar.[55]

The Triple Resynchronization in Paced Heart Failure Patients (TRIP-HF) study compared the effects of triple-site versus dual-site biventricular stimulation in 40 patients with permanent atrial fibrillation. No significant difference in ventricular resynchronization ratio, quality of life, and 6-min hall walk was observed between dual-site and triple-site pacing; however, significantly higher left ventricular ejection fraction (27% vs 35%) and smaller left ventricular end-systolic volume (157 vs 134) were observed with triple-site stimulation.[50] The V3 trial (Dual-Site LV Pacing in CRT Non Responders: Multicenter Randomized Trial) is evaluating the effect of multisite pacing in 100 nonresponders (randomized in multisite upgrade via addition of a second CS lead vs conventional groups), and the planned follow-up is 12 months. The MPP IDE study and MORE-CRT MPP studies are ongoing large, prospective randomized multicenter trials also comparing multipoint versus biventricular pacing.

Issues with multisite pacing include a technically more difficult implantation and potentially higher lead dislodgement rate (unless a quadripolar lead is used). Current CRT devices require adaptors to enable multisite pacing, and the higher current drain shortens battery life. At present, multisite pacing is technically feasible, but more results will be needed from prospective trials to evaluate its role in CRT.

SUMMARY

In spite of technical developments including preoperative imaging, multipolar LV leads, and better delivery tools, optimal targeting for LV lead pacing continues to be elusive. Routine use of preoperative advanced imaging tools (CTA, MRI) may not be feasible outside large centers. At present, transvenous implantation of the LV lead is mostly based on anatomic position, although several electrical and echocardiographic methods have been shown to improve CRT outcomes with targeted lead placement. Further studies are needed to develop reproducible and clinically feasible techniques for LV lead pacing segment selection to decrease the number of nonresponder patients.

REFERENCES

1. Baldasseroni S, Opasich C, Gorini M, et al. Left bundle-branch block is associated with increased 1-year sudden and total mortality rate in 5517 outpatients with congestive heart failure: a report from the Italian Network on Congestive Heart Failure. Am Heart J 2002;143:398–405.

2. Hawkins NM, Wang D, McMurray JJ, et al. Prevalence and prognostic impact of bundle branch block in patients with heart failure: evidence from the CHARM programme. Eur J Heart Fail 2007;9:510–7.

3. Leclercq C, Faris O, Tunin R, et al. Systolic improvement and mechanical resynchronization does not require electrical synchrony in the dilated failing heart with left bundle-branch block. Circulation 2002;106:1760–3.

4. Kass DA, Chen CH, Curry C, et al. Improved left ventricular mechanics from acute VDD pacing in patients with dilated cardiomyopathy and ventricular conduction delay. Circulation 1999;99:1567–73.

5. Prinzen FW, Hunter WC, Wyman BT, et al. Mapping of regional myocardial strain and work during ventricular pacing: experimental study using magnetic resonance imaging tagging. J Am Coll Cardiol 1999;33:1735–42.

6. Eschalier R, Ploux S, Ritter P, et al. Nonspecific intraventricular conduction delay: definitions, prognosis, and implications for cardiac resynchronization therapy. Heart Rhythm 2015;12:1071–9.

7. Noheria A, DeSimone CV, Lachman N, et al. Anatomy of the coronary sinus and epicardial coronary venous system in 620 hearts: an electrophysiology perspective. J Cardiovasc Electrophysiol 2013;24:1–6.

8. Da Costa A, Gate-Martinet A, Rouffiange P, et al. Anatomical factors involved in difficult cardiac resynchronization therapy procedure: a non-invasive study using dual-source 64-multi-slice computed tomography. Europace 2011;14(6):833–40.

9. Habib A, Lachman N, Christensen KN, et al. The anatomy of the coronary sinus venous system for the cardiac electrophysiologist. Europace 2009;11(Suppl 5):v15–21.

10. Saremi F, Muresian H, Sanchez-Quintana D. Coronary veins: comprehensive CT-anatomic classification and review of variants and clinical implications. Radiographics 2012;32:E1–32.

11. Blendea D, Shah RV, Auricchio A, et al. Variability of coronary venous anatomy in patients undergoing cardiac resynchronization therapy: a high-speed rotational venography study. Heart Rhythm 2007;4:1155–62.

12. Kaufmann J, Gerds-Li JH, Kriatselis C, et al. Three-dimensional rotational venography of the coronary sinus tree facilitates left ventricular lead implantation for CRT. J Interv Card Electrophysiol 2015;42:125–8.

13. Blendea D, Mansour M, Shah RV, et al. Usefulness of high-speed rotational coronary venous angiography during cardiac resynchronization therapy. Am J Cardiol 2007;100:1561–5.

14. Bilchick KC, Dimaano V, Wu KC, et al. Cardiac magnetic resonance assessment of dyssynchrony and myocardial scar predicts function class improvement following cardiac resynchronization therapy. JACC Cardiovasc Imag 2008;1:561–8.

15. Lam A, Mora-Vieira LF, Hoskins M, et al. Performance of 3D, navigator echo-gated, contrast-enhanced, magnetic resonance coronary vein imaging in patients undergoing CRT. J Interv Card Electrophysiol 2014;41:155–60.

16. Kawakubo M, Nagao M, Kumazawa S, et al. Evaluation of cardiac dyssynchrony with longitudinal strain analysis in 4-chamber cine MR imaging. Eur J Radiol 2013;82:2212–6.

17. European Heart Rhythm Association, European Society of Cardiology, Heart Rhythm Society, et al. 2012 EHRA/HRS expert consensus statement on cardiac resynchronization therapy in heart failure: implant and follow-up recommendations and management. Heart Rhythm 2012;9:1524–76.

18. Moss AJ, Hall WJ, Cannom DS, et al. Cardiac-resynchronization therapy for the prevention of heart-failure events. N Engl J Med 2009;361:1329–38.

19. Tang AS, Wells GA, Talajic M, et al. Cardiac-resynchronization therapy for mild-to-moderate heart failure. N Engl J Med 2010;363:2385–95.

20. van Rees JB, de Bie MK, Thijssen J, et al. Implantation-related complications of implantable cardioverter-defibrillators and cardiac resynchronization therapy devices: a systematic review of randomized clinical trials. J Am Coll Cardiol 2011;58: 995–1000.

21. Worley SJ. How to use balloons as anchors to facilitate cannulation of the coronary sinus left ventricular lead placement and to regain lost coronary sinus or target vein access. Heart Rhythm 2009;6:1242–6.

22. Jackson KP, Hegland DD, Frazier-Mills C, et al. Impact of using a telescoping-support catheter system for left ventricular lead placement on implant success and procedure time of cardiac resynchronization therapy. Pacing Clin Electrophysiol 2013;36: 553–8.

23. Behar JM, Bostock J, Zhu Li AP, et al. Cardiac resynchronization therapy delivered via a multipolar left ventricular lead is associated with reduced mortality and elimination of phrenic nerve stimulation: long-term follow-up from a multicenter registry. J Cardiovasc Electrophysiol 2015;26:540–6.

24. Soga Y, Ando K, Yamada T, et al. Efficacy of coronary venoplasty for left ventricular lead implantation. Circ J 2007;71:1442–5.

25. Worley SJ. Implant venoplasty: dilation of subclavian and coronary veins to facilitate device implantation: indications, frequency, methods, and complications. J Cardiovasc Electrophysiol 2008;19:1004–7.

26. Abben RP, Chaisson G, Nair V. Traversing and dilating venous collaterals: a useful adjunct in left ventricular electrode placement. J Invasive Cardiol 2010;22:E93–6.

27. Luedorff G, Grove R, Kranig W, et al. Different venous angioplasty manoeuvres for successful implantation of CRT devices. Clin Res Cardiol 2009; 98:159–64.

28. Geller L, Szilagyi S, Zima E, et al. Long-term experience with coronary sinus side branch stenting to stabilize left ventricular electrode position. Heart Rhythm 2011;8:845–50.

29. Maytin M, Carrillo RG, Baltodano P, et al. Multicenter experience with transvenous lead extraction of active fixation coronary sinus leads. Pacing Clin Electrophysiol 2012;35:641–7.

30. Nagele H, Hashagen S, Ergin M, et al. Coronary sinus lead fragmentation 2 years after implantation with a retained guidewire. Pacing Clin Electrophysiol 2007;30:438–9.

31. Brignole M, Auricchio A, Baron-Esquivias G, et al. 2013 ESC Guidelines on cardiac pacing and cardiac resynchronization therapy: the Task Force on cardiac pacing and resynchronization therapy of the European Society of Cardiology (ESC). Developed in collaboration with the European Heart Rhythm Association (EHRA). Eur Heart J 2013;34: 2281–329.

32. Singh JP, Klein HU, Huang DT, et al. Left ventricular lead position and clinical outcome in the Multicenter Automatic Defibrillator Implantation Trial-Cardiac Resynchronization Therapy (MADIT-CRT) trial. Circulation 2011;123:1159–66.

33. Bristow MR, Saxon LA, Boehmer J, et al. Cardiac-resynchronization therapy with or without an implantable defibrillator in advanced chronic heart failure. N Engl J Med 2004;350:2140–50.

34. Linde C, Abraham WT, Gold MR, et al. Randomized trial of cardiac resynchronization in mildly symptomatic heart failure patients and in asymptomatic patients with left ventricular dysfunction and previous heart failure symptoms. J Am Coll Cardiol 2008;52: 1834–43.

35. Heist EK, Fan D, Mela T, et al. Radiographic left ventricular-right ventricular interlead distance predicts the acute hemodynamic response to cardiac resynchronization therapy. Am J Cardiol 2005;96:685–90.

36. Singh JP, Fan D, Heist EK, et al. Left ventricular lead electrical delay predicts response to cardiac resynchronization therapy. Heart Rhythm 2006;3: 1285–92.

37. Heist EK, Taub C, Fan D, et al. Usefulness of a novel "response score" to predict hemodynamic and clinical outcome from cardiac resynchronization therapy. Am J Cardiol 2006;97:1732–6.

38. Gepstein L, Hayam G, Ben-Haim SA. A novel method for nonfluoroscopic catheter-based electroanatomical mapping of the heart. In vitro and in vivo accuracy results. Circulation 1997;95:1611–22.

39. Schilling RJ, Peters NS, Davies DW. Simultaneous endocardial mapping in the human left ventricle using a noncontact catheter: comparison of contact and reconstructed electrograms during sinus rhythm. Circulation 1998;98:887–98.

40. Ryu K, D'Avila A, Heist EK, et al. Simultaneous electrical and mechanical mapping using 3D cardiac mapping system: novel approach for optimal cardiac resynchronization therapy. J Cardiovasc Electrophysiol 2010;21:219–22.

41. Pastore CA, Tobias N, Samesima N, et al. Ventricular electrical activation in cardiac resynchronization as characterized by body surface potential mapping. Arq Bras Cardiol 2007;88:251–7.

42. Ploux S, Eschalier R, Whinnett ZI, et al. Electrical dyssynchrony induced by biventricular pacing: implications for patient selection and therapy improvement. Heart Rhythm 2015;12:782–91.

43. Khan FZ, Virdee MS, Palmer CR, et al. Targeted Left Ventricular Lead Placement to Guide cardiac Resynchronization Therapy: the TARGET study: a randomized, controlled trial. J Am Coll Cardiol 2012; 59:1509–18.

44. Saba S, Marek J, Schwartzman D, et al. Echocardiography-guided left ventricular lead placement for cardiac resynchronization therapy: results of the Speckle Tracking Assisted Resynchronization Therapy for Electrode Region trial. Circ Heart Fail 2013; 6:427–34.

45. Petryka J, Misko J, Przybylski A, et al. Magnetic resonance imaging assessment of intraventricular dyssynchrony and delayed enhancement as predictors of response to cardiac resynchronization therapy in patients with heart failure of ischaemic and nonischaemic etiologies. Eur J Radiol 2012;81:2639–47.

46. de Roest GJ, Wu L, de Cock CC, et al. Scar tissue-guided left ventricular lead placement for cardiac resynchronization therapy in patients with ischemic cardiomyopathy: an acute pressure-volume loop study. Am Heart J 2014;167:537–45.

47. Brugada J, Brachmann J, Delnoy PP, et al. Automatic optimization of cardiac resynchronization therapy using SonR-rationale and design of the clinical trial of the SonRtip lead and automatic AV-VV optimization algorithm in the paradym RF SonR CRT-D (RESPOND CRT) trial. Am Heart J 2014;167:429–36.

48. Birnie D, Lemke B, Aonuma K, et al. Clinical outcomes with synchronized left ventricular pacing: analysis of the adaptive CRT trial. Heart Rhythm 2013;10:1368–74.

49. Baker JH 2nd, McKenzie J 3rd, Beau S, et al. Acute evaluation of programmer-guided AV/PV and VV delay optimization comparing an IEGM method and echocardiogram for cardiac resynchronization therapy in heart failure patients and dual-chamber ICD implants. J Cardiovasc Electrophysiol 2007;18: 185–91.

50. Leclercq C, Gadler F, Kranig W, et al. A randomized comparison of triple-site versus dual-site ventricular stimulation in patients with congestive heart failure. J Am Coll Cardiol 2008;51:1455–62.

51. Rogers DP, Lambiase PD, Lowe MD, et al. A randomized double-blind crossover trial of triventricular versus biventricular pacing in heart failure. Eur J Heart Fail 2012;14:495–505.

52. Thibault B, Dubuc M, Khairy P, et al. Acute haemodynamic comparison of multisite and biventricular pacing with a quadripolar left ventricular lead. Europace 2013;15:984–91.

53. Pappone C, Calovic Z, Vicedomini G, et al. Multipoint left ventricular pacing improves acute hemodynamic response assessed with pressure-volume loops in cardiac resynchronization therapy patients. Heart Rhythm 2014;11:394–401.

54. Shetty AK, Sohal M, Chen Z, et al. A comparison of left ventricular endocardial, multisite, and multipolar epicardial cardiac resynchronization: an acute haemodynamic and electroanatomical study. Europace 2014;16:873–9.

55. Niederer SA, Shetty AK, Plank G, et al. Biophysical modeling to simulate the response to multisite left ventricular stimulation using a quadripolar pacing lead. Pacing Clin Electrophysiol 2012;35:204–14.

Robotic-Assisted Left Ventricular Lead Placement

Advay G. Bhatt, MD[a], Jonathan S. Steinberg, MD[a,b],*

KEYWORDS

• Robotic • Epicardial leads • Cardiac resynchronization therapy

KEY POINTS

• The current endovascular approach for cardiac resynchronization is limited by anatomic constraints precluding accurate targeting of the optimal pacing site.
• Convention surgical left ventricular (LV) lead placement has been used as rescue therapy but with significant morbidity and similar limited precision for targeting the optimal pacing site.
• Robot-assisted surgery for LV lead placement allows for superior precision to target the optimal pacing site in conjunction with preoperative and intraoperative mapping techniques.
• Robot-assisted surgery for LV lead placement has been associated with comparable therapeutic efficacy of cardiac resynchronization as with leads via the coronary sinus.

INTRODUCTION

Cardiac resynchronization therapy (CRT) has been demonstrated by several randomized controls trial to improve exercise capacity, quality of life, hospitalizations for heart failure (HF), cardiac structure, and mortality in patients with symptomatic HF, impaired left ventricular (LV) systolic function, and wide QRS complex.[1–6] Dyssynchronous ventricular activation is the putative pathophysiologic mechanism that leads to detrimental hemodynamics, and structural and molecular changes associated with worse clinical outcomes and is the therapeutic target for CRT. Despite the marked disease modifying effect of the therapy on specific targeted populations, there is significant heterogeneity in individual response, such that approximately one-third of patients do not experience a clinical response or benefit from reverse remodeling.[7–9] A great deal of effort has been focused on refining patient selection to improve clinical response by identifying predictors of nonresponse or superresponse to CRT. The presence of echocardiographic dyssynchrony, myocardial scar burden, and optimal programming have all been evaluated with variable results. The most important clinical factors associated with response remain QRS width and morphology, in particular, left bundle branch block morphology with QRS duration of greater than 150 milliseconds. These factors signify substantial septal to posterior wall electromechanical delay that may be mitigated by CRT. However, the most important technical factors to achieving CRT are related to identifying the optimal pacing site and precise delivery of a pacing lead to that target region.

IDENTIFYING THE OPTIMAL PACING SITE

The early studies on CRT did not systematically evaluate the site of LV simulation, region of maximal electromechanical delay, or account

Disclosures: None (A.G. Bhatt); Consultant for and research support from Medtronic (J.S. Steinberg).
[a] Arrhythmia Institute, The Valley Health System, 223 North Van Dien Avenue, Ridgewood, NJ 07450, USA;
[b] University of Rochester School of Medicine and Dentistry, Rochester, NY, USA
* Corresponding author. Arrhythmia Institute, The Valley Health System, 223 North Van Dien Avenue, Ridgewood, NJ 07450.
E-mail address: steijo@valleyhealth.com

cardiacEP.theclinics.com

for variability in coronary sinus (CS) anatomy that could limit lead delivery. The traditional site of LV stimulation was subjectively determined fluoroscopically with greatest separation between the right and LV leads. Butter and colleagues[10] in 2001 demonstrated that contractile function significantly improved with LV free wall stimulation compared with anterior stimulation. The overall extent of the optimal stimulation site or "sweet spot" for CRT was determined in an animal model to be circumscribed by broad area centered in the mid to apical LV lateral wall; optimal CRT is better preserved with apical compared with basal pacing.[11] The core clinical trials of CRT demonstrated conflicting data in regards to lead placement. In the COMPANION, MADIT-CRT, and RAFT trials, anterior, posterior, or lateral LV stimulation sites had equivalent improvements in functional outcome and mortality[12–14]; however, apical lead position was associated with excess mortality.[13,14]

The clinical experience of implementing CRT lacks precision, but there is considerable research into quantitatively determining optimal pacing sites using echocardiography, cardiac MRI, and electrical mapping at the time of implant. The use of tissue Doppler imaging (TDI) to guide LV lead placement at the site of maximal delay is associated with the greatest improvement in cardiac structure and function.[15] Speckle-tracking 2-dimensional radial strain analysis to guide CRT has been shown to result in improvements in combined mortality or HF hospitalizations.[16,17] Cardiac MRI has similarly been used to assess strain and to guide lead placement away from regions of dense myocardial scar.[17–19] Maximal local electrical delay (QLV), a measure of dyssynchrony and assessed at the time of device implantation, is associated with acute hemodynamic response and reverse modeling and may serve as a simpler tool to map the optimal pacing site at implant.[20–22]

CONVENTIONAL APPROACH TO CARDIAC RESYNCHRONIZATION THERAPY

The standard technique for cannulating the CS includes using specialized lead delivery systems with different shapes to account for variations in right atrial anatomy and location of the CS ostium. The lead delivery system is used to guide either a J-tipped guidewire or diagnostic electrophysiologic catheter into the CS. Subselective sheaths and angioplasty wires may be used to facilitate access in difficult cases. The lead delivery sheath is then tracked over the wire or catheter into the CS. A balloon-occlusive venogram is performed to fully delineate CS anatomy and subjectively

identify a suitable branch to target for lead delivery.

In general, a posterolateral or lateral branch is chosen without consideration of whether the branch subtends the site of maximal electromechanical delay or the presence of myocardial scar. If a posterior or lateral branch is not available or technically feasible, then a more anterior branch may be selected given the results of the major clinical trials. A lead is then guided into the target branch with the aide of a stylet or an over-the-wire technique, at which point the presumed success of CRT is ascertained by angiographic lead position and stability with suitable pacing thresholds and absence of diaphragmatic stimulation. **Box 1** lists the several anatomic constraints that may limit successful cannulation of the CS, delivery of a pacing lead into the appropriate branch, or maintaining lead stability.[23]

Despite several different techniques and a multitude of specially designed tools for CS cannulation or lead delivery, up to 10% of attempts fail.[6] If these anatomic barriers are overcome, there remains the issue of suboptimal pacing thresholds, a high degree of latency limiting effective CRT in areas of myocardial scar, and phrenic nerve stimulation.

The technical challenge posed by these factors leads to prolonged procedure time, greater radiation exposure, greater exposure to iodinated

---

Box 1
Anatomic features limiting coronary sinus cannulation or lead delivery

Coronary sinus cannulation

Prominent sub-Eustachian pouch

Prominent Thebesian valve

Dilated right atrium distorting the coronary sinus os

Dilated left ventricle distorting the coronary sinus os

Lead delivery or stability within the coronary sinus

Coronary sinus stenosis

Coronary sinus spasm

Prominent valve of Vieussens

Tortuous coronary sinus body or branches

Persistent left superior vena cava

Small or absent posterolateral or lateral branches

Ectactic branches

contrast with potential for nephrotoxicity, greater risk of CS dissection or perforation, or a relatively high rate of lead migration or dislodgement needing early intervention.[24]

SURGICAL APPROACH TO CARDIAC RESYNCHRONIZATION THERAPY

When endovascular delivery of a lead for CRT is unsuccessful, the next recommendation is a surgical approach to access and deliver a lead on the LV posterolateral wall to facilitate resynchronization. The surgical options include an approach with median sternotomy, thoracotomy, and thoracoscopically with or without robotic assistance. These surgical approaches allow direct access to the LV surface for mapping the optimal pacing site and precise lead placement without the need for fluoroscopy or contrast.[25,26]

Surgical approaches to achieving CRT are used as a last resort given the risks associated with endotracheal intubation, single lung ventilation, general anesthesia, sternotomy or thoracotomy, and more prolonged convalescent period in debilitated patients with advanced HF and other comorbidities.

Lead Design and Performance

The technical problems associated with epicardial lead delivery includes difficult fixation owing to a beating heart and epicardial fat. These factors are associated with a greater incidence of sensing and capture problems as well as reduced longevity, as described in the pediatric population with early unipolar epicardial lead designs.[27,28] Lead fracture owing to high mechanical stress at contact points with the ribs and intercostal muscles may further limit longevity; care must be taken with lead tunneling and manipulation at the time of implant.

The development of steroid-eluting bipolar pacing electrodes designs has improved epicardial lead performance and longevity. There are currently 2 different steroid-eluting bipolar epicardial designs (**Fig. 1**): screw-in (MyoDex 1084T [St. Jude Medical, St. Paul, MN] or MyoPore 511212 [GreatBatch Medical, Clarence, NY]) and suture-on leads (Capture Epi 4968, Medtronic, Minneapolis, MN). Steroid-eluting sew-on leads are thought to have superior electrical and mechanical performance compared with screw-on leads, but require exposure of bare myocardium to achieve adequate pacing performance and require finer dexterity when placed thoracoscopically.[25] The screw-in leads are secured to the myocardium with specialized introducer tools.

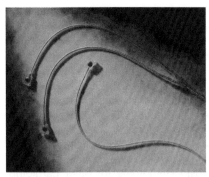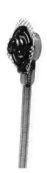

Fig. 1. Suture-on (*left*) and screw-in (*right*) and epicardial leads. On the left are unipolar and bipolar suture on leads. On the right is a bipolar screw-in lead. (*Courtesy of* St. Jude Medical, St. Paul, MN and Medtronic, Minneapolis, MN.)

Clinical data on the endurance and performance of epicardial LV leads for CRT in adults are limited. The 10-year survival of a screw-in lead (not steroid eluting) was reported as 92%, and 96% for a steroid-eluting suture-on lead.[25] A recent retrospective study compared steroid-eluting screw-in and suture-on lead designs for LV stimulation via different surgical approaches.[29] The study evaluated lead performance over a follow-up of 48 months of 130 consecutive patients undergoing surgical placement of an LV lead and found no difference in pacing thresholds (0.8 vs 1.1 V) or sensing (10–12 mV) in long-term follow-up. There was a moderate acute increase in pacing thresholds for screw-in leads that decreased over time and sensing showed an upward trend over the duration of follow-up for both types of leads. The only appreciable difference was that impedances for suture-on leads were higher compared with screw-in leads (710 vs 435 Ω).

Open Surgical Approach

The traditional surgical approach for epicardial lead placement was performed via median sternotomy, which affords the best exposure and access to the anterior aspect of the heart. This approach has been used historically in the pediatric population for right atrial and right ventricular epicardial pacing given concerns with long-standing endovascular leads or aberrant anatomy owing to congenital heart disease. However, significant cardiac manipulation is required to map and deliver a lead to the mid posterolateral LV wall; direct visualization or mapping may be limited.[25]

Median sternotomy leads to the largest scar with a greater risk of mediastinitis or osteomyelitis, prolonged operative time, slower recuperation, and increased mortality. This approach is more challenging in the face of prior cardiothoracic surgery given adhesions limiting dissection or visualization and difficulty identifying bypass grafts. In the same token, median sternotomy solely for CRT could produce pericardial and pleural adhesions and heighten risk should future cardiothoracic surgery be needed. Given these concerns other less invasive approaches have been developed, although there may be a limited role for concomitant epicardial lead implantation at the time of median sternotomy for other cardiothoracic surgery.[30]

Thoracotomy and Minimal Thoracotomy

Thoracotomy has been the most common approach for LV epicardial lead placement and allows direct access and visualization of the posterolateral LV wall without requiring significant cardiac manipulation.[25] The extensive rib-spreading procedure is associated with significant postoperative pain, prolonged recovery, postoperative HF exacerbations, and increased mortality.[25,31]

To minimize, the trauma and morbidity associated with full thoracotomy, a more limited or minimal thoracotomy approach allows access to the posterolateral LV for epicardial lead placement. For minimal thoracotomy, general anesthesia with double-lumen endotracheal intubation and single lung ventilation is established. The patient is placed at a 30° right lateral decubitus position and a 3- to 5-cm skin incision is made over the fourth or fifth left intercostal spaces anterior to the midaxillary line. A self-retaining retractor is used to allow adequate exposure.[32,33] Under single lung ventilation, the left lung is dissected from the pericardium and retracted posteriorly. A pericardiotomy is performed away from the phrenic nerve. The use of stay or traction sutures in the pericardium allows direct visualization of the myocardium. The epicardial lead is then placed while trying to avoid obtuse marginal branches and scar. Typically, screw-in leads are deployed given that special lead implant tools have been developed for fixation[34] and limited exposure does not allow sufficient maneuverability to apply sutures.[25] Once adequate sensing and capture are confirmed, the pericardium is closed around the lead. The lead is then tunneled to the preexisting subpectoral implant site. Chest tubes are variably required.

Minimal thoracotomy offers several advantages in that it is very well-tolerated with low complication rates; special equipment is not mandatory and the procedure may be performed in any surgical suite. The main disadvantage is limited exposure necessitating more expertise to secure a lead to the optimal pacing site. In particular, this approach may be more advantageous in patients with severe LV dilation and in those with prior cardiothoracic surgery given that thoracoscopic procedure would be more difficult and dangerous owing to limited space that restricts manipulation of surgical instruments.[32,33]

Video-Assisted Thoracoscopic Surgery

Minimally invasive endoscopic techniques are currently used in a wide range of surgical procedures and have been extended to cardiac and thoracic surgery with thoracoscopic techniques. Video-assisted thoracoscopic surgery (VATS) is accomplished with double-lumen endotracheal intubation and single-lung ventilation while the patient is placed at 45° to 60° right lateral decubitus position. There are a number of different port configurations described including anterolateral and posterolateral positions with most commonly 3 ports; 2-port configurations have also been successful.[25,32,35–37] With a 3-port configuration, there is a primary working port for instrumentation, a second grasping port, and a third endoscope port. The procedure technique then is similar to minimal thoracotomy: pericardiotomy, mapping, and delivery of a screw-on lead through the working port with a specialized lead implant tool. Once adequate sensing and capture have been confirmed, the lung is reinflated gradually with sufficient intrathoracic slack on the pacing lead to account for reinflation. The proximal end of the lead is the directed through the most cranial port and then tunneled to the preexisting subpectoral implant site.

VATS allows for smaller incisions and superior visualization of the heart and thorax without spreading the ribs.[35–37] This leads to an enhanced ability to map the optimal pacing site and lead delivery while resulting in less trauma, better pain control, faster recovery, and a better cosmetic result.[35] VATS is reported to better preserve pulmonary mechanics and is associated wither fewer respiratory complications.[37]

Manipulation of instruments in a confined space with only 2-dimensional visualization can lead to inadvertent damage to the epicardium, coronary arteries, and lung that would require conversion to full thoracotomy. Marked LV dilation may make port positioning difficult and the procedure technically challenging owing to limited maneuverability.[35–37] The presence of pleural and/or pericardial adhesions limit visualization and may be more difficult to manage thoracoscopically, especially after coronary artery bypass grafting. VATS require single lung ventilation or insufflation of carbon dioxide, which may not be hemodynamically tolerated in patients with advanced cardiopulmonary disease.

There is a significant learning curve to obtain the advanced skills to successfully accomplish VATS for LV lead placement including pericardiotomy, experience dealing with pleural and pericardial adhesions if considered in patients with prior cardiothoracic surgery, and avoiding prior coronary artery bypass grafts.[33,36]

Robot-assisted Surgery (the da Vinci Surgical System)

Robot-assisted surgery was developed to combine the advantages of open and minimally invasive surgical approaches while allowing for superior visualization, dexterity, and precision with an optimum ergonomic design.[25,38–40] The da Vinci Surgical System (Intuitive Surgical, Inc., Sunnyvale, CA) is composed of a surgeon console and a patient-side instrument cart with 4 articulated and interactive robotic arms controlled from the console (**Fig. 2**). The 4 arms incorporate a high performance vision system and up to 3 proprietary "EndoWrist" microinstruments, including scalpels, scissors, forceps, or electrocautery (**Fig. 3**).

The console consists of 2 separate video screens, 1 for each eye, 2 controllers that actuate finger and wrist motion to the robotic instruments, and foot pedals to control camera focus, field movement clutch, and electrocautery. Unlike standard thoracoscopic instruments with 4° of freedom, the EndoWrist microinstruments have 7° of freedom[25] leading to a range of motion that is superior to the human wrist with true ambidextrous

function (**Fig. 4**).[38–40] Finger and wrist movements are registered by the computer system where processing allows for motion scaling and elimination of inherent human tremor that coupled with the enhanced range of motion allow for precise micromovements. The clutch and other safety mechanisms allow for readjustment of hand position and avoidance of unintended movements.[38] Visualization is performed through an endoscope with 2 cameras in parallel, one channeled to each eye, that allow for real-time stereoscopic 3-dimensional vision with depth perception and high-power ($\times$10) magnification.[38–40]

Robot-assisted lead implantation for CRT is similarly performed with double-lumen endotracheal intubation and single-lung ventilation, but with the patient placed in a full posterolateral thoracotomy position to allow for easy access to the posterolateral wall of the LV. Three incisions are made along the posterior axillary line: the 10-mm camera port is placed in the seventh intercostal space, the 8-mm left arm port in the ninth intercostal space, and the 8-mm right arm port in the fifth intercostal space (**Fig. 5**). Another 10-mm working port is inserted posterior to the camera port and is used for lead delivery and sutures. The port positions should be adjusted to individually account for differences in thoracic wall geometry and cardiac anatomy.[32] The left chest is insufflated with carbon dioxide to expand the working space between the heart and thoracic wall. A pericardiotomy is performed posterior to the phrenic nerve and the obtuse marginal branches are identified.[25,32,33,38–40] Most often a screw-in lead is introduced through the working port, electrical mapping is performed, and the lead is fixed to the optimal pacing site. Ventilation may be held during lead fixation to maximize working space. Once the lead is

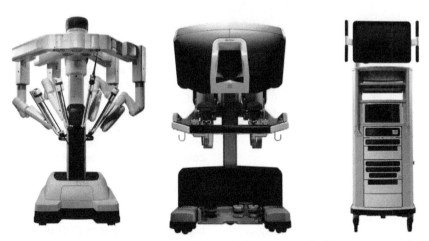

Fig. 2. The da Vinci System showing the patient side articulating arm unit (*left*), surgeon console (*middle*), and vision cart (*right*). (Copyright © 2015 Intuitive Surgical, Inc., Sunnyvale, CA.)

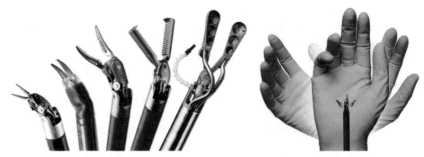

Fig. 3. EndoWrist microinstruments (*left*) and range of motion in response to wrist movements (*right*). (Copyright © 2015 Intuitive Surgical, Inc., Sunnyvale, CA.)

fixed to the myocardium, the pericardium is closed and supports fixation. The proximal end of the lead is withdrawn through the right arm port and tunneled to a counterincision in the axilla. A chest tube is placed through the left arm port to evacuate air and is then removed. The port sites are then closed and the patient is placed in a supine position.[38] The lead is then tunneled to the preexisting subpectoral implant site.

Left Ventricular Mapping Techniques

Robot-assisted CRT allows for superior access and visualization of the posterior aspect of the

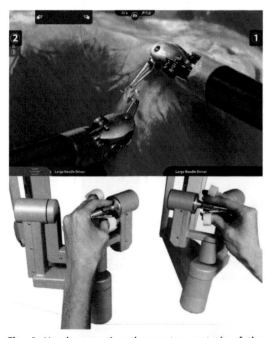

Fig. 4. Hands operating the master controls of the surgeon console and the operative screen. Wrist and finger movements are actuated to precise micromovements with superior dexterity and range of motion. (Copyright © 2015 Intuitive Surgical, Inc., Sunnyvale, CA.)

LV and affords the ability to perform detailed mapping to optimize lead performance and precisely target the optimal pacing site, generally found between the mid to apical posterolateral wall. The optimal pacing site generally corresponds to the site of maximal electromechanical delay and may be assessed formally with several different techniques alone or in combination, including TDI, electrical mapping, or pressure–volume loops.[15–17,25,41,42]

TDI correlating LV lead position to the site of latest mechanical activation is associated with improvement in LV function and geometry.[15] The technique is limited because it measures only longitudinal myocardial velocity parallel to the direction of the ultrasound beam and is unable to distinguish between passive or active motion. This may be overcome by assessing tissue deformation with strain rate imaging. However, circumferential or radial strain may be more sensitive for the assessment of dyssynchrony.[43] Three small studies using echocardiographic measures to assess lead concordance with the latest activated site were mixed. The use of tissue Doppler alone did not demonstrate benefit.[44] The incorporation of 2-dimensional speckle tracking to assess circumferential strain was associated with improvement in LV performance and geometry.[45,46] The use of speckle tracking to prospectively guide LV lead placement is associated with a net clinical benefit in HF or mortality based on results from 2 randomized, controlled trials.[16,17]

As previously described, assessment of QLV from within the CS predicts acute hemodynamic response and reverse remodeling. Polasek and colleagues[42] used this technique with a surgical epicardial approach by passing a decapolar electrophysiologic catheter through 1 port to map the latest activated site compared with QRS duration. The authors were able to target the site with the highest ratio of QLV to QRS duration that tended to be more favorable compared with an empiric implant site. The point to point mapping afforded

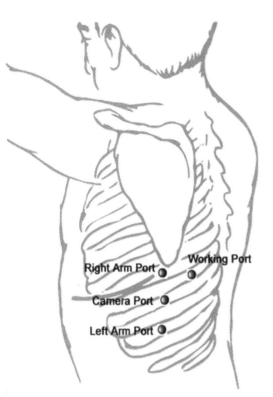

Fig. 5. Port placement for robotic left ventricular epicardial lead placement. The ports are placed in line with the tip of the scapula, allowing for posterior access to the left ventricular surface. (*From* DeRose JJ, Ashton RC, Belsley S, et al. Robotically assisted left ventricular epicardial lead implantation for biventricular pacing. J Am Coll Cardiol 2003;41:1417; with permission.)

with this technique allowed for greater spatial resolution owing to ability to sample more than 50 sites,[41] whereas TDI is limited to 12 segments.

Intraoperative assessment of hemodynamic response to pacing from multiple different epicardial sites may be performed with the use of a conductance catheter advanced to the LV via a retrograde aortic approach to optimize pressure-volume loops for stroke work and dP/dt.[41] This technique remains experimental and needs further study to be incorporated into clinical practice.

Benefits of Robot-Assisted Cardiac Resynchronization Therapy

Robot-assisted CRT contributes above and beyond the small incision, less trauma, better visualization, shorter recovery, and better cosmetic result than that afforded with standard VATS. As described, robot assistance allows for 3-dimensional visualization, elimination of tremor, and superior dexterity. The precision of the system

allows for detailed access and mapping of the entire epicardial surface to avoid scar and achieve long-term lead performance and durability.

Limitations of Robot-Assisted Cardiac Resynchronization Therapy

Despite the impressive technology augmenting and enhancing surgical lead implantation for CRT, there are several technical, clinical, and administrative considerations. The technical limitations of the da Vinci Surgical System include the following.[40]

1. Incomplete and delayed motion tracking: The inherent latency in the system owing to processing and mechanical transduction may limit dexterity and has been shown to increase errors in novices to the technique.
2. Lack of haptic or tactile feedback: Operators must rely on visual cues of tissue deformation to assess contact, suturing, and lead fixation.
3. More prolonged operative time: Owing to the need for configuring and deploying the robotic system, operative times are longer compared with minimal thoracotomy or VATS.

The clinical limitations relate to the need for general anesthesia, single lung ventilation, and potential for complications given the need to work in confined spaces. Moreover, there is no clinical evidence of superiority in reverse remodeling, morbidity, or mortality despite the perception that lead placement more precisely targets the optimal pacing site.

There are considerable costs associated with robot-assisted surgery, including the large initial capital outlay for the da Vinci Surgical System, as well as ongoing costs for reusable and disposable equipment. Given the cost issues, this system is limited to only a few specialized centers. As such, there is a steep learning curve and limited opportunities to develop and enhance the needed robotic skills.

Clinical Trials and Case Series with Robot-assisted Cardiac Resynchronization Therapy

The literature on surgical epicardial lead placement includes largely small case series of patients in whom lead placement via the CS was unsuccessful. Several observational studies evaluated surgical LV lead implant via either minimal thoracotomy or VATS in a total of 325 patients without standardization of surgical approach, lead design, or site of lead fixation.[35–37,47–51] These approaches were found to be feasible with near 100% lead implant success rates, low operative morbidity, and low operative mortality. One study suggested that surgical epicardial lead performance was superior to CS leads.[48] TDI to map the optimal pacing site, in 1 study, was not associated with evidence of reverse remodeling, although the patient population had advanced HF with a 14% mortality rate during 6 months of follow-up.[47] Long-term clinical response was not assessed in the remaining studies. Ailawadi and colleagues[52] demonstrated that, in 45 patients requiring surgical lead implant, mortality and readmission for HF was comparable with patients with leads placed via the CS.

Mair and colleagues[51] performed robot-assisted lead placement in 33 of 80 patients, which was associated with prolonged procedure time, 15% conversion rate to thoracotomy, and lead performance comparable with the other operative techniques. Bhamidipati and colleagues[53] compared robotic assistance with minimal thoracotomy in a total of 24 patients and found no difference in lead performance and negligible difference in cost, although procedure time and duration of mechanical ventilation was more prolonged with robotic assistance; duration of stay was comparable.

With the obvious advantages and precision associated with robot-assisted lead placement, the technique has been evaluated with more rigor over short-, medium- and long-term follow-up.[54–58] Between 2002 and 2007, 78 patient underwent robot-assisted LV lead placement. **Box 2** lists the reason for epicardial lead implant of decreasing frequency, 70 of which were performed after lead delivery via the CS was unsuccessful. Two cases (2.6%) required conversion to minimal thoracotomy owing to complications. Mean operative time was 51 minutes and decreased to 45 minutes with additional experience. All patients were extubated in the operating room and median duration of stay was 1.5 days.[25]

Lead implant success rate was 100% and the optimal pacing set was selected by TDI in the last 48 patients. Lead performance was excellent in long-term follow-up. Mean threshold at the time of implant was 1.0 V, 2.1 V at 4 months, and 2.3 V at 44 months. Mean impedance at the time of implant was 1010 Ω, 491 Ω at 4 months, and 451 Ω at 44 months. Three leads (3.8%) failed and required intervention.

There was an 81% response rate at 3 months, more favorable than seen in CRT trials, which then decreased to 71% at the time of maximum follow-up (**Fig. 6**). Clinical response and reverse remodeling were evident at 12 months with improvement in functional class, LV diastolic dimension, LV systolic dimension, and LV ejection fraction. The observed mortality rate of the cohort was 11% at 12 months, 18% at 24 months, and 22% at 36 months.

A randomized, controlled trial of CRT via the CS compared with robot-assisted lead implant that was performed by our group in 21 patients demonstrated 100% successful lead implant with robot assistance and 83% via the endovascular approach.[58] There were 2 cases of diaphragmatic stimulation in the endovascular group and 2 cases of pocket hematomas in the surgical group. LV performance, functional class, and other measures of HF severity improved equivalently in both groups. The notable difference was that epicardial lead performance was worse compared with CS leads at 6 and 12 months follow-up: the threshold was 4.0 V versus 1.2 V at 6 months and 5.0 V versus 1.3 V at 12 months.

> **Box 2**
> **Indications for epicardial left ventricular lead implant**
>
> Inability to cannulate the coronary sinus
>
> Primary epicardial lead implant (eg, concomitant cardiac surgery)
>
> Unsuitable target branches of the coronary sinus
>
> Coronary sinus dissection or perforation
>
> Coronary sinus lead failure
>
> Phrenic nerve stimulation
>
> Subclavian vein occlusion
>
> Right ventricular perforation

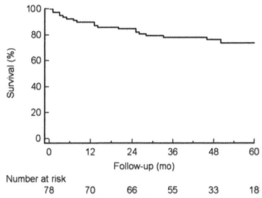

Number at risk

78	70	66	55	33	18

Fig. 6. Cumulative survival of patients undergoing cardiac resynchronization with robot-assisted left ventricular lead implant over a mean follow-up of 44 months. (*From* Kamath GS, Balaram S, Choi A, et al. Long-term outcome of leads and patients following robotic epicardial left ventricular lead placement for cardiac resynchronization therapy. Pacing Clin Electrophysiol 2011;34:239; with permission.)

Challenges and Unanswered Questions

Despite the technical and clinical advantages afforded by robot-assisted LV lead placement for CRT, including preoperative or intraoperative mapping of the optimal pacing site, the net clinical benefit remains similar to the traditional endovascular approach via the CS and the nonresponder rate remains significant. This lack of demonstrable superiority despite the presumption of achieving an optimal pacing site suggests that further refinement of the technique is needed or that there are other determinants of response, including age, QRS duration, HF duration, severity of LV dysfunction and adverse remodeling, and myocardial scar burden.

TDI was used for mapping but speckle tracking may be a more sensitive way to assess mechanical delay and has been shown to predict improvement in clinical outcomes. Another question that arises is whether any 1 mapping technique is sufficient or should a combination of techniques be used. Perhaps preoperative speckle tracking may narrow the region of interest to the latest mechanically activated segment and then allow for more focused and detailed assessment of the latest electrically activated (QLV) segment to further fine tune the site of lead implantation.

Lead performance and durability seems to be adequate, but ongoing surveillance is needed given that indications for CRT have expanded to the population of patients with mild HF. Accordingly, as CRT implants increase there will likely be growth in the need for surgical lead implantation. This population would be expected to have improved response to CRT and improved survival compared with the population of patient with advanced HF treated with robot-assisted lead implantation; epicardial leads would need to perform over much longer periods of time.

SUMMARY

Robot-assisted LV lead implantation for CRT is a feasible and safe technique with superior visualization, dexterity, and precision to target the optimal pacing site. The technique has been associated with clinical response and beneficial reverse remodeling comparable with the conventional approach via the CS. The lack of clinical superiority and a residual high nonresponder rate suggest that the appropriate clinical role for the technique remains as rescue therapy after a failed attempt or inadequate results with a transvenous implant.

REFERENCES

1. Cazeau S, Leclercq C, Lavergne T, et al, Multisite Stimulation in Cardiomyopathies (MUSTIC) Study Investigators. Effects of multisite biventricular pacing in patients with heart failure and intraventricular conduction delay. N Engl J Med 2001;344:873–80.
2. Auricchio A, Stellbrink C, Sack S, et al, Pacing Therapies in Congestive Heart Failure (PATH-CHF) Study Group. Long-term clinical effect of hemodynamically optimized cardiac resynchronization therapy in patients with heart failure and ventricular conduction delay. J Am Coll Cardiol 2002;39:2026–33.
3. Abraham WT, Fisher WG, Smith AL, et al, MIRACLE Study Group Multicenter InSync Randomized Clinical Evaluation. Cardiac resynchronization in chronic heart failure. N Engl J Med 2002;346:1845–53.
4. Bristow MR, Saxon LA, Boehmer J, et al, Comparison of Medical Therapy Pacing and Defibrillation in Heart Failure COMPANION Investigators. Cardiac-resynchronization therapy with or without an implantable defibrillator in advanced chronic heart failure. N Engl J Med 2004;350:2140–50.
5. Cleland JGF, Daubert J-C, Erdmann E, et al, Cardiac Resynchronization-Heart Failure CARE-HF Study Investigators. The effect of cardiac resynchronization on morbidity and mortality in heart failure. N Engl J Med 2005;352:1539–49.
6. Moss AJ, Hall WJ, Cannom DS, et al, MADIT-CRT Trial Investigators. Cardiac-resynchronization therapy for the prevention of heart-failure events. N Engl J Med 2009;361:1329–38.
7. Stellbrink C, Breithardt OA, Franke A, et al. Impact of cardiac resynchronization therapy using hemodynamically optimized pacing on left ventricular remodeling in patients with congestive heart failure and ventricular conduction disturbances. J Am Coll Cardiol 2001;38:1957–65.
8. Yu CM, Fung JW, Zhang Q, et al. Tissue Doppler imaging is superior to strain rate imaging and postsystolic shortening on the prediction of reverse remodeling in both ischemic and nonischemic heart failure after cardiac resynchronization therapy. Circulation 2004;110:66–73.
9. Yu C-M, Wing-hong Fung J, Zhang Q, et al. Understanding nonresponders of cardiac resynchronization therapy–current and future perspectives. J Cardiovasc Electrophysiol 2005;16:1117–24.
10. Butter C, Auricchio A, Stellbrink C, et al, Pacing Therapy for Chronic Heart Failure II Study Group. Effect of resynchronization therapy stimulation site on the systolic function of heart failure patients. Circulation 2001;104:3026–9.
11. Helm RH, Byrne M, Helm PA, et al. Three-dimensional mapping of optimal left ventricular pacing site for cardiac resynchronization. Circulation 2007;115:953–61.
12. Saxon LA, Olshansky B, Volosin K, et al. Influence of left ventricular lead location on outcomes in the companion study. J Cardiovasc Electrophysiol 2009;20:764–8.

13. Singh JP, Klein HU, Huang DT, et al. Left ventricular lead position and clinical outcome in the multicenter automatic defibrillator implantation trial-cardiac resynchronization therapy (MADIT-CRT) trial. Circulation 2011;123:1159–66.

14. Wilton SB, Exner DV, Healey JS, et al. Left ventricular lead position and outcomes in the resynchronization-defibrillation for ambulatory heart failure trial (RAFT). Can J Cardiol 2014;30:413–9.

15. Ansalone G, Giannantoni P, Ricci R, et al. Doppler myocardial imaging to evaluate the effectiveness of pacing sites in patients receiving biventricular pacing. J Am Coll Cardiol 2002;39:489–99.

16. Khan FZ, Virdee MS, Palmer CR, et al. Targeted left ventricular lead placement to guide cardiac resynchronization therapy: the TARGET study: a randomized, controlled trial. J Am Coll Cardiol 2012; 59:1509–18.

17. Saba S, Marek J, Schwartzman D, et al. Echocardiography-guided left ventricular lead placement for cardiac resynchronization therapy: results of the speckle tracking assisted resynchronization therapy for electrode region trial. Circ Heart Fail 2013; 6:427–34.

18. Heydari B, Jerosch-Herold M, Kwong RY. Imaging for planning of cardiac resynchronization therapy. JACC Cardiovasc Imaging 2012;5:93–110.

19. Leyva F, Foley PWX, Chalil S, et al. Cardiac resynchronization therapy guided by late gadolinium-enhancement cardiovascular magnetic resonance. J Cardiovasc Magn Reson 2011;13:29.

20. Gold MR, Birgersdotter-Green U, Singh JP, et al. The relationship between ventricular electrical delay and left ventricular remodelling with cardiac resynchronization therapy. Eur Heart J 2011;32:2516–24.

21. Gold MR, Yu Y, Singh JP, et al. The effect of left ventricular electrical delay on AV optimization for cardiac resynchronization therapy. Heart Rhythm 2013;10:988–93.

22. Gold MR, Leman RB, Wold N, et al. The effect of left ventricular electrical delay on the acute hemodynamic response with cardiac resynchronization therapy. J Cardiovasc Electrophysiol 2014;25:624–30.

23. Morgan JM, Delgado V. Lead positioning for cardiac resynchronization therapy: techniques and priorities. Europace 2009;11(Suppl 5):v22–8.

24. van Rees JB, de Bie MK, Thijssen J, et al. Implantation-related complications of implantable cardioverter-defibrillators and cardiac resynchronization therapy devices: a systematic review of randomized clinical trials. J Am Coll Cardiol 2011;58:995–1000.

25. Balaram SK, DeRose JJ, Steinberg JS. Surgical approaches to epicardial left ventricular lead implantation for biventricular pacing. In: Yu C, Hayes DL, Auricchio A, editors. Cardiac resynchronization therapy. 2nd edition. Hoboken, NJ: Wiley-Blackwell; 2009. p. 239–49.

26. Steinberg JS, Derose JJ. The rationale for nontransvenous leads and cardiac resynchronization devices. Pacing Clin Electrophysiol 2003;26:2211–2.

27. Cohen MI, Bush DM, Vetter VL, et al. Permanent epicardial pacing in pediatric patients: seventeen years of experience and 1200 outpatient visits. Circulation 2001;103:2585–90.

28. Tomaske M, Gerritse B, Kretzers L, et al. A 12-year experience of bipolar steroid-eluting epicardial pacing leads in children. Ann Thorac Surg 2008;85: 1704–11.

29. Burger H, Kempfert J, van Linden A, et al. Endurance and performance of two different concepts for left ventricular stimulation with bipolar epicardial leads in long-term follow-up. Thorac Cardiovasc Surg 2012;60:70–7.

30. Mellert F, Schneider C, Esmailzadeh B, et al. Implantation of left ventricular epicardial leads in cardiosurgical patients with impaired cardiac function–a worthwhile procedure in concomitant surgical interventions? Thorac Cardiovasc Surg 2012;60:64–9.

31. Daoud EG, Kalbfleisch SJ, Hummel JD, et al. Implantation techniques and chronic lead parameters of biventricular pacing dual-chamber defibrillators. J Cardiovasc Electrophysiol 2002;13:964–70.

32. Navia JL, Atik FA. Minimally invasive surgical alternatives for left ventricle epicardial lead implantation in heart failure patients. Ann Thorac Surg 2005;80: 751–4.

33. Mihalcz A, Kassai I, Geller L, et al. Alternative techniques for left ventricular pacing in cardiac resynchronization therapy. Pacing Clin Electrophysiol 2014; 37:255–61.

34. Doll N, Opfermann UT, Rastan AJ, et al. Facilitated minimally invasive left ventricular epicardial lead placement. Ann Thorac Surg 2005;79:1023–5.

35. Gabor S, Prenner G, Wasler A, et al. A simplified technique for implantation of left ventricular epicardial leads for biventricular re-synchronization using video-assisted thoracoscopy (VATS). Eur J Cardiothorac Surg 2005;28:797–800.

36. Jutley RS, Waller DA, Loke I, et al. Video-assisted thoracoscopic implantation of the left ventricular pacing lead for cardiac resynchronization therapy. Pacing Clin Electrophysiol 2008;31:812–8.

37. Papiashvilli M, Haitov Z, Fuchs T, et al. Left ventricular epicardial lead implantation for resynchronisation therapy using a video-assisted thoracoscopic approach. Heart Lung Circ 2011;20:220–2.

38. Derose JJ, Kypson AP. Robotic arrhythmia surgery and resynchronization. Am J Surg 2004; 188:104S–11S.

39. Woo YJ. Robotic cardiac surgery. Int J Med Robot 2006;2:225–32.

40. Modi P, Rodriguez E, Chitwood WR. Robot-assisted cardiac surgery. Interact Cardiovasc Thorac Surg 2009;9:500–5.

41. Dekker ALAJ, Phelps B, Dijkman B, et al. Epicardial left ventricular lead placement for cardiac resynchronization therapy: optimal pace site selection with pressure-volume loops. J Thorac Cardiovasc Surg 2004;127:1641–7.

42. Polasek R, Skalsky I, Wichterle D, et al. High-density epicardial activation mapping to optimize the site for video-thoracoscopic left ventricular lead implant. J Cardiovasc Electrophysiol 2014;25:882–8.

43. Helm RH, Leclercq C, Faris OP, et al. Cardiac dyssynchrony analysis using circumferential versus longitudinal strain: implications for assessing cardiac resynchronization. Circulation 2005;111:2760–7.

44. Fung JWH, Lam Y-Y, Zhang Q, et al. Effect of left ventricular lead concordance to the delayed contraction segment on echocardiographic and clinical outcomes after cardiac resynchronization therapy. J Cardiovasc Electrophysiol 2009;20:530–5.

45. Becker M, Franke A, Breithardt OA, et al. Impact of left ventricular lead position on the efficacy of cardiac resynchronisation therapy: a two-dimensional strain echocardiography study. Heart 2007;93: 1197–203.

46. Bedi M, Suffoletro M, Tanabe M, et al. Effect of concordance between sites of left ventricular pacing and dyssynchrony on acute electrocardiographic and echocardiographic parameters in patients with heart failure undergoing cardiac resynchronization therapy. Clin Cardiol 2006;29:498–502.

47. Navia JL, Atik FA, Grimm RA, et al. Minimally invasive left ventricular epicardial lead placement: surgical techniques for heart failure resynchronization therapy. Ann Thorac Surg 2005;79:1536–44 [discussion: 1536–44].

48. Mair H, Sachweh J, Meuris B, et al. Surgical epicardial left ventricular lead versus coronary sinus lead placement in biventricular pacing. Eur J Cardiothorac Surg 2005;27:235–42.

49. Atoui R, Essebag V, Wu V, et al. Biventricular pacing for end-stage heart failure: early experience in surgical vs. transvenous left ventricular lead placement. Interact Cardiovasc Thorac Surg 2008;7: 839–44.

50. Quigley RL. A hybrid approach to cardiac resynchronization therapy. Ann Thorac Cardiovasc Surg 2011;17:273–6.

51. Mair H, Jansens J-L, Lattouf OM, et al. Epicardial lead implantation techniques for biventricular pacing via left lateral mini-thoracotomy, video-assisted thoracoscopy, and robotic approach. Heart Surg Forum 2003;6:412–7.

52. Ailawadi G, LaPar DJ, Swenson BR, et al. Surgically placed left ventricular leads provide similar outcomes to percutaneous leads in patients with failed coronary sinus lead placement. Heart Rhythm 2010;7:619–25.

53. Bhamidipati CM, Mboumi IW, Seymour KA, et al. Robotic-assisted or minithoracotomy incision for left ventricular lead placement: a single-surgeon, single-center experience. Innovations (Phila) 2012;7: 208–12.

54. DeRose JJ, Ashton RC, Belsley S, et al. Robotically assisted left ventricular epicardial lead implantation for biventricular pacing. J Am Coll Cardiol 2003;41: 1414–9.

55. Joshi S, Steinberg JS, Ashton RC, et al. Follow-up of robotically assisted left ventricular epicardial leads for cardiac resynchronization therapy. J Am Coll Cardiol 2005;46:2358–9.

56. Derose JJ, Balaram S, Ro C, et al. Midterm follow-up of robotic biventricular pacing demonstrates excellent lead stability and improved response rates. Innovations (Phila) 2006;1:105–10.

57. Kamath GS, Balaram S, Choi A, et al. Long-term outcome of leads and patients following robotic epicardial left ventricular lead placement for cardiac resynchronization therapy. Pacing Clin Electrophysiol 2011;34:235–40.

58. Garikipati NV, Mittal S, Chaudhry F, et al. Comparison of endovascular versus epicardial lead placement for resynchronization therapy. Am J Cardiol 2014;113:840–4.

Coronary Sinus Lead Extraction

Edmond M. Cronin, MB BCh BAO, FHRS, CCDS[a],*, Bruce L. Wilkoff, MD, FHRS, CCDS[b]

KEYWORDS

• Lead extraction • Cardiac resynchronization therapy • Coronary sinus

KEY POINTS

- Coronary sinus (CS) lead extraction presents unique challenges because of the complex anatomy of the coronary venous system.
- Most sites of fibrous adhesions are found outside of the CS; however, a variety of tools and approaches are used once this structure is reached.
- Success rates and complications are comparable to those of other leads in experienced centers.
- Reimplantation may be limited by CS or branch occlusion postextraction.
- Active fixation CS leads present significant challenges to extraction, although limited series have reported acceptable success and morbidity.

INTRODUCTION

Transvenous lead extraction of CS leads presents unique challenges. Indications for cardiac resynchronization therapy (CRT) have recently expanded, in response to several landmark clinical trials, to patients with mild heart failure and frequent ventricular pacing.[1,2] Therefore, it is anticipated that extraction of CS leads will also be required more frequently, especially because patients with CRT are among those at the highest risk of cardiac implantable electronic device (CIED)-related complications.[3] This article reviews the approach, techniques, and outcomes of CS lead extraction.

INDICATIONS FOR CORONARY SINUS LEAD EXTRACTION

The indications for CS lead extraction in general mirror those for other leads, as outlined in a Heart Rhythm Society expert consensus document.[4] Because the risk of developing system infection

is higher for patients with multiple leads (such as CRT systems) than for single-chamber or dual-chamber CIEDs,[5] infectious indications for extraction of CS leads are likely more common than for other leads. Extraction and reimplantation due to lead dysfunction are also likely more common, because it may be difficult to implant more than 1 lead in the confined space of the CS and its branches. The prevalence of subclavian or superior caval venous occlusion is increased with multiple leads and, therefore, is seen more commonly with CRT systems.[6–8] This precludes abandonment and replacement of a dysfunctional lead, making lead extraction necessary if ipsilateral access is to be maintained. Specific indications for CS lead extraction not often seen with other leads include extraction due to phrenic nerve stimulation and increased threshold due to changes in underlying myocardium, such as increased epicardial fat or progressive fibrosis. Indications for lead extraction with an emphasis on CS leads are summarized in **Box 1**.

Conflicts of Interest: None (E.M. Cronin); Consultant and Advisor for: Medtronic, Boston Scientific, St. Jude Medical, and Spectranetics (B.L. Wilkoff).
[a] Division of Cardiology, Hartford Hospital, 80 Seymour Street PO Box 5037, Hartford CT 06102, USA;
[b] Department of Cardiovascular Medicine, Cleveland Clinic, 9500 Euclid Avenue, Cleveland OH 44195, USA
* Corresponding author.
E-mail address: edmond.cronin@hhchealth.org

Card Electrophysiol Clin 7 (2015) 661–671
http://dx.doi.org/10.1016/j.ccep.2015.08.020
1877-9182/15/$ – see front matter © 2015 Elsevier Inc. All rights reserved.

Box 1
Indications for lead extraction that pertain to coronary sinus leads

Infection

Class I

1. Definite CIED system infection (level of evidence B)
2. CIED pocket infection (level of evidence B)
3. Valvular endocarditis without definite lead involvement (level of evidence B)
4. Occult gram-positive bacteremia (level of evidence B)

Class IIa

1. Persistent occult gram-negative bacteremia (level of evidence B)

Class III (not recommended)

1. Superficial infection without involvement of the device and/or leads (level of evidence C)
2. Chronic bacteremia due to a source other than the CIED, when long-term suppressive antibiotics are required (level of evidence C)

Chronic Pain

Class IIa

1. Severe chronic pain (level of evidence C)

Thrombosis or Venous Stenosis

Class I

1. Thromboembolic events associated with thrombus on a lead or a lead fragment (level of evidence C)
2. Bilateral subclavian vein or SVC occlusion precluding implantation of a needed transvenous lead (level of evidence C)
3. Planned stent deployment in a vein already containing a transvenous lead, to avoid entrapment of the lead (level of evidence C)
4. SVC stenosis or occlusion with limiting symptoms (level of evidence C)
5. Ipsilateral venous occlusion preventing placement of an additional lead with a contraindication to the contralateral side (level of evidence C)

Class IIa

1. Ipsilateral venous occlusion preventing placement of an additional lead, without a contraindication to the contralateral side (level of evidence C)

Functional Leads

Class I

1. Life-threatening arrhythmias secondary to retained leads (level of evidence B)
2. Leads that, due to their design or their failure, may pose an immediate threat to the patients if left in place (level of evidence B)
3. Leads that interfere with the operation of implanted cardiac devices (level of evidence B)
4. Leads that interfere with the treatment of a malignancy (level of evidence C)

Class IIb

1. Abandoned functional lead that poses a risk of interference with the operation of the active CIED system (level of evidence C)
2. Functioning leads that due to their design or their failure pose a potential future threat to the patient if left in place (level of evidence C)
3. Leads that are functional but not being used (level of evidence C)
4. To enable MRI when there is no other available imaging alternative for the diagnosis (level of evidence C)
5. To permit the implantation of an MRI conditional CIED system (level of evidence C)

Class III

1. Functional but redundant leads if patients have a life expectancy of less than 1 year (level of evidence C)
2. Known anomalous placement of leads or through a systemic venous atrium or systemic ventricle (level of evidence C)

Nonfunctional Leads

Class I

1. Life-threatening arrhythmias secondary to retained leads or lead fragments (level of evidence B)
2. Leads that, due to their design or their failure, may pose an immediate threat to the patients if left in place (level of evidence B)
3. Leads that interfere with the operation of implanted cardiac devices (level of evidence B)
4. Leads that interfere with the treatment of a malignancy (level of evidence C)

Class IIa

1. Leads that due to their design or their failure pose a threat to the patient, that is, not immediate or imminent if left in place (level of evidence C)
2. If a CIED implantation would require more than 4 leads on 1 side or more than 5 leads through the SVC (level of evidence C)
3. To enable MRI when there is no other available imaging alternative for the diagnosis (level of evidence C)

Class IIb

1. At the time of an indicated CIED procedure in patients with nonfunctional leads (level of evidence C)
2. To permit the implantation of an MRI conditional CIED system (level of evidence C)

Class III

1. Patients with nonfunctional leads and a life expectancy of less than 1 year (level of evidence C)
2. Known anomalous placement of leads or through a systemic venous atrium or systemic ventricle (level of evidence C)

Adapted from Wilkoff BL, Love CJ, Byrd CL, et al. Transvenous lead extraction: Heart Rhythm Society expert consensus on facilities, training, indications, and patient management. Heart Rhythm 2009;6:1095–7; with permission.

TRAINING AND FACILITIES

The standards outlined in the Heart Rhythm Society expert consensus document[4] apply to CS lead extraction as to other leads. Although in the authors' experience CS leads are extracted more frequently with manual traction than are other leads of similar implant duration, anatomic considerations may render these leads more complex to extract than atrial or ventricular leads. Furthermore, patients receiving CRT devices are often among the most medically complex of CIED patients, and reimplantation procedures are among the most technically challenging; therefore, considerable expertise is required.

PREPROCEDURAL CONSIDERATIONS

The risks and benefits of lead extraction should be fully discussed, and patients should be advised of all options, including the risk of hemodynamic decline with loss of cardiac resynchronization and the potential inability to reimplant in the same or other veins to restore cardiac resynchronization. Patients who are frail or with limited life expectancy may benefit from a conservative approach, although these patients already have 3 leads and there is less space available to add transvenous leads without extraction. Informed consent should be obtained and documented in the medical record. Metabolic and hemodynamic status should be optimized. A great majority of patients with CS leads have heart failure; therefore, appropriate management of volume status is crucial. Anticoagulant drugs should be withheld until coagulation measures have returned to normal or, in the case of the novel anticoagulants, for approximately 48 hours. For infectious indications, these measures should be balanced against the need to remove the source of infection as expeditiously as possible.

FACILITY REQUIREMENTS

- Sterile environment (electrophysiology laboratory or operating room)

- Good-quality fluoroscopy
- On-site, immediately (<5 minutes) available cardiothoracic surgery support
- Open chest cart available, including sternal saw
- Anesthesia support, either for the entire case or available
- Blood cross-matched and available (the authors maintain 4 units in the room or operating room refrigerator)
- Large-bore venous access, preferably right femoral vein, to allow temporary pacing and use of femoral tools if required
- Continuous arterial pressure monitoring
- Echo machine turned on and ready
- Range of extraction tools, including stylets, powered and manual sheaths, and femoral tools
- Full range of implant tools if case involves reimplantation

TECHNIQUE OF CORONARY SINUS LEAD EXTRACTION

In general, the authors' approach is as follows:

- The lead is freed up from its tie-down sleeve and pocket fibrosis.
- A standard stylet is inserted.
- Low force traction is applied – this may remove the lead itself and demonstrates the location of fibrotic adhesions.
- The lead is cut proximally to expose the lead components.
- A locking stylet (Liberator [Cook Medical, Bloomington, Indiana] or Lead Locking Device [Spectranetics, Colorado Springs, Colorado]) is inserted to the tip and locked in place. Because the locking stylet can protrude past the end hole of the conductor, care must be taken to prevent this from occurring.
- Further low force traction is then applied.
- The lead components (insulation and conductors) are secured to the locking stylet with sutures to prevent elongation of the lead during extraction.
- A 12F excimer laser sheath (GlideLight [Spectranetics]) is advanced over the lead with laser activation at sites of adhesion. At times, 14F or 16F sheaths are used due to use on implantable cardioverter-defibrillator (ICD) or right ventricular (RV) or right atrial leads or to provide additional support for countertraction.
- An outer sheath may be useful to provide support and additional mechanical disruption of adhesions.

- The bevel of the laser and outer sheaths are maintained away from the lateral aspect of the superior vena cava (SVC).
- Sufficient tension is continuously applied to the lead to provide a rail over which to advance the laser sheath.
- On reaching the CS os, countertraction is applied with the laser sheath while traction is applied to the lead.
- The sheath may be advanced within the CS if necessary for more distal countertraction.
- Laser activation within the CS should almost never be used because mechanical dissection is safer due to the complex angulation of the CS and its thin walls.

Other tools and techniques are also used. Mechanical dilation sheaths may be used, either from the implant vein, the femoral vein, or the (right) internal jugular vein, as described by Bongiorni and colleagues.[9] Furthermore, rotating threaded tip sheaths (Evolution [Cook Medical] and TightRail [Spectranetics]) also may be used, especially for lysis of fibrous binding sites in the great vessels; however, experience with these specifically for CS lead extraction is limited. An inferior vein approach using standard femoral tools also may be useful (**Fig. 1**). This offers specific advantages and disadvantages:

- CS leads may be grasped from the femoral vein and removed from this approach.
- The Needle's Eye Snare (Cook Medical) can grasp the course of the CS lead in the right atrium.
- A free-floating lead may be grasped using the Amplatz GooseNeck Snare (ev3 Endovascular, Plymouth, Minnesota) or the EN Snare Endovascular Snare System (Merit Medical Systems, South Jordan, Utah).
- The direction of traction from the femoral vein aligns more closely with the course of the lead in the CS than that from the superior vein.
- Binding sites are most commonly found in the superior veins, which may be more easily approached from above.[10]
- The femoral vein does not provide a reimplant route in the case of an occluded implant vein, unless a femoral drag-through technique is used.[11]

The sites of fibrous adhesion have been characterized by Bongiorni and colleagues,[10] as shown in **Fig. 2**. These data are derived from extraction of passive fixation CS leads using mechanical dissection sheaths. Only 10% of patients had evidence of fibrous adhesions within the CS or its

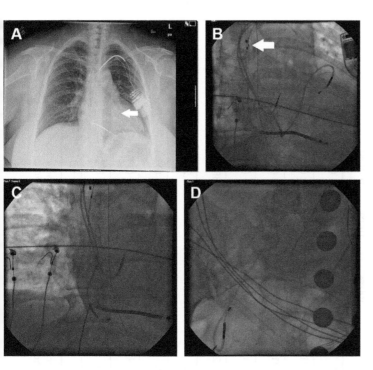

Fig. 1. CS lead extraction using the femoral approach. The patient had undergone CRT-D implant for nonischemic cardiomyopathy and left bundle branch block 9 years prior. Her device history was complex involving atrial lead extraction and reimplant for fracture after a fall, extraction of a Riata 1581 lead (St Jude Medical, Sylmar, California) for insulation abrasion causing atrial oversensing, extraction of a CS lead that became dislodged from a posterolateral branch during the ICD lead extraction, and reimplantation into an anterolateral branch (*arrow* [A]). This dislodged and was found to have migrated into the anterior interventricular vein on follow-up (B). The left subclavian vein was occluded. Due to the presence of the distal tip of the previous CS lead, which broke and became lodged in the brachiocephalic vein (*arrow* [B]), a femoral approach was used. The lead was dislodged from the CS with manual traction. This was then grasped in the right atrium with a 25-mm Gooseneck Snare, providing a means to preserve vascular access from the implant vein while extracting the lead (C).[11] The lead broke during extraction, with the distal portion along with conductor wire shown in the iliac vein prior to removal (D).

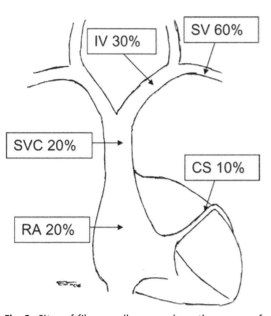

Fig. 2. Sites of fibrous adherence along the course of CS leads. IV, innominate vein; SV, subclavian vein; SVC, superior vena cava; RA, right atrium. (*From* Bongiorni MG, Zucchelli G, Soldati E, et al. Usefulness of mechanical transvenous dilation and location of areas of adherence in patients undergoing coronary sinus lead extraction. Europace 2007;9:72; with permission.)

branches, suggesting that the sites generic to other intracardiac leads are likely to present most difficulty during CS lead extraction.

RESULTS OF CORONARY SINUS LEAD EXTRACTION

Several single-center, and 1 multicenter, experiences[10,12–24] have been published describing the results of CS lead extraction, which are summarized in **Table 1**. These cover a total of 664 leads with implant durations varying from 0 to 27 years. A variety of tools were used according to the extractor's preference, but a trend toward requiring more tools and powered sheaths can be seen in leads with longer implant duration, consistent with experience in other lead types. In the largest published experience, in which the indication was infection in all cases, 76.9% of CS leads were removed with traction alone compared with 71.7% of ventricular leads requiring a laser sheath. This is consistent with clinical experience that CS leads are removed more often with traction than atrial or ventricular leads. This may be due to thinner lead diameter, leading to less surface area for fibrous adhesions, lack of defibrillation coils (except for CS defibrillation leads, described later), and lack of either active or passive fixation

Table 1
Summary of published series of coronary sinus lead extraction

Author	No. Leads	Mean (Range) Implant Duration, Months	Traction Only	Mechanical Sheath	Powered Sheath	Femoral Approach	Complete Success	Clinical Success	Major Procedural Complications	Transvenous Reimplant Success
Tyers et al,[12] 2003	13[a]	67.8 (0.3–320.4)	3/13	3/13	8/13	0	100%	100%	0 (0%)	2/3
Kasravi et al,[13] 2005	14	17 (2–43)	11/14	0	0	3/14	100%	100%	0 (0%)	13/14
De Martino et al,[14] 2005	12	13.9 (3–46)	12/12	0	0	0	100%	100%	0 (0%)	12/12
Burke et al,[15] 2005	10[a]	10.5 (3–59)	6/10	0	4/10	0	100%	100%	0 (0%)	7/10
Williams et al,[16] 2011	60[a]	35.8 (1–116)	54/60	0	6/60	1	98%	98%	1 (1.4%)	43/43
di Cori et al,[17] 2012	147	29	103/147	44/147	0	4/147	99%	99%	1 (0.7%)	NR
Maytin et al,[18] 2012	12[b]	14.2 (2.3–23.6)	0/12	3/12	10/12	3/12	92%	92%	0 (0%)	NR
Sheldon et al,[19] 2012	125	18.5 (0.26–98.9)	114/125	0	6/125	3/125	99%	99%	9 (7.2%)	95/103
Chu et al,[20] 2012	24	29.5 (3–78)	16/24	4/24	0	4/24	95.8%	100%	NR	NR
Rickard et al,[21] 2012	173	22.3	133/173	0	40/173	0	97.7%	100%	1.2%	88/107
Lisy et al,[22] 2013	41	17.2 (0–104.9)	13/41	17/41	5/41	0	100%	100%	0 (0%)	NR
Starck et al,[23] 2013	27	33.3 (1–76)	NR	NR	NR	NR	94.7%	100%	0 (0%)	7/7
Kypta et al,[24] 2015	6[b]	46.5	0	0	6/6	0	100%	100%	1 (16.6%)	NR
Total	664	—	—	—	—	—	98%	99%	2.1%	89.3%

Several overlapping reports have been omitted, with the largest series from each center included. Complications reported are due to CS lead extraction only, as far as it was possible to ascertain. Due to different definitions of complications used in each report, the numbers presented here may differ slightly to those in individual reports.

[a] Includes CS defibrillation coils.

[b] Series of Attain Starfix 4195 extractions. A single lead is also included in di Cori et al.[17]

mechanisms in most CS leads. The distribution of fibrous adhesion sites, as described by Bongiorni and colleagues[10] (see **Fig. 2**), suggests that the CS may be less likely to promote fibrous adhesions, although with the multiplicity of potential confounding factors this is not certain. In totality, the complete and clinical success rates are comparable to or better than those seen in general lead extraction experiences (for instance, these were 96.5% and 97.7% in the LExICon study[25]).

COMPLICATIONS OF CORONARY SINUS LEAD EXTRACTION

When adjudicating complications, it may be difficult to ascertain whether an event was due to CS lead or other lead extraction, because many procedures involve extraction of other leads. That said, the incidence of major adverse events as presented in **Table 1**, is similar to the 1.4% seen in LExICon.[25] Adverse events during CS lead extraction may include

- CS avulsion or dissection – which may cause tamponade or a smaller pericardial effusion or may complicate access for reimplantation
- CS branch dissection or closure, leading to failure to reimplant a new lead
- Cardiac tear in the right atrial course of the lead

- Vascular avulsion or tear – in the SVC or brachiocephalic or subclavian veins
- Arteriovenous fistula[26]
- Pulmonary embolism, including of fragmented lead material or fibrous tissue
- Anesthetic complications
- Pocket or lead infection
- Stroke
- Death
- Hematoma
- Subclavian (or other implant vein) thrombosis
- Air embolism
- Hemorrhage, blood transfusion
- Pneumothorax

These adverse events should be classified as intraprocedure and postprocedure, and major and minor, as outlined in the expert consensus document.[4]

REIMPLANTATION

Many patients should undergo reimplant after CS lead extraction. The indications for implant and current appropriateness, however, should be thoroughly reviewed at this stage. Extraction of a nonfunctional CS lead to replace it is inappropriate, for instance, if the patient is a CRT nonresponder. This may be appropriate without reimplant in other circumstances (**Fig. 3**). Reimplantation is carried

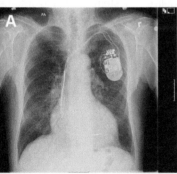
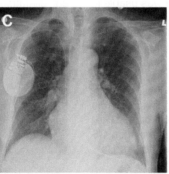
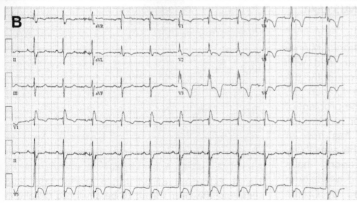

Fig. 3. Extraction of a CS lead without reimplantation. The patient was referred for extraction of a CRT-D system due to pocket infection (*A*). The quadripolar CS lead was extracted using manual traction. Intraprocedural recordings showed the RV and LV electrograms almost simultaneous. He was a clinical nonresponder to CRT, however, and his ECG postextraction showed right bundle branch block (*B*). A single-chamber ICD was implanted on the contralateral side after 6 weeks of antibiotic therapy (*C*).

out during the same procedure if the indication for extraction is noninfectious, and, on the contralateral side, after postextraction blood cultures are negative for at least 72 hours, if the indication is infection. The authors generally reimplant during the same hospitalization if the patient is pacemaker dependent or at high risk of appropriate therapies and delay reimplantation until a prolonged course of antibiotics has been completed otherwise. Involvement of an infectious disease specialist is useful to determine the appropriate duration of therapy postextraction.

The growth of fibrous tissue surrounding the lead in the CS branch and/or avulsion of part of the wall of the vessel may cause closure of the branch or dissection of the main CS, rendering reimplantation challenging. This accounts for the less than 100% reimplant rate seen in **Table 1**. Reimplantation after extraction for infection is also typically carried out from the right side, which many operators may be less familiar with and, therefore, may be associated with a lower success rate. In the authors' series of 173 patients extracted for infection, reimplantation was attempted from the contralateral side in 107 patients and was unsuccessful in 19 (17.2%) patients, largely due to absence of appropriate CS branches.[21]

Burke and colleagues[15] performed CS venograms after lead extraction in 10 patients and reported that the original implant vein was usable in only 50%. Reimplantation was unsuccessful in 2/7 (29%) due to occlusion of all branch veins or the main CS. Reimplantation after CS lead extraction was examined by the Pisa group[17] in 90 patients, with successful reimplant in 86 (95.6%). Failure was due to no available CS branches in 2 patients, CS occlusion in 1 patient, and unacceptable thresholds and phrenic stimulation in 1 patient. Reimplantation after extraction of active fixation CS leads is of particular concern (discussed later).

ACTIVE FIXATION CORONARY SINUS LEAD EXTRACTION

The Attain Starfix model 4195 (Medtronic, Minneapolis, Minnesota) is a 5F unipolar lead with extendable fixation lobes and is currently the only commercially available active fixation CS lead. It was introduced to combat the problem of lead dislodgement and the need for reoperation for repositioning, a problem that has now at least partially been addressed by the availability of quadripolar leads. Several reports have described significant complexity and difficulty in extracting these leads (summarized by Cronin and colleagues[27]). In the authors' experience of

4 leads, implant duration 392 to 1029 days, only the proximal fixation lobes retracted completely, and in 1 case, not at all.[27,28] This has also been found by other investigators.[18] The excimer laser sheath was required in each case, and in 3 cases, was advanced past the CS os to remove the lead (**Fig. 4**). Extraction was, however, successful in all 4 cases. Reimplantation was complicated by subtotal or total occlusion of the branch vein in 3 cases but successful in another branch: in the fourth case, the main CS was occluded in its midportion without any more proximal branches and the patient underwent epicardial left ventricular (LV) lead placement. A multicenter report of 12 leads at 6 centers also found that extraction sheaths were uniformly required and were advanced into the CS, or even into a branch vessel, in three-quarters. One failure (8.3%) led to surgical extraction. Reimplantation outcomes were not addressed in this report. These data are concerning given the short implant duration of the leads (2.3–23.6 months in the multicenter report).

Other techniques have been described in the extraction of Starfix leads. Bongiorni and colleagues[29] used a CS delivery system (Attain Command [Medtronic, Minneapolis, Minnesota]), using its preformed shape to provide countertraction support within the CS. Curnis and colleagues[30] used a variety of approaches, including mechanical dilatation, delivery system, and a bioptome from the femoral approach, but eventually a thoracoscopic surgical procedure was necessary to remove the broken distal portion of the lead from

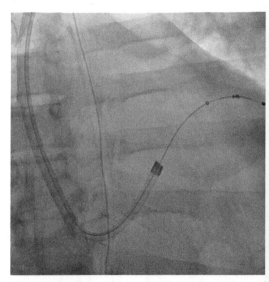

Fig. 4. Extraction of an Attain Starfix 4195 lead requiring the laser sheath to be advanced distally in the CS to remove the lead.

the coronary venous branch. Kypta and colleagues[24] reported outcomes of 6 procedures using the Evolution rotating threaded tip sheath in leads with implant duration of 3 to 7.5 years. Similar to previous experiences, the fixation lobes could not be retracted in any case. The extraction sheath was advanced into the CS branch as far as the lead tip in the first 2 cases (an aggressive maneuver). Both patients developed pericardial effusion, 1 treated with sternotomy and the other conservatively. The operators then modified their technique to include less distal position of the extraction sheath and the use of countertraction and used the second-generation Evolution RL for the next 4 cases without further complications. This experience highlights the complexity of extraction of these leads and reinforces the traction/countertraction principle generic to extraction of other leads – it is the authors' practice not to advance any extraction sheath beyond the ring electrode.

In the authors' experience, the density of fibrous adhesions surrounding the fixation lobes of the Starfix lead has been much greater than that found with passive fixation leads, especially allowing for the shorter implant duration, and correlates with extraction difficulty. This may be due to local injury of the CS branch vessel wall during deployment of the lobes, with resulting fibrous reaction (**Fig. 5**). Starfix leads should only be implanted as a last resort, in patients unfit for epicardial lead placement, and especially avoided in younger patients or those at higher risk of device infection (**Box 2**).

CORONARY SINUS DEFIBRILLATION COILS

Defibrillation coils were implanted in the CS in the 1990s as part of atrial defibrillator systems no longer available and as part of ICD systems in patients with high defibrillation threshold.[31] It was demonstration of facilitated extraction of medical adhesive backfilled defibrillation coils and ePTFE-covered coils versus bare CS coils in an ovine model that led to the widespread adoption of coil treatments in current RV ICD leads.[32] Some of the early CS lead experiences included extraction of CS defibrillation coils.[12,15,16] Perhaps surprisingly, the limited literature on extraction of these coils has reported successful extractions without complications, using excimer laser,[12,15,16,33] manual traction,[12] and mechanical dilation using a femoral workstation.[34] Again it must be emphasized that these are expected to be complex extraction procedures and should be undertaken only after careful weighing of risk and benefit and by operators familiar with a variety of techniques.

ALTERNATIVES TO CORONARY SINUS LEAD EXTRACTION

For patients or leads deemed too high risk for extraction, alternatives may include

- Implantation of a new CS lead alongside a nonfunctional lead—may be difficult because the existing lead may obstruct access to the CS or its side branches
- Epicardial LV lead placement with abandonment of the transvenous lead
- Direct His bundle pacing
- Transseptal LV endocardial pacing

FUTURE DIRECTIONS

The need for CS lead extraction has increased substantially over recent years and is expected

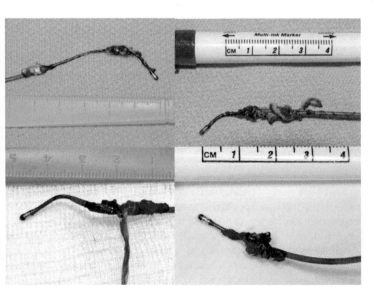

Fig. 5. Vigorous fibrous tissue ingrowth surrounding the active fixation lobes of 4 extracted Attain Starfix 4195 leads. (*From* Cronin EM, Ingelmo CP, Rickard J, et al. Active fixation mechanism complicates coronary sinus lead extraction and limits subsequent reimplantation targets. J Interv Card Electrophysiol 2013;36:83; with permission.)

to continue to grow for the medium term, given the expansion of indications for CRT-D and CRT-P[1,2] and the increasing incidence of CIED infection.[35] The advent of quadripolar leads may act against this trend by increasing options for electronic repositioning and reducing the number of procedures needed for noninfectious indications. Continued evolution in extraction tools is expected to make lead extraction even safer and more effective than at present. Eventually, leadless pacing may extend to CRT, leading to a reduced need for CS leads, but likely new challenges in electrode placement and extraction.

REFERENCES

1. Epstein AE, DiMarco JP, Ellenbogen KA, et al. 2012 ACCF/AHA/HRS focused update incorporated into the ACCF/AHA/HRS 2008 guidelines for device-based therapy of cardiac rhythm abnormalities: a report of the American College of Cardiology Foundation/American Heart Association Task Force on Practice Guidelines and the Heart Rhythm Society. J Am Coll Cardiol 2013;61(3):e6–75.

2. Curtis AB, Worley SJ, Adamson PB, et al. Biventricular pacing for atrioventricular block and systolic dysfunction. N Engl J Med 2013;368(17):1585–93.

3. Poole JE, Gleva MJ, Mela T, et al. Complication Rates associated with pacemaker or implantable cardioverter-defibrillator generator replacements and upgrade procedures: results from the REPLACE registry. Circulation 2010;122:1553–61.

4. Wilkoff BL, Love CJ, Byrd CL, et al. Transvenous lead extraction: heart rhythm society expert consensus on facilities, training, indications, and patient management. Heart Rhythm 2009;6:1085–104.

5. Sohail MR, Uslan DZ, Khan AH, et al. Risk factor analysis of permanent pacemaker infection. Clin Infect Dis 2007;45(2):166–73.

6. van Rooden CJ, Molhoek SG, Rosendaal FR, et al. Incidence and risk factors of early venous thrombosis associated with permanent pacemaker leads. J Cardiovasc Electrophysiol 2004;15(11):1258–62.

7. Haghjoo M, Nikoo MH, Fazelifar AF, et al. Predictors of venous obstruction following pacemaker or implantable cardioverter-defibrillator implantation: a contrast venographic study on 100 patients admitted for generator change, lead revision, or device upgrade. Europace 2007;9(5):328–32.

8. Korkeila P, Nyman K, Ylitalo A, et al. Venous obstruction after pacemaker implantation. Pacing Clin Electrophysiol 2007;30(2):199–206.

9. Bongiorni MG, Soldati E, Zucchelli G, et al. Transvenous removal of pacing and implantable cardiac defibrillating leads using single sheath mechanical dilatation and multiple venous approaches: high success rate and safety in more than 2000 leads. Eur Heart J 2008;29:2886–93.

10. Bongiorni MG, Zucchelli G, Soldati E, et al. Usefulness of mechanical transvenous dilation and location of areas of adherence in patients undergoing coronary sinus lead extraction. Europace 2007;9:69–73.

11. Rogers DP, Lambiase PD, Chow AW. Successful coronary sinus lead replacement despite total venous occlusion using femoral pull through, two operator counter-traction and subclavian venoplasty. J Interv Card Electrophysiol 2007;19(1):69–71.

12. Tyers GF, Clark J, Wang Y, et al. Coronary sinus lead extraction. Pacing Clin Electrophysiol 2003;26(1 Pt 2):524–6.

13. Kasravi B, Tobias S, Barnes MJ, et al. Coronary sinus lead extraction in the era of cardiac resynchronization therapy: single center experience. Pacing Clin Electrophysiol 2005;28(1):51–3.

14. De Martino G, Orazi S, Bisignani G, et al. Safety and feasibility of coronary sinus left ventricular leads extraction: a preliminary report. J Interv Card Electrophysiol 2005;13(1):35–8.

15. Burke MC, Morton J, Lin AC, et al. Implications and outcome of permanent coronary sinus lead extraction and reimplantation. J Cardiovasc Electrophysiol 2005;16(8):830–7.

16. Williams SE, Arujuna A, Whitaker J, et al. Percutaneous lead and system extraction in patients with cardiac resynchronization therapy (CRT) devices and coronary sinus leads. Pacing Clin Electrophysiol 2011;34(10):1209–16.

17. di Cori A, Bongiorni MG, Zucchelli G, et al. Large, single-center experience in transvenous coronary sinus lead extraction: procedural outcomes and predictors for mechanical dilatation. Pacing Clin Electrophysiol 2012;35(2):215–22.

18. Maytin M, Carrillo RG, Baltodano P, et al. Multicenter experience with transvenous lead extraction of active fixation coronary sinus leads. Pacing Clin Electrophysiol 2012;35(6):641–7.

19. Sheldon S, Friedman PA, Hayes DL, et al. Outcomes and predictors of difficulty with coronary sinus lead removal. J Interv Card Electrophysiol 2012;35(1):93–100.

20. Chu XM, Li XB, Zhang P, et al. Percutaneous extraction of leads from coronary sinus vein and branch by modified techniques. Chin Med J (Engl) 2012;125(20):3707–11.

21. Rickard J, Tarakji K, Cronin E, et al. Cardiac venous left ventricular lead removal and reimplantation following device infection: a large single-center experience. J Cardiovasc Electrophysiol 2012;23:1213–6.

22. Lisy M, Kornberger A, Schmid E, et al. Application of intravascular dissection devices for closed chest coronary sinus lead extraction: an interdisciplinary approach. Ann Thorac Surg 2013;95(4):1360–5.

23. Starck CT, Caliskan E, Klein H, et al. Results of transvenous lead extraction of coronary sinus leads in patients with cardiac resynchronization therapy. Chin Med J (Engl) 2013;126:4703–6.

24. Kypta A, Blessberger H, Saleh K, et al. Removal of active-fixation coronary sinus leads using a mechanical rotation extraction device. Pacing Clin Electrophysiol 2015;38:302–5.

25. Wazni O, Epstein LM, Carillo RG, et al. Lead extraction in the contemporary setting: the LExICon study. J Am Coll Cardiol 2010;55:579–86.

26. Cronin EM, Brunner MP, Tan CD, et al. Incidence, management, and outcomes of the arteriovenous fistula complicating transvenous lead extraction. Heart Rhythm 2014;11:404–11.

27. Cronin EM, Ingelmo CP, Rickard J, et al. Active fixation mechanism complicates coronary sinus lead extraction and limits subsequent reimplantation targets. J Interv Card Electrophysiol 2013;36(1):81–6.

28. Baranowski B, Yerkey M, Dresing T, et al. Fibrotic tissue growth into the extendable lobes of an active fixation coronary sinus lead can complicate extraction. Pacing Clin Electrophysiol 2011;34(7):e64–5.

29. Bongiorni MG, Di Cori A, Zucchelli G, et al. A modified transvenous single mechanical dilatation technique to remove a chronically implanted active-fixation coronary sinus pacing lead. Pacing Clin Electrophysiol 2011;34(7):e66–9.

30. Curnis A, Bontempi L, Coppola G, et al. Active-fixation coronary sinus pacing lead extraction: a hybrid approach. Int J Cardiol 2012;156:e51–2.

31. Faheem O, Padala A, Kluger J, et al. Coronary sinus shocking lead as salvage in patients with advanced CHF and high defibrillation thresholds. Pacing Clin Electrophysiol 2010;33(8):967–72.

32. Wilkoff BL, Belott PH, Love CJ, et al. Improved extraction of ePTFE and medical adhesive modified defibrillation leads from the coronary sinus and great cardiac vein. Pacing Clin Electrophysiol 2005;28:205–11.

33. Hamid S, Arujuna A, Rinaldi CA. A shocking lead in the coronary sinus. Europace 2009;11:833–4.

34. Van Gelder B, Bracke F. Extraction of a coronary sinus atrioverter and a dual-coil ventricular shock lead from the same patient: a tailored approach. Europace 2011;13:756–7.

35. Greenspon AJ, Patel JD, Lau E, et al. 16-year trends in the infection burden for pacemakers and implantable cardioverter-defibrillators in the United States 1993 to 2008. J Am Coll Cardiol 2011;58(10):1001–6.

Indication for CRT Implantation

Cardiac Resynchronization Therapy: An Overview on Guidelines

Giuseppe Boriani, MD, PhD[a],*, Martina Nesti, MD[b], Matteo Ziacchi, MD, PhD[a], Luigi Padeletti, MD[c]

KEYWORDS

- Atrial fibrillation • Bundle branch block • Cardiac resynchronization therapy • Guidelines
- Heart failure • QRS interval

KEY POINTS

- Cardiac resynchronization therapy (CRT) is included in international consensus guidelines as a treatment with proven efficacy in well-selected patients on top of optimal medical therapy. Although all the guidelines strongly recommend CRT for LBBB with QRS duration greater than 150 milliseconds, lower strength of recommendation is reported for QRS duration of 120 to 150 milliseconds, especially if not associated with LBBB. CRT is not recommended for a QRS of less than 120 milliseconds.
- The process of translating consensus guidelines into "real-world" practice is incomplete. Efforts should be dedicated to "synchronize" the competence and expertise of many physicians in order to deliver this treatment to the right patient, at the right time, and in the appropriate setting.

INTRODUCTION

Clinical guidelines are systematically developed statements and recommendations regarding clinical decision making to help practitioners and patients to make the most appropriate decisions about management and treatment of specific clinical conditions and diseases. Clinical guidelines are produced on the basis of a systematic revision process of the medical literature and opinion of experts and should provide extensive, critical, and well-balanced information on the benefits and limitations of a series of therapeutic and diagnostic choices to assist in taking decisions in individual cases. Application of guidelines to the management of individual patients always requires rational judgment and informed considerations, even when guidelines recommendations are properly linked to evidence.

Since the mid 1980s, national and international guidelines focused on different diseases have been developed. The reasonable expectation included an improvement in the process of health care provision by making it more effective and efficient. Despite the great efforts dedicated to development and implementation of evidence-based guidelines, contradictory results emerge by analysis of guidelines implementation and medical decisions in the "real world." A series of surveys indicate that around 30% to 40% of patients do not receive treatments based on scientific evidence, and around 20% to 25% receive treatments that may be unnecessary and sometimes even harmful.[1]

With regard to pacemaker and implantable electrical devices, the American College of Cardiology, the American Heart Association, and the Heart Rhythm Society (formerly the North American

a Institute of Cardiology, Department of Experimental, Diagnostic and Specialty Medicine, University of Bologna, S. Orsola-Malpighi University Hospital, Via Giuseppe Massarenti 9, Bologna 40138, Italy; b Electrophysiology and Pacing Centre, Heart and Vessels Department, University of Firenze, Largo Brambilla 3, Firenze 50134, Italy; c Specialty School in Cardiovascular Diseases, University of Firenze, Largo Brambilla 3, Firenze 50134, Italy
* Corresponding author.
E-mail address: giuseppe.boriani@unibo.it

Card Electrophysiol Clin 7 (2015) 673–693
http://dx.doi.org/10.1016/j.ccep.2015.08.015
1877-9182/15/$ – see front matter © 2015 Elsevier Inc. All rights reserved.

Society of Cardiac Pacing and Electrophysiology) published the first guidelines for the implantation of cardiac pacemakers and antiarrhythmia devices in 1984.[2] Since that time, major advancements in technology and clinical evidence of benefit occurred with regard to device therapy and these developments have led to periodic updating of the guidelines in 1991, 1998, 2002, 2008, and 2012.[3] The European Society of Cardiology released the first document including recommendations on use of implantable cardioverter defibrillators in 1992[4] and then released guidelines on pacing and cardiac resynchronization therapy (CRT) in 2006 and 2013.[5,6]

CARDIAC RESYNCHRONIZATION THERAPY AS AN EFFECTIVE TREATMENT IN HEART FAILURE

CRT was proposed as the result of pioneering experiences performed in France around 20 years ago.[7–9] CRT is an electrical treatment based on biventricular or left ventricular-only pacing that was initially applied as a last resort therapeutic solution for patients with severe heart failure (HF) associated with left bundle branch block (LBBB). Despite the novelty of the approach and the technical limitations of implantable leads in the first phases of clinical use, the evaluation of CRT moved rapidly from isolated case reports and small case series or uncontrolled studies to randomized controlled trials (Table 1). Multisite Stimulation in Cardiomyopathy (MUSTIC) was the first randomized study on CRT[21] and was followed by a randomized controlled trial with blinded assessment of the effects, namely, the Multicenter InSync Randomized Clinical Evaluation (MIRACLE) study.[10,11] The MIRACLE trial included implant of a CRT device followed by randomization to biventricular pacing "on" or "off" for 6 months with blinded assessment of the presence/absence of improvement in symptoms, HF status, and quality of life.[10] A paradigm shift in obtaining solid evidence in favor of CRT use in patients with moderate to severe HF were the Cardiac Resynchronization—Heart Failure (CARE HF) and the Comparison of Medical Therapy, Pacing, and Defibrillation in Heart Failure (COMPANION) trials[13,14] that randomized patients to optimal medical therapy versus CRT (with a pacemaker in CARE HF, with or without a defibrillator in COMPANION), using "hard endpoints"[13,14] as primary endpoints of efficacy (all-cause mortality or hospitalization).

As a result of the randomized controlled trials performed in the last 15 years (see Table 1), CRT has been proposed by all the international consensus guidelines as a treatment with proven efficacy in improving symptoms, reducing hospitalizations, inducing reverse remodeling, and reducing mortality in well-selected patients with wide QRS (and LBBB), left ventricular dysfunction, and moderate to severe (New York Heart Association [NYHA] class III-IV) or mild (NYHA class II) HF, on top of optimal medical therapy.[6] More recently, patients with conventional indications for pacing, a left ventricular ejection fraction of 50% or less and NYHA class I to III resulted to benefit from biventricular pacing in a relatively long follow-up,[19] although with a number needed to treat, much higher than that of others CRT trials.[22]

GUIDELINES ON CARDIAC RESYNCHRONIZATION THERAPY

In the present review, we analyze the recommendations for CRT implant included in the guidelines on pacing and CRT delivered by the European Society of Cardiology and in the guidelines by the American College of Cardiology, the American Heart Association, and the Heart Rhythm Society, as well as the recommendations for CRT included guidelines on HF delivered by the same societies. Moreover, we analyze the guidelines on CRT delivered by the Canadian Cardiovascular Society and by National Institute for Health and Care Excellence (NICE; Table 2). These guidelines have some differences with regard to the grading of recommendations (see Table 2), which is very explicit and associated with a predefined wording of recommendations in both European and American guidelines. Conversely, NICE does not report in the guidance specific explanations focused on grading of recommendations, implying that the reader can find some information in another NICE publication.[27] The recent NICE guidelines on implantable cardioverter defibrillators (ICDs) and CRT are in some way unique, because they are based on individual patient data network meta-analyses, based on 12,638 patients from 13 clinical trials, taking into account not only evidence but also cost-effectiveness estimates.[28] The approach of NICE of considering cost effectiveness is quite original because, even if economic evaluations are an important aspect of health technology assessment,[29–32] economic estimates were deliberately excluded from clinical recommendations in guidelines delivered by the European Society of Cardiology[33] and has never been considered in guidelines from North America.

We analyze the recommendations delivered from these guidelines with regard to class of recommendation and level of evidence, if available, taking into account different categories of patients, on the basis of clinical aspects (severity

Table 1
Randomized clinical trials on cardiac resynchronization therapy enrolling more than 100 patients: patient population and main findings

Trial	No. of Patients	Trial Design (Follow-up Duration)	NYHA Class	LVEF (%)	QRS Duration (ms)	Primary Endpoints	Secondary Endpoints	Main Findings
MIRACLE[10]	453	Double-blind, randomized trial CRT vs OMT (6 mo)	III–IV	≤35	≥130	NYHA class, exercise capacity, QoL	Peak Vo₂, LVEDD, LVEF, clinical composite response	CRT-P improved NYHA class, QoL, exercise capacity and LVEDD, and increased LVEF
MIRACLE-ICD[11]	369	Double-blind, randomized trial CRT-D vs ICD (6 mo)	III–IV	<35	≥130	NYHA class, exercise capacity, QoL	Peak Vo₂, LVEDD, LVEF, clinical composite response	CRT-D improved NYHA class, QoL, peak Vo₂
CONTAK CD[12]	490	Double-blind, randomized trial CRT-D vs ICD (6 mo)	II–III–IV	≤35	≥120	NYHA class, exercise capacity, QoL	LV volume, LVEF composite of mortality, VT/VF, hospitalizations	CRT-D improved exercise capacity, NYHA class, QoL, reduced LV volumes and increased LVEF

(continued on next page)

Table 1
(continued)

Trial	No. of Patients	Trial Design (Follow-up Duration)	NYHA Class	LVEF (%)	QRS Duration (ms)	Primary Endpoints	Secondary Endpoints	Main Findings
CARE-HF[13]	813	Double-blind, randomized trial OMT vs CRT-P (29.4 mo)	III–IV	≤35	≥120	All-cause mortality or hospitalization	All-cause mortality, NYHA class, QoL	CRT-P decreased all-cause mortality and hospitalizations and improved NYHA class and QoL
COMPANION[14]	1520	Double-blind, randomized trial OMT vs CRT-P/or vs CRT-D (15 mo)	III–IV	≤35	≥120	All-cause mortality or hospitalization	All-cause mortality, cardiac mortality	CRT-P and CRT-D decreased all-cause mortality or hospitalizations
MIRACLE-ICD II[15]	186	Double-blind, randomized trial CRT-D vs ICD (6 mo)	II	≤35	≥130	Peak V_{O_2}	VE/VCO₂, NYHA, QoL, functional capacity, LV volumes and LVEF, composite clinical endpoint	CRT-D improved NYHA, VE/CO₂ and LV volumes and improved LVEF
REVERSE[16]	610	Double-blind, randomized trial CRT on vs CRT off (12 mo)	I–II	≤40	≥120	Worsening of clinical composite endpoint	LVESV index, HF hospitalizations and all-cause mortality	CRT-P/CRT-D did not improve the primary endpoint and did not reduce all-cause mortality but decreased LVESV index and HF hospitalizations

Trial	N	Study design	NYHA	LVEF	QRS	Primary endpoint	Secondary endpoint	Results
MADIT-CRT[17]	1820	Single-blind, randomized trial CRT-D vs ICD (12 mo)	I–II	≤30	≥130	All-cause mortality or HF hospitalization	All-cause mortality or LVESV	CRT-D decreased the endpoint of HF hospitalizations or all-cause mortality; LVESV was reduced; CRT-D did not reduce all-cause mortality
RAFT[18]	1798	Double-blind, randomized trial CRT-D vs ICD (40 mo)	II–III	≤30	≥120	All-cause mortality or HF hospitalizations	All-cause mortality and cardiovascular death	CRT-D decreased the endpoint all-cause mortality or HF hospitalizations; in NYHA III, CRT-D only decreased all-cause mortality
BLOCK HF[19]	918	Double-blind, randomized trial RV vs BIV pacing (37 mo)	I–II–III	≤50	123–125 (mean value)	All-cause mortality, acute HF, increase in LVESV >15%	Composite endpoint of death from any cause, acute HF, death from any causes, hospitalizations	BIV pacing was superior to RV pacing in patients with atrioventricular block, mild-to-moderate HF and abnormal LV systolic function
ECHO CRT[20]	1680	Multicenter, randomized trial, CRT in patients with echo dyssynchrony (19, 4 mo)	I–II–III–IV	≤35	<130	Composite endpoint (death from any cause and hospitalization for worsening HF)	Death from any cause and hospitalization for HF	CRT did not decrease hospitalizations for HF or death from any cause; CRT increased mortality in patients with LVEF ≤35% and narrow QRS

Abbreviations: BIV, biventricular; BLOCK HF, Biventricular versus Right Ventricular Pacing in Heart Failure Patients with Atrioventricular Block; CARE-HF, Cardiac Resynchronization—Heart Failure; COMPANION, Comparison of Medical Therapy, Pacing, and Defibrillation in Heart Failure; CRT, cardiac resynchronization therapy; CRT-D, cardiac resynchronization therapy with a defibrillator; CRT-P, cardiac resynchronization therapy with a pacemaker; ECHO CRT, Echocardiography Guided Cardiac Resynchronization Therapy; HF, heart failure; ICD, implantable cardioverter defibrillator; LV, left ventricular; LVEDD, left ventricular end diastolic diameter; LVEF, left ventricular ejection fraction; LVESV, left ventricular end-systolic volume; MADIT-CRT, Multicenter Automatic Defibrillator Implantation With Cardiac Resynchronization Therapy; MIRACLE, Multicenter InSync Randomized Clinical Evaluation; MIRACLE-ICD, The Multicenter InSync ICD Randomized Clinical Evaluation; NYHA, New York Heart Association; OMT, optimal medical therapy; QoL, quality of life; RAFT, Resynchronization–Defibrillation for Ambulatory Heart Failure Trial; REVERSE, Resynchronization Reverses Remodeling in Systolic Left Ventricular Dysfunction; RV, right ventricular.
Data from Refs.[10–20]

Table 2
Comparison of grading of recommendations

Recommendations	ESC Guidelines on Cardiac Pacing and CRT 2013[6]	ACCF/AHA/HRS Guidelines for Device-based Therapy 2012[3]	ESC Guidelines HF 2012[23]	ACCF/AHA/HRS Guidelines HF 2013[24]	Canadian Cardiovascular Society Guidelines on the Use of CRT 2013[25]	NICE 2014[26]
Class of recommendations						
Evidence and/or general agreement that given treatment or procedure is beneficial, useful, effective.	Class I	Class I	Class I	Class I	Strong recommendations	Based on evidence plus cost-effectiveness estimates
Conflicting evidence and/or a divergence of opinion about the usefulness/efficacy of the given treatment or procedure. Weight of evidence/opinion is in favor of usefulness/efficacy.	Class IIa	Class IIa	Class IIa	Class IIa	Weak recommendations	—
Conflicting evidence and/or a divergence of opinion about the usefulness/efficacy of the given treatment or procedure. Usefulness/efficacy is less well-established by evidence/efficacy.	Class IIb	Class IIb	Class IIb	Class IIb	Weak recommendations	—

Evidence or general agreement that the given treatment or procedure is not useful/effective.	Class III	Class III no benefit	Class III	Class III no benefit	No recommendations	—
Evidence or general agreement that the given treatment or procedure in some cases may be harmful.	Class III	Class III harmful	Class III	Class III harmful	No recommendations	—
Levels of evidence						
Data derived from multiple randomized clinical trials or metaanalyses.	Level of evidence A	Level of evidence A	Level of evidence A	Level of evidence A	High quality of evidence	—
Data derived from a single randomized clinical trial or large nonrandomized studies.	Level of evidence B	Level of evidence B	Level of evidence B	Level of evidence B	Low quality of evidence	—
Consensus of opinion of the experts and/or small studies, retrospective studies, registries.	Level of evidence C	Level of evidence C	Level of evidence C	Level of evidence C	No evidence	—

Abbreviations: ACCF, American College of Cardiology Foundation; AHA, American Heart Association; CRT, cardiac resynchronization therapy; ESC, European Society of Cardiology; HF, heart failure; HRS, Heart Rhythm Society; NICE, National Institute for Health and Care Excellence.

Data from Refs.[3,6,23–26]

of HF, sinus rhythm or atrial fibrillation, electrocardiographic aspects, etc). We also consider potential indications to apply CRT with a pacemaker or a defibrillator.

RECOMMENDATIONS FOR CARDIAC RESYNCHRONIZATION THERAPY WITH REGARD TO PATIENTS IN SINUS RHYTHM WITH MODERATE TO SEVERE HEART FAILURE

Table 3 shows, in parallel, the recommendation for implanting a CRT device in patients in sinus rhythm with moderate to severe HF (NYHA functional class III-IV). Although all the guidelines strongly recommend CRT in case of LBBB with a QRS duration of greater than 150 milliseconds, lower strength of recommendations, with some heterogeneity, appears when QRS duration is 120 to 150 milliseconds, especially if not associated with LBBB. Of note, for all the guidelines CRT is not recommended or not considered in case of a QRS duration of less than 120 milliseconds and, specifically, no indication emerges for guiding the implant on the basis of echocardiographic evaluation of dyssynchrony.

RECOMMENDATIONS FOR CARDIAC RESYNCHRONIZATION THERAPY WITH REGARD TO PATIENTS IN SINUS RHYTHM WITH MILD HEART FAILURE

Table 4 shows, in parallel, the recommendation for implanting a CRT device in patients in sinus rhythm with mild HF (NYHA functional class II). Although all the guidelines strongly recommend CRT in case of LBBB with a QRS duration of greater than 150 milliseconds, lower strength of recommendations, with some heterogeneity, appears when there is not a LBBB and the QRS is 120 to 150 milliseconds.

RECOMMENDATIONS FOR CARDIAC RESYNCHRONIZATION THERAPY WITH REGARD TO PATIENTS WITH PERMANENT ATRIAL FIBRILLATION AND LEFT VENTRICULAR DYSFUNCTION/HEART FAILURE

Table 5 shows, in parallel, the recommendation for implanting a CRT device in patients with permanent atrial fibrillation and left ventricular dysfunction or HF. The use of CRT in this setting has never been object of a dedicated, randomized clinical trial targeted on hard endpoints. Therefore, no class I recommendation were delivered by the specific guidelines on CRT (see Table 5).

PATIENTS ALREADY IMPLANTED WITH A CONVENTIONAL PACEMAKER OR IMPLANTABLE CARDIOVERTER DEFIBRILLATOR: INDICATIONS FOR UPGRADE TO A CARDIAC RESYNCHRONIZATION THERAPY DEVICE

Use of CRT in these cases is related to patients presenting with HF, but also to patients with atrial fibrillation with uncontrolled heart rate who are candidates for AV junction ablation. As shown in Table 6, no major differences can be found in guidelines recommendations. A corrigendum was delivered on HF guidelines delivered by the European Society of Cardiology on this topic.[34]

PATIENTS WITH CONVENTIONAL PACEMAKER INDICATIONS AND LEFT VENTRICULAR DYSFUNCTION/HEART FAILURE: INDICATIONS FOR IMPLANT OF A CARDIAC RESYNCHRONIZATION THERAPY DEVICE

Use of CRT in these cases is covered by the guidelines according to the recommendations shown in Table 7. This indication has been object of a controlled trial, Biventricular versus Right Ventricular Pacing in Heart Failure Patients with Atrioventricular Block (BLOCK HF),[19] published in April 2013, so a key factor in interpreting the variable level of evidence coupled with delivered recommendations is the date of guidelines drafting and delivery. In general, a class IIa recommendation is delivered by most guidelines for this type of indication.

INDICATIONS TO IMPLANT A CARDIAC RESYNCHRONIZATION THERAPY PACEMAKER VERSUS A CARDIAC RESYNCHRONIZATION THERAPY DEFIBRILLATOR DEVICE IN CANDIDATES TO CARDIAC RESYNCHRONIZATION THERAPY IN THE SETTING OF PRIMARY PREVENTION OF SUDDEN DEATH

This issue has been object of several controversies and debates and has relevance in view of the financial impact of choosing a pacemaker versus a defibrillator,[35,36] also with implications on reimbursement.[37] Table 8 reports in parallel the different approaches proposed by the guidelines we analyzed.

Patient profile, costs, expected patient longevity, and risk of complications are all variables to be considered in clinical decision making.[38–40] In this regard, both the European Society of Cardiology Guidelines on cardiac pacing and CRT 2013[6] and the American College of Cardiology Foundation/American Heart Association/Heart Rhythm Society guidelines on HF

Table 3
Patients in sinus rhythm with moderate to severe HF (NYHA III-IV): indications for implant of a CRT device

Indication	ESC Guidelines on Cardiac Pacing and CRT 2013[6]	ACCF/AHA/HRS Guidelines for Device-based Therapy 2012[3]	ESC Guidelines HF 2012[23]	ACCF/AHA/HRS Guidelines HF 2013[24]	Canadian Cardiovascular Society Guidelines on the Use of CRT 2013[25]	NICE 2014[26]
LBBB with QRS duration >150 ms	CRT is recommended in chronic HF patients and LVEF ≤35% who remain in NYHA functional class III and ambulatory IV despite adequate medical treatment Class I Level of evidence A	CRT is indicated for patients who have LVEF ≤35% NYHA class III, or ambulatory IV symptoms on guideline-directed medical therapy Class I Level of evidence A	CRT is recommended in patients with LVEF ≤35% in NYHA functional class III and ambulatory IV despite adequate medical treatment, who are expected to survive with good functional status for >1 y Class I Level of evidence A	CRT is recommended in patients with LVEF ≤35% in NYHA functional class III and ambulatory IV despite adequate medical treatment Class I Level of evidence A	CRT is recommended in chronic HF patients and LVEF ≤35% who remain in NYHA functional class III and ambulatory IV despite adequate medical treatment Strong recommendation High quality evidence	CRT is recommended

(continued on next page)

Table 3
(continued)

Indication	ESC Guidelines on Cardiac Pacing and CRT 2013[6]	ACCF/AHA/HRS Guidelines for Device-based Therapy 2012[3]	ESC Guidelines HF 2012[23]	ACCF/AHA/HRS Guidelines HF 2013[24]	Canadian Cardiovascular Society Guidelines on the Use of CRT 2013[25]	NICE 2014[26]
LBBB with QRS duration 120–150 ms	CRT is recommended in chronic HF patients and LVEF ≤35% who remain in NYHA functional class III and ambulatory IV despite adequate medical treatment Class I Level of evidence B	CRT is indicated for patients who have LVEF ≤35% NYHA class III, or ambulatory IV symptoms on guideline-directed medical therapy Class IIa Level of evidence B	CRT is recommended in patients with LVEF ≤35% in NYHA functional class III and ambulatory IV despite adequate medical treatment, who are expected to survive with good functional status for >1 y Class I Level of evidence A	CRT is recommended in patients with LVEF ≤35% in NYHA functional class III and ambulatory IV despite adequate medical treatment Class IIa Level of evidence B	CRT is recommended in chronic HF patients and LVEF ≤35% who remain in NYHA functional class III and ambulatory IV despite adequate medical treatment Strong recommendation High quality evidence	CRT is recommended
Non–LBBB with QRS duration >150 ms	CRT should be considered in chronic HF patients and LVEF ≤35% who remain in NYHA functional class III and ambulatory IV despite adequate medical treatment Class IIa Level of evidence B	CRT is indicated for patients who have LVEF ≤35% NYHA class III, or ambulatory IV symptoms on guideline-directed medical therapy Class IIa Level of evidence A	CRT should be considered in patients with LVEF ≤35% in NYHA functional class III and ambulatory IV despite adequate medical treatment, who are expected to survive with good functional status for >1 y Class IIa Level of evidence A	CRT is recommended in patients with LVEF ≤35% in NYHA functional class III and ambulatory IV despite adequate medical treatment Class IIa Level of evidence A	CRT is recommended in chronic HF patients and LVEF ≤35% who remain in NYHA functional class III and ambulatory IV despite adequate medical treatment Weak recommendation Low quality evidence	CRT is recommended

Non–LBBB with QRS duration 120–150 ms	CRT may be considered in chronic HF patients and LVEF ≤35% who remain in NYHA functional class III and ambulatory IV despite adequate medical treatment; Class IIb; Level of evidence B	CRT is indicated for patients who have LVEF ≤35% NYHA class III, or ambulatory IV symptoms on guideline-directed medical therapy; Class IIb; Level of evidence B	CRT is not considered	CRT is recommended in patients with LVEF ≤35% in NYHA functional class III and ambulatory IV despite adequate medical treatment; Class IIb; Level of evidence B	There is no clear evidence of benefit with CRT among patients with QRS duration <150 ms because of non–LBBB conduction; No recommendation; Low-quality evidence	CRT is not considered
QRS duration <120 ms	CRT in chronic HF patients and LVEF ≤35% is not recommended; Class III; Level of evidence B	CRT is not considered	CRT is not considered	CRT in chronic HF patients and LVEF ≤35% is not recommended; Class III; Level of evidence B	There is no clear evidence of benefit with CRT among patients with QRS duration <150 ms because of non–LBBB conduction; No recommendation; Low-quality evidence	CRT is not considered

Abbreviations: ACCF, American College of Cardiology Foundation; AHA, American Heart Association; CRT, cardiac resynchronization therapy; ESC, European Society of Cardiology; HF, heart failure; HRS, Heart Rhythm Society; LBBB, left bundle branch block; LVEF, left ventricular ejection fraction; NICE, National Institute for Health and Care Excellence; NYHA, New York Heart Association.

Data from Refs.[3,6,23–26]

Table 4
Patients in sinus rhythm with mild HF (NYHA II): indications for implant of a CRT device

Indication	ESC Guidelines on Cardiac Pacing and CRT 2013[6]	ACCF/AHA/HRS Guidelines for Device-based Therapy 2012[3]	ESC Guidelines HF 2012[23]	ACCF/AHA/HRS Guidelines HF 2013[24]	Canadian Cardiovascular Society Guidelines on the Use of CRT 2013[25]	NICE 2014[26]
LBBB with QRS duration > 150 ms	CRT is recommended in chronic HF patients and LVEF ≤35% who remain in NYHA functional class II. Class I. Level of evidence A	CRT is indicated for patients who have LVEF ≤35% NYHA class II. Class I. Level of evidence B	CRT is recommended in patients with LVEF ≤35% in NYHA functional class II who are expected to survive with good functional status for >1 y. Class I. Level of evidence A	CRT is recommended in patients with LVEF ≤35% in NYHA functional class II. Class I. Level of evidence B	CRT is recommended in chronic HF patients and LVEF ≤35% who remain in NYHA functional class II. Strong recommendation. High-quality evidence	CRT is recommended
LBBB with QRS duration 120–150 ms	CRT is recommended in chronic HF patients and LVEF ≤35% who remain in NYHA functional class II. Class I. Level of evidence B	CRT is indicated for patients who have LVEF ≤35% NYHA class II. Class IIa. Level of evidence B	CRT is recommended in patients with LVEF ≤35% in NYHA functional class II, who are expected to survive with good functional status for >1 y. Class I. Level of evidence A	CRT is recommended in patients with LVEF ≤35% in NYHA functional class II. Class IIa. Level of evidence B	CRT is recommended in chronic HF patients and LVEF ≤35% who remain in NYHA functional class II. Strong recommendation. High-quality evidence	CRT is recommended
Non–LBBB with QRS duration >150 ms	CRT should be considered in chronic HF patients and LVEF ≤35% who remain in NYHA functional class II. Class IIa. Level of evidence B	CRT is indicated for patients who have LVEF ≤35% NYHA class II. Class IIb. Level of evidence B	CRT should be considered in patients with LVEF ≤35% in NYHA functional class II, who are expected to survive with good functional status for >1 y. Class IIa. Level of evidence A	CRT is recommended in patients with LVEF ≤35% in NYHA functional class II. Class IIb. Level of evidence B	CRT is recommended in chronic HF patients and LVEF ≤35% who remain in NYHA functional class II. Weak recommendation. Low-quality evidence	CRT is recommended

Non–LBBB with QRS duration 120–150 ms	CRT may be considered in chronic HF patients and LVEF ≤35% who remain in NYHA functional class II. Class IIb. Level of evidence B	CRT is indicated for patients who have LVEF ≤35% NYHA class II. Class III. Level of evidence B	CRT is not considered	CRT is not recommended in patients with LVEF ≤35% in NYHA functional class II. Class III. Level of evidence B	There is no clear evidence of benefit with CRT among patients with QRS duration <150 ms because of non–LBBB conduction. No recommendation. Low-quality evidence	CRT is not considered
QRS duration <120 ms	CRT in chronic HF patients and LVEF ≤35% is not recommended. Class III. Level of evidence B	CRT is not considered	CRT is not considered	CRT in chronic HF patients and LVEF ≤35% is not recommended. Class III. Level of evidence B	There is no clear evidence of benefit with CRT among patients with QRS duration <150 ms because of non–LBBB conduction. No recommendation. Low-quality evidence	CRT is not considered

Abbreviations: ACCF, American College of Cardiology Foundation; AHA, American Heart Association; CRT, cardiac resynchronization therapy; ESC, European Society of Cardiology; HF, heart failure; HRS, Heart Rhythm Society; LBBB, left bundle branch block; LVEF, left ventricular ejection fraction; NICE, National Institute for Health and Care Excellence; NYHA, New York Heart Association.

Data from Refs.[3,6,23–26]

Table 5
Patients with permanent atrial fibrillation and LV dysfunction/HF: indications for implant of a CRT device

Indication	ESC Guidelines on Cardiac Pacing and CRT 2013[6]	ACCF/AHA/HRS Guidelines for Device-based Therapy 2012[3]	ESC Guidelines HF 2012[23]	ACCF/AHA/HRS Guidelines HF 2013[24]	Canadian Cardiovascular Society Guidelines on the Use of CRT 2013[25]	NICE 2014[26]
Patients with HF, wide QRS, and reduced LVEF	CRT should be considered in chronic HF patients, intrinsic QRS ≥120 ms, and LVEF ≤35% who remain in NYHA class III and ambulatory IV despite adequate medical treatment, provided that a BIV pacing as close to 100% as possible can be achieved. Class IIa. Level of evidence B	CRT can be useful in patients with atrial fibrillation and LVEF ≤35% despite adequate medical treatment if the patients requires ventricular pacing or otherwise meets CRT criteria. Class IIa. Level of evidence B	CRT-P/CRT-D should be considered in patients in NYHA functional class III or ambulatory class IV with a QRS duration ≥120 ms and an EF ≤35%, who are expected to survive with good functional status for >1 y, to decrease the risk of HF worsening if the patient is pacemaker dependent as a result of AV nodal ablation. Class IIa. Level of evidence B CRT-P/CRT-D may be considered in patients in NYHA functional class III or ambulatory class IV with a QRS duration ≥120 ms and an EF ≤35%, who are expected to survive with good functional status for >1 y, to reduce the risk of HF worsening if the patient requires pacing because of an intrinsically slow ventricular rate or the patient's ventricular rate is ≤60 bpm at rest and ≤90 bpm during exercise. Class IIb. Level of evidence C	CRT can be useful in patients with atrial fibrillation and LVEF ≤35% despite adequate medical treatment if the patients requires ventricular pacing or otherwise meets CRT criteria. Class IIa. Level of evidence B	CRT may be considered for patients in permanent AF who are otherwise suitable for this therapy. Weak recommendation. Low-quality Evidence	CRT is recommended

| Patients with uncontrolled heart rate who are candidates for AV junction ablation | CRT should be considered in patients with reduced LVEF who are candidates for AV junction ablation for rate control

Class IIa
Level of evidence B | CRT can be useful in patients with atrial fibrillation and LVEF ≤35% despite adequate medical treatment if AV nodal ablation or pharmacologic rate control will allow near 100% ventricular pacing with CRT

Class IIa
Level of evidence B | CRT may be considered in patients in NYHA class III or ambulatory IV, with a QRS ≥120 ms and LVEF ≤35% who are expected to survive with good functional status for >1 y, to reduce the risk of HF worsening if the patients will be pacemaker dependent as a result of AV nodal ablation

Class IIa
Level of evidence B | CRT can be useful in patients with atrial fibrillation and LVEF ≤35% despite adequate medical treatment if AV nodal ablation or pharmacologic rate control will allow near 100% ventricular pacing with CRT

Class IIa
Level of evidence B | Not considered | Not considered |
|---|---|---|---|---|---|---|

Abbreviations: ACCF, American College of Cardiology Foundation; AHA, American Heart Association; AV, atrioventricular; CRT, cardiac resynchronization therapy; CRT-D, cardiac resynchronization therapy with a defibrillator; CRT-P, cardiac resynchronization therapy with a pacemaker; ESC, European Society of Cardiology; HF, heart failure; HRS, Heart Rhythm Society; IV, intravenous; LVEF, left ventricular ejection fraction; NICE, National Institute for Health and Care Excellence; NYHA, New York Heart Association.

Data from Refs.[3,6,23–26]

Table 6
Patients already implanted with a conventional pacemaker or ICD: indications for upgrade to a CRT device

Indication	ESC Guidelines on Cardiac Pacing and CRT 2013[6]	ACCF/AHA/HRS Guidelines for Device-based Therapy 2012[3]	ESC Guidelines HF 2012[23]	ACCF/AHA/HRS Guidelines HF 2013[24]	Canadian Cardiovascular Society Guidelines on the Use of CRT 2013[25]	NICE 2014[26]
Previous pacemaker or ICD implant	CRT is indicated in HF patients with LVEF <35% and high percentage of ventricular pacing who remain in NYHA class III and ambulatory IV despite adequate medical treatment Class I Level of evidence B	Patients with LV dysfunction in the setting of chronic RV pacing, and possibly as a result of RV pacing AF patients who experience HF after AV junction ablation and RV pacing Class IIa Level of evidence B	Not considered	CRT can be useful for patients on GDMT who have LVEF ≤35% and are undergoing replacement device implantation with ventricular pacing (>40%). Class IIa Level of evidence C	CRT may be considered for patients with chronic RV pacing or who are likely to be chronically paced, have signs and/or symptoms of HF, and an LVEF value ≤35% Weak recommendation, low-quality evidence	Not considered

Abbreviations: ACCF, American College of Cardiology Foundation; AF, atrial fibrillation; AHA, American Heart Association; CRT, cardiac resynchronization therapy; ESC, European Society of Cardiology; GDMT, guideline determined medical therapy; HF, heart failure; HRS, Heart Rhythm Society; ICD, implantable cardioverter defibrillator; LV, left ventricular; LVEF, left ventricular ejection fraction; NICE, National Institute for Health and Care Excellence; NYHA, New York Heart Association; RV, right ventricular.
Data from Refs.[3,6,23–26]

Table 7
Patients with conventional pacemaker indications and LV dysfunction/HF: indications for implant of a CRT device

Indication	ESC Guidelines on Cardiac Pacing and CRT 2013[6]	ACCF/AHA/HRS Guidelines for Device-based Therapy 2012[3]	ESC Guidelines HF 2012[23]	ACCF/AHA/HRS Guidelines HF 2013[24]	Canadian Cardiovascular Society Guidelines on the Use of CRT 2013[25]	NICE 2014[26]
Candidate to permanent pacing	CRT should be considered in HF patients, reduced EF and expected high percentage of ventricular pacing to decrease the risk of worsening HF Class IIa Level of evidence B	Regardless of the duration of the native QRS complex, patients with LV dysfunction who have a conventional indication for pacing and in whom ventricular pacing is expected to predominate may benefit from biventricular pacing Class IIa Level of evidence B	In patients with an indication for conventional pacing and no other indication for CRT who are expected to survive with good functional status for >1 y: CRT should be considered in those in NYHA functional class III or IV with an EF ≤35%, irrespective of QRS duration, to decrease the risk of worsening of HF Class IIa Level of evidence C CRT may be considered in those in NYHA functional class II with an EF ≤35%, irrespective of QRS duration, to reduce the risk of worsening of HF Class IIb Level of evidence C	CRT can be useful for patients on GDMT who have LVEF ≤35% and are undergoing new device implantation with anticipated ventricular pacing percent of >40. Class IIa Level of evidence C CRT can be useful in patients with AF and LVEF ≤35% on GDMT if (1) the patient requires ventricular pacing and (2) AV nodal ablation or rate control allows near 100% ventricular pacing with CRT Class IIa Level of evidence B	Not considered	Not considered

Abbreviations: ACCF, American College of Cardiology Foundation; AF, atrial fibrillation; AHA, American Heart Association; AV, atrioventricular; CRT, cardiac resynchronization therapy; EF, ejection fraction; ESC, European Society of Cardiology; GDMT, guideline directed medical therapy; HF, heart failure; HRS, Heart Rhythm Society; LVEF, left ventricular ejection fraction; NICE, National Institute for Health and Care Excellence; NYHA, New York Heart Association.
Data from Refs.[3,6,23–26]

Table 8
Indications to implant CRT-P versus CRT-D device in candidates to CRT in the setting of primary prevention of sudden death

Indication	ESC Guidelines on Cardiac Pacing and CRT 2013[6]	ACCF/AHA/HRS Guidelines for Device-based Therapy 2012[3]	ESC Guidelines HF 2012[23]	ACCF/AHA/HRS Guidelines HF 2013[24]	Canadian Cardiovascular Society Guidelines on the Use of CRT 2013[25]	NICE 2014[26]
Factors favoring CRT-D	Life expectancy >1 y, stable HF, NYHA II, ischemic heart disease (low and intermediate MADIT risk score) Lack of comorbidities Class IIa Level of evidence B	All patients without factors favoring CRT-P	Not considered	HF ≥40 d post-myocardial infarction with LVEF <35%, NYHA class II/III symptoms on chronic medical therapy, expected to live >1 y Class I Level of evidence A High risk of nonsudden death, such as frequent hospitalizations, frailty, or severe comorbidities Class IIb Level of evidence B	Patients who are suitable for resynchronization therapy and for an ICD Strong recommendation, high-quality evidence	Patients in NYHA II with: • 120–149 ms with LBBB • ≥150 ms with or without LBBB Patients in NYHA I with: • ≥150 milliseconds with or without LBBB
Factors favoring CRT-P	Advanced HF Severe renal insufficiency or dialysis Other major comorbidities Frailty Cachexia Class IIa Level of evidence B	Elderly patients with important comorbidities	Not considered	Not considered	Patients who are suitable for resynchronization therapy, but not for an ICD Strong recommendation, moderate-quality evidence	Patients in NYHA IV with: • 120–149 ms without LBBB • 120–149 ms with LBBB • ≥150 ms with or without LBBB

Abbreviations: ACCF, American College of Cardiology Foundation; AHA, American Heart Association; CRT, cardiac resynchronization therapy; CRT-D, cardiac resynchronization therapy with a defibrillator; CRT-P, cardiac resynchronization therapy with a pacemaker; ESC, European Society of Cardiology; HF, heart failure; HRS, Heart Rhythm Society; ICD, implantable cardioverter defibrillator; LBBB, left bundle branch block; LVEF, left ventricular ejection fraction; NICE, National Institute for Health and Care Excellence; NYHA, New York Heart Association.

Data from Refs.[3,6,23–26]

2013[24] offer a clinically oriented approach that takes into account comorbidities and patients' profiles before implantation.

BEYOND GUIDELINES: DEFINITION OF APPROPRIATE USE CRITERIA FOR CARDIAC RESYNCHRONIZATION THERAPY

The process of delivering guidelines recommendations is usually responsibility of a committee of well-respected leaders who rigorously review available data from the literature, adding clinical experience and consensus among experts in the field when evidence is lacking (this is the case of level of evidence C recommendations). Because there are many clinical decisions that need to be taken in the absence of trial data, the American College of Cardiology in collaboration with the Heart Rhythm Society recently proposed a different approach: the definition of appropriate use criteria for CRT for prespecified clinical scenarios.[41,42] In detail, a review of common clinical scenarios where ICDs and CRT devices are considered was performed, resulting in coverage of several aspects related to secondary prevention, primary prevention, comorbidities, device replacements, CRT, and other. As a result, 369 clinical scenarios related to use and management of ICDs and CRT devices were developed by a multidisciplinary writing group and scored by an independent technical panel of experts, involved in a modified Delphi exercise, with delivery of scenario-specific scores on a scale of 1 to 9 to designate care that is appropriate (median, 7–9), may be appropriate (median, 4–6), and is rarely appropriate (median, 1–3). The results of this process in terms of final ratings delivered by 17 technical panel members were that 45% of the indications were rated as appropriate, 33% were rated as may be appropriate, and 22% were rated as rarely appropriate. In general, the judgment appropriate was assigned to scenarios for which clinical trial evidence and/or clinical experience was available and supported device implantation.[41]

It is premature to evaluate how much the approach of appropriate use criteria can substantially help physician decision making, also improving the complex process of health care delivery, coverage, and reimbursement. This approach has yet to be proposed in Europe.

FROM GUIDELINES TO "THE REAL WORLD": HETEROGENEITY IN USE OF CARDIAC RESYNCHRONIZATION THERAPY

CRT is an effective treatment, if appropriately targeted, but the process of translating consensus guidelines into "real-world" practice is incomplete. Many data indicate that CRT is underused and there is great heterogeneity in its implementation, both in North America and Europe, with marked variability in implant rates either when cross-country or within country analysis are performed.[43–47]

SUMMARY

Renewed and improved efforts should be dedicated to "synchronize" the competence and expertise of many physicians including cardiologists, electrophysiologists, HF specialists, physicians of cardiac imaging departments, physicians involved in the practice of internal medicine and general practitioners to deliver this effective treatment at the right patient, at the right time and in the appropriate setting.[48] Consensus guidelines are the first step in the complex process of health care delivery, which involves many stakeholders and important policy decisions; only joint efforts can improve appropriate access to effective treatments such as CRT.[29]

REFERENCES

1. Grol R, Grimshaw J. From best evidence to best practice: effective implementation of change. Lancet 2003;362:1225–30.
2. Frye RL, Collins JJ, DeSanctis RW, et al. Guidelines for permanent cardiac pacemaker implantation, May 1984. A report of the Joint American College of Cardiology/American Heart Association Task Force on Assessment of Cardiovascular Procedures (Subcommittee on pacemaker implantation). Circulation 1984;70:331A–9A.
3. Epstein AE, DiMarco JP, Ellenbogen KA, et al. American College of Cardiology Foundation; American Heart Association Task Force on Practice Guidelines; Heart Rhythm Society. 2012 ACCF/AHA/HRS focused update incorporated into the ACCF/AHA/HRS 2008 guidelines for device-based therapy of cardiac rhythm abnormalities: a report of the American College of Cardiology Foundation/American Heart Association Task Force on Practice Guidelines and the Heart Rhythm Society. J Am Coll Cardiol 2013;61:e6–75.
4. Guidelines for the use of implantable cardioverter defibrillators. A task force of the Working Groups on Cardiac Arrhythmias and Cardiac Pacing of the European Society of Cardiology. Eur Heart J 1992; 13:1304–10.
5. Vardas PE, Auricchio A, Blanc JJ, et al, European Society of Cardiology, European Heart Rhythm Association. Guidelines for cardiac pacing and cardiac resynchronization therapy: The Task Force for

Cardiac Pacing and Cardiac Resynchronization Therapy of the European Society of Cardiology. Developed in collaboration with the European Heart Rhythm Association. Eur Heart J 2007;28:2256–95.

6. Brignole M, Auricchio A, Baron-Esquivias G, et al. 2013 ESC Guidelines on cardiac pacing and cardiac resynchronization therapy: the Task Force on Cardiac Pacing and Resynchronization Therapy of the European Society of Cardiology (ESC). Developed in collaboration with the European Heart Rhythm Association (EHRA). Eur Heart J 2013;34: 2281–329.

7. Cazeau S, Ritter P, Bakdach S, et al. Four chamber pacing in dilated cardiomyopathy. Pacing Clin Electrophysiol 1994;17:1974–9.

8. Leclercq C, Cazeau S, Ritter P, et al. A pilot experience with permanent biventricular pacing to treat advanced heart failure. Am Heart J 2000;140:862–70.

9. Boriani G, Biffi M, Martignani C, et al. Cardiac resynchronization by pacing: an electrical treatment of heart failure. Int J Cardiol 2004;94:151–61.

10. Abraham WT, Fisher WG, Smith AL, et al. Cardiac resynchronization in chronic heart failure. N Engl J Med 2002;346:1845–53.

11. Young JB, Abraham WT, Smith AL, et al. Combined cardiac resynchronization and implantable cardioversion defibrillation in advanced chronic heart failure: the MIRACLE ICD Trial. JAMA 2003;289:2685–94.

12. Higgins SL, Hummel JD, Niazi IK, et al. Cardiac resynchronization therapy for the treatment of heart failure in patients with intraventricular conduction delay and malignant ventricular tachyarrhythmias. J Am Coll Cardiol 2003;42:1454–9.

13. Cleland JG, Daubert JC, Erdmann E, et al. The effect of cardiac resynchronization on morbidity and mortality in heart failure. N Engl J Med 2005;352:1539–49.

14. Bristow MR, Saxon LA, Boehmer J, et al, Comparison of Medical Therapy, Pacing, and Defibrillation in Heart Failure (COMPANION) Investigators. Cardiac-resynchronization therapy with or without an implantable defibrillator in advanced chronic heart failure. N Engl J Med 2004;350:2140–50.

15. Abraham WT, Young JB, Leon AR, et al. Effects of cardiac resynchronization on disease progression in patients with left ventricular systolic dysfunction, an indication for an implantable cardioverter-defibrillator, and mildly symptomatic chronic heart failure. Circulation 2004;110:2864–8.

16. Linde C, Abraham WT, Gold MR, et al. Randomized trial of cardiac resynchronization in mildly symptomatic heart failure patients and in asymptomatic patients with left ventricular dysfunction and previous heart failure symptoms. J Am Coll Cardiol 2008;52: 1834–43.

17. Moss AJ, Hall WJ, Cannom DS, et al. Cardiac-resynchronization therapy for the prevention of heart-failure events. N Engl J Med 2009;361: 1329–38.

18. Tang AS, Wells GA, Talajic M, et al. Cardiac-resynchronization therapy for mild-to-moderate heart failure. N Engl J Med 2010;363:2385–95.

19. Curtis AB, Worley SJ, Adamson PB, et al, Biventricular versus Right Ventricular Pacing in Heart Failure Patients with Atrioventricular Block (BLOCK HF) Trial Investigators. Biventricular pacing for atrioventricular block and systolic dysfunction. N Engl J Med 2013;368:1585–93.

20. Ruschitzka F, Abraham WT, Singh JP, et al. Cardiac-resynchronization therapy in heart failure with a Narrow QRS complex. N Engl J Med 2013;369:1395–405.

21. Cazeau S, Leclercq C, Lavergne T, et al. Effects of multisite biventricular pacing in patients with heart failure and intraventricular conduction delay. N Engl J Med 2001;344:873–80.

22. Boriani G, Ziacchi M, Diemberger I, et al. BLOCK HF: how far does it extend indications for cardiac resynchronization therapy? J Cardiovasc Med (Hagerstown) 2014. [Epub ahead of print].

23. McMurray JJ, Adamopoulos S, Anker SD, et al. ESC guidelines for the diagnosis and treatment of acute and chronic heart failure 2012: the Task Force for the Diagnosis and Treatment of Acute and Chronic Heart Failure 2012 of the European Society of Cardiology. Developed in collaboration with the Heart Failure Association (HFA) of the ESC. Eur J Heart Fail 2012; 14:803–69.

24. Yancy CW, Jessup M, Bozkurt B, et al. 2013 ACCF/AHA guideline for the management of heart failure: a report of the American College of Cardiology Foundation/American Heart Association Task Force on Practice Guidelines. Circulation 2013;128:e240–327.

25. Exner DV, Birnie DH, Moe G, et al. Canadian Cardiovascular Society guidelines on the use of cardiac resynchronization therapy: evidence and patient selection. Can J Cardiol 2013;29:182–95.

26. The National Institute for Health and Care Excellence. (NICE). Implantable cardioverter defibrillators and cardiac resynchronisation therapy for arrhythmias and heart failure (review of TA95 and TA120). Issued: June 2014. NICE technology appraisal guidance 314 guidance. Available at: nice.org.uk/ta314. Accessed May 22, 2015.

27. The National Institute for Health and Care Excellence. (NICE). The guidelines manual. 2012. Available at: http://publications.nice.org.uk/pmg6. Accessed May 22, 2015.

28. Leyva F, Plummer CJ. National Institute for Health and Care Excellence 2014 guidance on cardiac implantable electronic devices: health economics reloaded. Europace 2015;17:339–42.

29. Boriani G, Maniadakis N, Auricchio A, et al. Health technology assessment in interventional

electrophysiology and device therapy: a position paper of the European Heart Rhythm Association. Eur Heart J 2013;34:1869–74.

30. Fattore G, Maniadakis N, Mantovani LG, et al. Health technology assessment: what is it? Current status and perspectives in the field of electrophysiology. Europace 2011;13(Suppl 2):ii49–53.

31. Maniadakis N, Vardas P, Mantovani LG, et al. Economic evaluation in cardiology. Europace 2011; 13(Suppl 2):ii3–8.

32. Boriani G, Diemberger I, Biffi M, et al. Cost-effectiveness of cardiac resynchronisation therapy. Heart 2012;98:1828–36.

33. Priori SG, Klein W, Bassand JP, ESC Committee for Practice Guidelines 2002-2004, ESC Committee for Practice Guidelines 2000-2002, European Society of Cardiology 2002-2004. Medical practice guidelines. Separating science from economics. Eur Heart J 2003;24:1962–4.

34. McMurray JJV, Adamopoulos S, Anker SD, et al. Corrigendum to: 'ESC Guidelines for the diagnosis and treatment of acute and chronic heart failure 2012' [Eur J Heart Fail 2012;14: 803–869]. Eur J Heart Fail 2013;15:361–2.

35. Daubert JC, Leclercq C, Mabo P. There is plenty of room for cardiac resynchronization therapy devices without back-up defibrillators in the electrical treatment of heart failure. J Am Coll Cardiol 2005;46: 2204–7.

36. Boriani G, Mantovani LG, Biffi M, et al. Cardiac resynchronization therapy: a cost or an investment? Europace 2011;13(Suppl 2):ii32–8.

37. Boriani G, Burri H, Mantovani LG, et al. Device therapy and hospital reimbursement practices across European countries: a heterogeneous scenario. Europace 2011;13(Suppl 2):ii59–65.

38. Padeletti L, Mascioli G, Perini AP, et al. Critical appraisal of cardiac implantable electronic devices: complications and management. Med Devices (Auckl) 2011;4:157–67.

39. Daubert JC, Saxon L, Adamson PB, et al. 2012 EHRA/HRS expert consensus statement on cardiac resynchronization therapy in heart failure: implant and follow-up recommendations and management. Europace 2012;14:1236–86.

40. Boriani G, Ziacchi M, Diemberger I, et al. Cardiac resynchronization therapy: the conundrum of predicting response in the individual patient. J Cardiovasc Med (Hagerstown) 2014;15:269–72.

41. Russo AM, Stainback RF, Bailey SR, et al. ACCF/HRS/AHA/ASE/HFSA/SCAI/SCCT/SCMR 2013 appropriate use criteria for implantable cardioverter-defibrillators and cardiac resynchronization therapy: a report of the American College of Cardiology Foundation appropriate use criteria task force, Heart Rhythm Society, American Heart Association, American Society of Echocardiography, Heart Failure Society of America, Society for Cardiovascular Angiography and Interventions, Society of Cardiovascular Computed Tomography, and Society for Cardiovascular Magnetic Resonance. Heart Rhythm 2013;10:e11–58.

42. Fogel RI, Epstein AE, Mark Estes NA 3rd, et al. The disconnect between the guidelines, the appropriate use criteria, and reimbursement coverage decisions: the ultimate dilemma. J Am Coll Cardiol 2014;63:12–4.

43. Piccini JP, Hernandez AF, Dai D, et al, Get With the Guidelines Steering Committee and Hospitals. Use of cardiac resynchronization therapy in patients hospitalized with heart failure. Circulation 2008;118: 926–33.

44. Curtis AB, Yancy CW, Albert NM, et al. Cardiac resynchronization therapy utilization for heart failure: findings from IMPROVE HF. Am Heart J 2009;158: 956–64.

45. Boriani G, Berti E, Biffi M, et al. Implantable electrical devices for prevention of sudden cardiac death: data on implant rates from a 'real world' regional registry. Europace 2010;12:1224–30.

46. Boriani G, Berti E, Belotti LM, et al. Cardiac resynchronization therapy: implant rates, temporal trends and relationships with heart failure epidemiology. J Cardiovasc Med (Hagerstown) 2014;15:147–54.

47. Arribas F, Auricchio A, Boriani G, et al. Statistics on the use of cardiac electronic devices and electrophysiological procedures in 55 ESC countries: 2013 report from the European Heart Rhythm Association (EHRA). Europace 2014;16(Suppl 1):i1–78.

48. Boriani G, Diemberger I, Biffi M, et al. Cardiac resynchronization therapy in clinical practice: need for electrical, mechanical, clinical and logistic synchronization. J Interv Card Electrophysiol 2006;17: 215–24.

Why the Authors Use Cardiac Resynchronization Therapy with Defibrillators

Edward Sze, MD[a], James P. Daubert, MD[b],*

KEYWORDS

- Cardiac resynchronization therapy • Heart failure • Systolic • Defibrillators • Implantable • Death
- Sudden

KEY POINTS

- Randomized trial evidence directly comparing cardiac resynchronization therapy (CRT) with a pacemaker (CRT-P) and with an implantable defibrillator (CRT-D) is not available.
- Indirect evidence suggests that CRT-D may reduce mortality to a greater degree because of greater sudden death reduction.
- CRT-D is more costly and possibly subject to more complications than CRT-P.

INTRODUCTION

Powerful Therapies for an Increasing Incidence of Heart Failure

One irony of modern cardiology is that our success in treating patients with acute cardiovascular disease has led to an increasing incidence of chronic left ventricular (LV) dysfunction.[1–3] As patients with cardiovascular disease live longer, their decreased mortality has translated to an increased opportunity for heart failure progression. We now face an expanding population of patients who meet the criteria for an intracardiac device.[4–7]

Two therapies indicated for patients with heart failure include cardiac resynchronization (CRT) and implantable-cardioverter defibrillators (ICDs). Both have been proven to benefit patients with chronic LV systolic dysfunction.[8–15] ICDs decrease the rate of sudden cardiac death (SCD) by attempting to terminate potentially fatal ventricular tachyarrhythmia (VTA). CRT seeks to improve LV function by decreasing mechanical dyssynchrony typically brought on by chronic right ventricular pacing or left bundle branch block (LBBB).

Although there is natural overlap in the patient populations indicated to receive either therapy, there are no randomized controlled trials (RCTs) that directly compare CRT only (CRT-P) to CRT plus defibrillator (CRT-D) (**Fig. 1**). When deciding which device or combination of devices to offer patients, a clinician must rely on indirect evidence. This review seeks to present data that will provide guidance to device placement for this growing population of patients.

E. Sze reports a pending research grant with Medtronic > $10,000. J.P. Daubert reports the following relationships with industry: (1) research grants to Duke University from Biosense Webster, Medtronic, Boston Scientific, and Gilead (all are >$10,000); (2) honoraria for lectures, advisory board, or consultation from ARCA Biopharma, Biosense-Webster, Biotronik, Boston Scientific, Cardiofocus, Gilead, Medtronic, Orexigen, St. Jude, and Vytronus (all are <$10,000); (3) fellowship support to Duke University provided by Biosense-Webster, Boston Scientific, Medtronic, and St. Jude (all are >$10,000).
[a] Clinical Cardiac Electrophysiology, Cardiology Division, Department of Medicine, Duke University Medical Center, Durham, NC 27710, USA; [b] Cardiac Electrophysiology, Duke University Medical Center, Box 3174, Durham, NC 27710, USA
* Corresponding author.
E-mail address: james.daubert@duke.edu

Card Electrophysiol Clin 7 (2015) 695–707
http://dx.doi.org/10.1016/j.ccep.2015.08.017

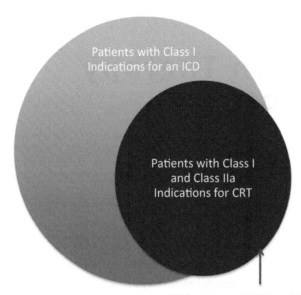

EF between 50% and 35% with
AV block & need for pacing

Fig. 1. The substantial but not complete overlap of indications for implantable defibrillator therapy and for CRT. AV, atrioventricular; EF, ejection fraction. (*Adapted from* Brignole M, Auricchio A, Baron-Esquivias G, et al. 2013 ESC Guidelines on cardiac pacing and cardiac resynchronization therapy: the Task Force on cardiac pacing and resynchronization therapy of the European Society of Cardiology (ESC). Developed in collaboration with the European Heart Rhythm Association (EHRA). Eur Heart J 2013;34(29):2281–329; and Tracy CM, Epstein AE, Darbar D, et al. 2012 ACCF/AHA/HRS focused update of the 2008 guidelines for device-based therapy of cardiac rhythm abnormalities: a report of the American College of Cardiology Foundation/American Heart Association Task Force on Practice Guidelines. Circulation 2012;126(14):1784–800.)

The Case for Cardiac Resynchronization Therapy Only

The logic for implanting CRT-P is straightforward. First, if CRT-P is effective in inducing LV reverse remodeling, a patient's ejection fraction (EF) may improve to the point that it obviates ICD therapy. This reasoning is supported by an echocardiogram substudy from Multicenter Automatic Defibrillator Implantation Trial-Cardiac Resynchronization Therapy (MADIT-CRT) that reported significantly less VTA in patients determined to be high responders to CRT (defined as a >25% reduction to LV end-systolic volume [LVESV]).[16]

Second, in certain populations, such as those with nonischemic cardiomyopathy (NICM), the benefit of ICDs is less clear. In DEFINITE (Defibrillators in Non-Ischemic Cardiomyopathy Treatment Evaluation), the largest RCT to examine the effect of ICDs in patients with NICM, ICDs provided a highly significant reduction of SCD but did not demonstrate an overall survival benefit.[17,18] Furthermore, an analysis from SCD-HeFT examined the benefits of ICDs in patients with NICM and found a nonsignificant survival benefit.[8] Both of these trials had relatively limited follow-up times, potentially obscuring the long-term benefits of ICD therapy. A meta-analysis from 2004 evaluated the efficacy of ICDs in patients with NICM by reviewing 5 prospective RCTs for primary prevention and 3 prospective RCTs for secondary prevention.[19] This study found a significant benefit for primary prevention (relative risk [RR] 0.69, $P = .002$) but an insignificant benefit for secondary prevention

(RR 0.69, $P = .22$).[19] Nevertheless, the question arises: if these patients received CRT, would any effect have been seen with ICD implantation?

Researchers from the University of Pittsburgh addressed the question of relative benefit of CRT-D in patients with NICM when they conducted a retrospective study of 157 patients. Their study followed patients who had LVEF of 35% or less, were pacemaker dependent, had no prior VTA, but were all upgraded to CRT-D. Among the 82 who had NICM, only 1 patient received an appropriate shock in 5 years of follow-up. This finding compared with 11 appropriate shocks in the 75 patients with ischemic disease.[17] The seemingly small risk of SCD in nonischemic patients suggests that, in the right population, we should consider the benefits of implanting CRT-P instead of CRT-D: less upfront costs to implantation; a smaller device size and smaller pocket size; less risk for implantation complications; longer average battery life; and zero risk for inappropriate shocks, shown in Multicenter Automatic Defibrillator Implantation Trial-Reduction in Inappropriate Therapy (MADIT-RIT) to be detrimental to cardiovascular outcomes.[17,20]

THE CASE FOR CARDIAC RESYNCHRONIZATION THERAPY PLUS DEFIBRILLATOR
Greater Protection from Sudden Cardiac Death

The obvious benefit of CRT-D is greater protection from SCD. Data from Cardiac Resynchronization—Heart Failure (CARE-HF), which compared the efficacy of CRT with optimal medical therapy (OMT) in patients with advanced heart failure symptoms (New York Heart Association III or IV), EF of 35% or less, QRS of 120 milliseconds or greater, and signs of mechanical dyssynchrony on echo, reported significant all-cause mortality reduction with CRT.[12] CRT therapy was also associated with a 22% reduction in SCD (29 SCD among 82 deaths in the CRT arm vs 38 SCD among 120 deaths in the OMT arm).[12] This reduction was better elaborated in the extended follow-up study of CARE-HF, where CRT demonstrated a significant decrease in SCD (34 SCD vs 54 SCD, 2.5% per annum vs 4.3% per annum, hazard ratio 0.54, $P = .005$)[21] (**Fig. 2**). Despite the significant reduction in SCD, the investigators hypothesized that there would be greater clinical benefit with the addition of ICD therapy. They noted the persistence of 34 SCDs in the CRT arm, and they observed that the bulk of the reduction in SCD seemed to occur in the last 8 months of follow-up (see **Fig. 2**).

Comparison of Medical Therapy, Pacing, and Defibrillation in Heart Failure (COMPANION) partially examined the hypothesized greater clinical benefit of CRT-D. In this large RCT, investigators compared OMT with either CRT-P or CRT-D in 1520 patients with severe LV dysfunction, advanced heart failure symptoms, and prolonged QRS duration. COMPANION showed that for the secondary end point of all-cause mortality, CRT-D yielded improved survival over CRT-P when both were compared with OMT (CRT-P reduced mortality by 24%; CRT-D reduced mortality by 36%)[13] (**Fig. 3**). COMPANION also found that, though both CRT-P and CRT-D trended toward significant reductions of pump failure deaths compared with OMT (29%, $P = .11$ and 27%, $P = .14$ respectively), only CRT-D significantly reduced SCD (56%, $P = .02$).[22] This finding supports the logical inference that CRT-D offers an incremental benefit for reduction of SCD. It should be noted that, although COMPANION offers direct comparison between CRT-P and CRT-D, it was not powered to show differences between the two modalities.

Last, Al-Majed and colleagues[23] performed a meta-analysis of 25 RCTs that assessed the efficacy of CRT. They found that in the 12 trials that reported the mode of death, the mortality benefit was driven largely by a reduction of heart failure–related deaths (RR 0.64, $I^2 = 0\%$). When assessing the effect of CRT on SCD, they were unable to find a significant reduction compared with control groups (RR 1.04, $I^2 = 0\%$).[23] Again, this suggests that the addition of an ICD would benefit mortality by reducing SCD (**Fig. 4**).

Potential for Proarrhythmia Associated with Cardiac Resynchronization Therapy

Although CRT may decrease the risk of SCD in patients who respond to therapy, it may actually increase the risk in those who do not. The same MADIT-CRT subanalysis that showed reduction in VTA among CRT responders, also showed that nonresponders had 25% more VTA when compared to patients who did not receive CRT.[16] The authors hypothesized that LV pacing may alter ventricular repolarization by reversing the normal sequence of activation, thereby predisposing the myocardium to either re-entry or early after depolarization.

These arrhythmogenic findings in MADIT-CRT were similar to those seen in REVERSE (REsynchronization reVErses REmodeling in Systolic left vEntricular dysfunction). In REVERSE, 508 patients received CRT-D and were randomized to either CRT-On or CRT-Off. Within the CRT-On group, the rate of VTA was 18.7% over 2 years, compared with 21.9% in the CRT-OFF group ($P = .84$).[24] However, within the CRT-On group, those who had signs of reverse remodeling (decrease in LVESV index $\geq 15\%$) exhibited a VTA rate of 5.6% (hazard ratio [HR] 0.31, $P = .001$).[24] These findings again suggest that, though reverse remodeling may have an antiarrhythmic effect, LV pacing without reverse remodeling is potentially proarrhythmic.

CRT-P may also increase risk in patients who have non-LBBB patterns on electrocardiogram (ECG). An analysis from MADIT-CRT showed that CRT was significantly associated with a reduction in VTA in patients with LBBB (HR 0.58, $P<.001$) but had no significant effect on non-LBBB patterns (right bundle branch block and intraventricular conduction delay; HR 1.05, $P = .82$).[25] However, CRT was found to be significantly associated with recurrent VTA in patients with non-LBBB patterns (HR 3.62, $P = .002$).

The possibility of CRT causing harm is further supported by evidence from a single-center retrospective study whereby 5 of 145 patients receiving CRT experienced incessant VTA shortly after implantation.[26] In this study, all patients with incessant VTA were successfully treated with discontinuation of LV pacing and initiation of an antiarrhythmic medication. Thus, in terms of proarrhythmia, it seems that there is the very rare patient with incessant VTA that clearly depends on the LV pacing as well as a tendency for nonresponders to have more VTA over time, as seen in MADIT-CRT and REVERSE.

Ability to Predict Cardiac Resynchronization Therapy Responders Is Imperfect

Given the potential increased risk of VTA induced by CRT, it becomes increasingly important to

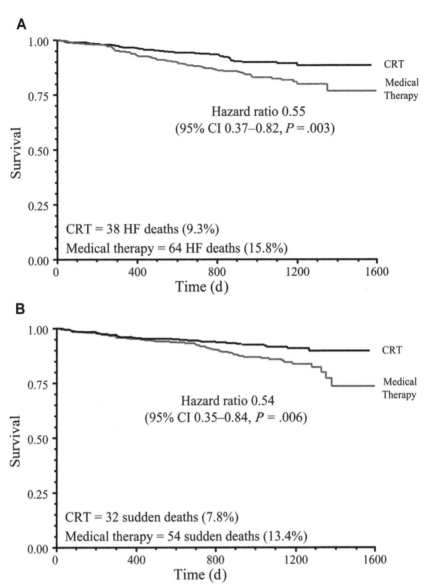

Fig. 2. Panel (A) shows the survival free from heart failure (HF) death in the long-term follow-up from the CARE-HF trial.[21] Note the divergence in the curves at about 200 to 300 days of follow-up. Panel (B) shows survival free from sudden death. Note that the curves are superimposed until about 500 to 600 days of follow-up. Nevertheless, statistically, the proportional hazard for the occurrence of sudden death was not found to differ throughout the course of the trial. CI, confidence interval. (*From* Cleland JG, Daubert JC, Erdmann E, et al. Longer-term effects of cardiac resynchronization therapy on mortality in heart failure [the CArdiac REsynchronization-Heart Failure (CARE-HF) trial extension phase]. Eur Heart J 2006;27:1930; with permission.)

predict which patients will be CRT responders. Unfortunately, determining who will benefit from CRT remains imperfect. Under the current CRT implantation criteria, the proportion of responders is in the range of 57% to 67%.[27–29] Certain clinical characteristics may help predict response. An analysis from MADIT-CRT examined 752 patients within the CRT arm who had paired echocardiograms 12 months apart. Investigators found that

6 factors were associated with a super-response to CRT (defined as patients in the top quartile of LVEF improvement). These factors included the following:

1. Female sex (odds ratio [OR] 1.96, P = .001)
2. No prior myocardial infarction (OR 1.80, P = .005)
3. LBBB (OR 2.05, P = .006)

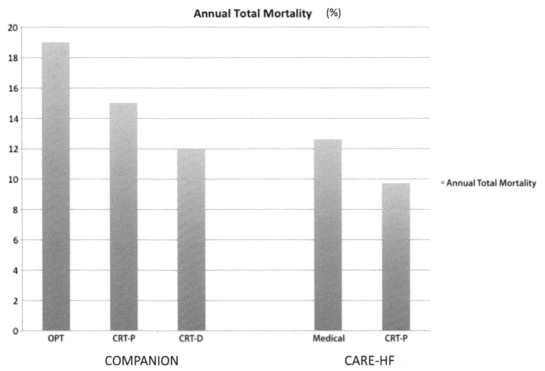

Fig. 3. Bar graph of 1-year all-cause mortality in the COMPANION trial[13] and the CARE-HF trial.[12] In COMPANION, the 1-year mortality is shown for optimal pharmacologic therapy group (OPT), optimal pharmacologic therapy plus CRT-P, and for optimal pharmacologic therapy plus CRT-D.

4. QRS duration of 150 milliseconds or greater (OR 1.79, $P = .007$)
5. Body mass index (BMI) less than 30 kg/m² (OR 1.51, $P = .035$)
6. Smaller baseline left atrial volume index (defined as 1 standard deviation [SD] less than the mean left atrial volume index; OR: 1.47, $P = .001$)

Despite knowledge of these highly significant predictors, it should be noted that their presence still did not confer clinical certainty. Within the hyporesponder group in MADIT-CRT (LVEF change <7.9%), 17% were women, 43% had no prior myocardial infarction, 56% had LBBB, 56% had a QRS duration of 150 milliseconds or greater, 64% had a BMI less than 30 kg/m², and the average LV atrial volume index was 44.5 mL/m² (compared with 43.7 mL/m² in the super-responder group).[30]

Highlighting the complexity of predicting which patients benefit from CRT, a second analysis from MADIT-CRT showed that clinical characteristics associated with reverse remodeling might also be affected by the cause of cardiomyopathy. In this study, patients were stratified by whether they had ischemic cardiomyopathy (ICM) or NICM. Both groups were seen to have significant benefit with CRT, but patients with NICM were on average seen to have a greater clinical response (44% reduction of heart failure hospitalization or death, $P = .002$ vs 34% reduction, $P = .001$) as well as greater echo response ([+SD] 37% ±16% reduction in LVESV for NICM vs 29% ±14% for ICM).[31] In the NICM group, female sex, LBBB, and diabetes predicted a favorable clinical response, whereas in the ICM group, a QRS duration of 150 milliseconds or greater, systolic blood pressure less than 115 mm Hg, and LBBB predicted a favorable clinical response.[31] This study further demonstrated that clinically significant factors in one population might not be significant in others.

The cardiology imaging literature has also shed light on potential predictors of CRT response. One analysis examined the nuclear single-photon emission computed tomography scans of 51 patients with ICM and LV dyssynchrony who were undergoing CRT. This study found that among patients with a transmural scar in the region of the implanted LV lead, none showed a response to CRT in 6 months of follow-up.[32] Bleeker and colleagues[33] also reported that among 40 patients with ICM and candidates for CRT, those with a transmural posterolateral scar seen on MRI

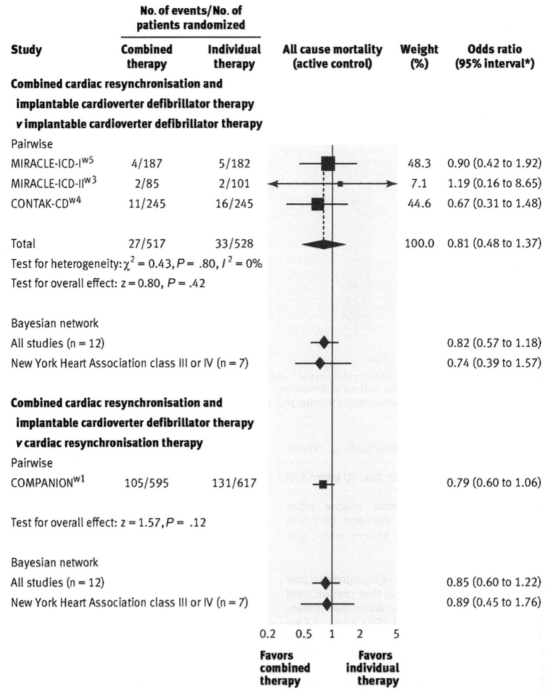

Fig. 4. The lower half of this image shows the comparative benefit on all-cause mortality of the combination of CRT-D compared with CRT-P by a Bayesian analysis.[61] For reference, the upper half shows the comparative benefit on all-cause mortality of combination of CRT-D compared with cardiac defibrillator (without CRT) by a Bayesian analysis. *95% confidence interval for pairwise comparison, 95% credible interval for Bayesian network comparison. (*From* Lam SK, Owen A. Combined resynchronisation and implantable defibrillator therapy in left ventricular dysfunction: Bayesian network meta-analysis of randomised controlled trials. BMJ 2007;335:925; with permission.)

(defined as >50% LV wall thickness) had a significantly decreased rate of echocardiographic response at 6 months compared with those without a scar (14% vs 81%, respectively, $P = .05$). Bilchick and colleagues[34] also found that dyssynchrony identified by global strain on MRI, absence of scar at the LV lead placement, prolonged QLV interval (duration of electrical activation from the onset of the ECG QRS to LV lead), and delayed LV contraction at the LV lead placement were all highly predictive of CRT response (defined as an LVESV decrease by 15% at 6 months by echocardiogram).

Despite all of these reported predictors for response, it should be noted that many of the studies used limited patient numbers and took place in single centers. This point raises the question of the generalizability of these findings and recalls the shadow of PROSPECT (Predictors of Response to CRT). PROSPECT was a multicenter study that sought to confirm the success of initial single-center studies but ultimately concluded that no echocardiographic sign of dyssynchrony could be recommended to help improve patient selection for CRT.[35] For now, much work remains in finding ways to accurately predict response to CRT, and no golden model exists.

Time to Response Is Not Immediate

Even among patients who do become CRT responders, time to LV reverse remodeling is not immediate. The echocardiographic substudy analysis from CARE-HF reviewed the echocardiograms of 365 patients who received OMT and CRT and 370 patients who received OMT. Echocardiograms were performed at 3, 9, and 18 months and study conclusion (mean follow-up 29 months). The results showed steady progression of LV remodeling, which by study end averaged a decrease in LVESV by more than 55.1 mL when compared with the control (95% confidence interval 67.2–42.9 mL, $P<.0001$). Although the study showed continued improvement in LV reverse remodeling over time, the most marked effects of CRT were seen in the first 3 to 9 months after implantation[36] (**Fig. 5**). These findings are comparable with the 12-month echo follow-up in MADIT-CRT that showed an average decrease in LVESV of 57 mL from baseline for CRT-D.[15] They are also similar to REVERSE, whereby serial echoes showed continuous improvement of the LVESV index at 6, 12, 18, and 24 months (101.5 mL/m², 87.7 mL/m², 83.5 mL/m², 74.4 mL/m², 72.2 mL/m², respectively).[24] Because the full effect of the CRT response is not seen immediately, these data

imply a period of ongoing risk for SCD in the peri-implantation period for potential responders and also raise the possibility that nonresponders may not be identified promptly.

Atrial Fibrillation May Inhibit Cardiac Resynchronization Therapy Effects

Atrial fibrillation is a common comorbidity in patients with LV dysfunction.[37] Its chaotic nature often leads to electrical stimulation of the LV through a patient's native conduction system, thereby decreasing the percentage of biventricular pacing. Data from MADIT-CRT have shown that even seemingly marginal decreases in the percentage of biventricular pacing correlate with a significant loss of response to CRT.[38] Similarly, in the Resynchronization for Ambulatory Heart Failure Trial (RAFT), atrial fibrillation was significantly associated with less benefit to CRT.[39] Consequently, the inability to maintain sinus rhythm may be a significant barrier to effective CRT therapy; its unexpected occurrence may prove problematic for predicting CRT response.

Lead Placement

The technical challenges of CRT should not be underestimated. Because of anatomic variants, such as a prominent thebesian valve covering the os of the coronary sinus or an unexpectedly large valve of Vieussens at the meeting of the great cardiac vein and vein of Marshall, achieving appropriate placement of a lead in the coronary sinus may not always be feasible.[40,41] In MADIT-CRT and RAFT, failure for placement of LV leads ranged between 7.5% and 10%.[14,15] Furthermore, although lead placement may not be guaranteed, neither is lead security. In a systematic review of 6 large trials of CRT, the overall lead dislodgement rate has been reported to be 5.7%.[42]

Issues with lead placement and security may only be part of the problem. There are data that argue that suboptimal placement of an LV lead may not decrease the risk of VTA despite signs of reverse remodeling. In 2013, Kutyifa and colleagues[43] analyzed data from MADIT-CRT and reported that LV lead placement in the posterior or lateral position was significantly associated with reduction in VTA compared with placement in the anterior position despite similar rates of remodeling (HR 0.57, $P = .006$). Still, patients with an LV lead in the anterior position had a similar rate of VTA as compared with patients with ICD only (HR 1.04, $P = .837$). Kutyifa and colleagues[43] also found no difference in VTA rates when comparing apical lead placement with nonapical sites.[43]

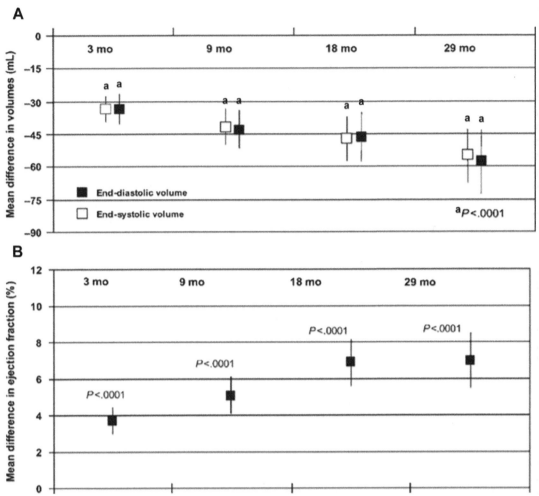

Fig. 5. Data on LV remodeling from the CARE-HF trial[36] show the time course after implementation of CRT on top of OMT as compared with the control arm treated with OMT alone. In panel (*A*), the end-diastolic and end-systolic volumes over time are plotted. Panel (*B*) shows the EF at baseline, 3, 9, 18, and 29 months. Mean values for the difference and standard deviations are displayed. (*From* Ghio S, Freemantle N, Scelsi L, et al. Long-term left ventricular reverse remodeling with cardiac resynchronization therapy: results from the CARE-HF trial. Eur J Heart Fail 2009;11:482; with permission.)

The importance of lead placement is also emphasized in the STARTER trial (Speckle Tracking Assisted Resynchronization Therapy for Electrode Region). Here echocardiographic strain patterns were used to identify the latest activating LV wall before CRT implantation. In this trial, 108 patients underwent CRT using strain guidance, whereas 75 underwent routine implantation. The strain-guided group had superior clinical results. They were more likely to have less VTA (HR 0.64, $P = .038$) and more likely to resynchronize their LV (defined as decreased to time-to-peak strain patterns; 72% vs 48% traditional implantation, $P = .006$). Patients whose LV resynchronized did better than those whose LV did not (HR 0.49, $P = .012$).[44]

Overall, the data regarding lead placement suggest that, in addition to clinical characteristics significantly associated with response to CRT, the technical skill of the implanting physician needs to be considered. Improper placement of a lead may lead to impaired response to CRT.

Cardiac Resynchronization Therapy Is Cost-effective

The initial up-front cost of CRT-D is higher than CRT-P. Over time, however, the incremental survival benefit and decreased need for CRT-D upgrade likely makes it cost-effective. In a 2005 economic analysis within COMPANION, investigators estimated the initial implantation costs to be $20,500 for CRT-P and $29,500 for CRT-D.[45,46] Postimplantation costs over 7 years were then estimated to be $39,400 for CRT-P and $52,700 for CRT-D. These costs then totaled $59,900 for CRT-P and $82,200 for CRT-D and were applied to an intention-to-treat analysis that looked at heart failure hospitalization and mortality over a 7-year period. Because of the follow-up of COMPANION averaging approximately 2 years, the final 5 years were extrapolated using projected event rates. The investigators also stratified the patients into their 3 corresponding treatment groups (OMT, CRT-P, and CRT-D), noting all admissions for hospitalization during follow-up, and attempting to estimate the cost for each admission by using diagnosis-related group codes. The investigators weighed the cost of admissions with the survival rate and patient-perceived quality of life, as measured by the Minnesota Living with Heart Failure Questionnaire (collected before implantation, at 3 months, and at 6 months). By doing so, they were able to calculate the cost of CRT-P to be approximately $19,600 per quality-adjusted patient life year (QALY) and the cost of CRT-D to be approximately $43,000 per QALY. Previously set benchmarks for reasonable cost per QALY were reported as $50,000 to $100,000.[46] Consequently, both CRT-P and CRT-D were argued to be cost-effective.

Risk of Upgrade to Cardiac Resynchronization Therapy Plus Defibrillator

Given the potential for proarrhythmia with CRT-P, as well as the possibility of failure to respond, patients who undergo CRT-P may require a CRT-D upgrade at a later time. Unfortunately, an upgrade may not be simple because of potential venous stenosis or occlusion. Rozmus and colleagues[47] reported that stenosis of the superior vena cava and subclavian veins are common after pacemaker implantation. Rozmus and colleagues[47] noted data from single-center studies that observed venous stenosis rates of more than 60%, with severe or total occlusions occurring in the range of 6% to 21% for all patients.[47–52] Consequently, for many patients with CRT-P, a CRT-D upgrade may simply not be feasible.

Data from the REPLACE registry also suggest that upgrades are not without significant risk. REPLACE enrolled 1744 patients from multiple centers undergoing replacement of either a pacemaker or ICD generator. Patients were stratified into 2 groups. Cohort 1 consisted of patients who only underwent generator change, whereas cohort

2 consisted of patients who underwent or were planned to undergo generator change plus placement of an additional lead. Cohort 1 had a major complication rate of 4.0% compared with cohort 2's major complication rate of 15.3%. Major complications were defined as those that lead to hospitalization, substantive parenteral therapy, or need for surgical intervention. Although many of the major complications were related to the addition of an LV lead, complications were also significantly higher with ICD generator placement.[53]

Krahn and colleagues[54] also reported significant complication rates for ICD replacement. In their study, among 1081 patients undergoing ICD replacement, 4.3% had complications and 2.6% had major complications. Thus, there is real procedural risk in upgrading CRT-P to CRT-D; this should be considered before CRT-P implantation.

Modern Implantable-Cardioverter Defibrillators Programming Reduces Shocks

One argument for CRT-P over CRT-D is the potential burden of inappropriate or unnecessary shocks with defibrillator therapy. MADIT-RIT was an RCT that assigned 1500 patients with a primary-prevention indication for ICD with one of 3 programming configurations.[20] It compared conventional ICD settings with less aggressive settings: high-rate therapy activated only at greater than 200 beats per minute and delayed therapy with significantly increased waiting time before initiating ICD therapies.

The results of MADIT-RIT showed that over an average follow-up time of 1.4 years, when compared with conventional therapy, high rate and delayed settings were associated with a significant reduction in the first occurrence of inappropriate ICD therapies (HR 0.21, P<.001 for high rate; HR 0.24, P<.001 for delayed settings). Somewhat unexpectedly, these significant reductions in inappropriate therapy also corresponded with a significant reduction in all-cause mortality. High-rate therapy compared with conventional settings yielded a mortality hazard ratio of 0.45, P = .01. Delayed therapy compared with conventional settings yielded a mortality HR of 0.56, P = .06.[20] These findings demonstrated that adjustment of ICD settings to a more conservative approach offered significant improvement to the effectiveness of ICDs.

The results of MADIT-RIT were similar to those from ADVANCE-III (Avoid Delivering Therapies for Nonsustained Arrhythmias in ICD Patients III) and PROVIDE (Programming Implantable Cardioverter Defibrillators in Patients with Primary Prevention Indication). ADVANCE-III, another large RCT comparing ICD settings, also showed significantly reduced inappropriate therapies when ICDs were programmed to more conservative settings (Incidence Rate Ratio (IRR) 0.55, $P = .008$). However, ADVANCE-III did not report a significant mortality benefit.[55] PROVIDE, a third RCT, not only showed a reduction in inappropriate therapies (12.4% shock rate in the conservative arm vs 19.4% shock rate in the conventional arm, $P<.001$) but it also reported a mortality benefit (HR 0.70, $P = .036$).[56] Consequently, one reasonable inference from evaluating data from MADIT-RIT, ADVANCE-III, and PROVIDE, and from meta-analyses reviewing programming strategies, would be that all previous trials involving ICDs, which used the more aggressive programming for both antitachycardia pacing and defibrillation, may have understated the benefit of ICD therapy.[57] Thus, enhanced programming should make a more compelling case for the survival benefit associated with ICD therapy, in addition to potentially improving quality of life by avoiding (unnecessary) shocks.

When Might Cardiac Resynchronization Therapy with a Pacemaker Be Appropriate?

Having reviewed the cases for both CRT-P and CRT-D, it should be noted that there are times when it is completely appropriate to implant CRT-P (Table 1). First, in the wake of BLOCK-HF (Biventricular versus Right Ventricular Pacing in Heart Failure Patients with Atrioventricular Block), for patients with no history of VTA, have LVEFs between 35% and 50%, and require a high degree of ventricular pacing, CRT-P is the only indicated therapy.[58–60] Second, for patients who are less likely to benefit from greater SCD protection, CRT-P should also be considered. This population would include patients with a higher risk for noncardiac mortality, such as those with older age and those with multiple advanced comorbidities. Third, in patients who have a high likelihood for CRT response and who wish to avoid potential costs and complications of ICDs, CRT-P may be reasonable. This population may include women with NICM and LBBB or those who have multiple predictors of favorable CRT response.

SUMMARY

CRT-P may cause LV reverse remodeling that obviates ICD therapy. By forgoing CRT-D, patients may face less up-front costs to device implantation, fewer complications, and face zero risk of inappropriate (or appropriate) shocks. However, patients who undergo CRT-P may be at an ongoing risk and in some cases an increased risk for SCD. Not all patients respond to CRT-P, and our ability to predict which patients do is imperfect. Uncontrolled atrial fibrillation may inhibit the effects of CRT-P, and it is a common comorbidity in patients with LV dysfunction. For those patients who do not respond to CRT-P, there is also an increased risk for VTA. For patients who do respond to CRT-P, the timing of response is not immediate. Although CRT-D has higher up-front costs compared with CRT-P, economic analysis shows that its marginally increased costs are reasonable given the QALY it offers. The need for potential CRT-D upgrade bears additional procedural risk, and it should be considered in patients who may receive CRT-P. Recent improvements in ICD programming have heightened the benefit of ICDs, and they strengthen the case that ICDs offer an increased mortality benefit. CRT-P may be appropriate for select patient populations, especially those least likely to receive benefit from ICDs. However, when considering between the two therapies, because of the greater protection from SCD, potential proarrhythmia associated with CRT (albeit rare), and acceptable cost of CRT-D, for most patients the authors recommend CRT-D (Table 2).

Table 1
Patients the authors may favor for CRT-P

Patients with increased risk for noncardiac mortality	• Older age, multiple noncardiac comorbidities • Advanced renal insufficiency • With higher mortality, less likely to derive benefit from ICD therapy
Patients with high likelihood for CRT response	• Patients with multiple predictors for CRT response: LBBB, NICM, female sex, wider QRS duration, BMI <30, and so forth • Patients likely to have high BiV pacing percentage (no afib, PVCs) • Patients with EF >35%, not ICD candidates (BLOCK-HF)[60]
Patient preference	• Smaller device size • Avoid any risk for inappropriate shocks • Desire for palliative therapy

Abbreviations: afib, atrial fibrillation; BiV, biventricular; PVC, premature ventricular contractions.

Table 2
Advantages to CRT-D

Greater protection from SCD	• In some patients, CRT may be proarrhythmic. • CRT responders may still experience SCD. • CRT-D offers incremental protection from SCD.
Benefit does not depend on CRT response	• It is difficult to accurately predict CRT response. • Atrial fibrillation can mitigate CRT's positive effects. • Time to response for CRT is not immediate.
Cost-effective	• There is no need for CRT-D upgrade at a later date. • There is a reasonable cost for QALY.

REFERENCES

1. Bueno H, Ross JS, Wang Y, et al. Trends in length of stay and short-term outcomes among Medicare patients hospitalized for heart failure, 1993-2006. JAMA 2010;303:2141–7.
2. Ezekowitz JA, Kaul P, Bakal JA, et al. Trends in heart failure care: has the incident diagnosis of heart failure shifted from the hospital to the emergency department and outpatient clinics? Eur J Heart Fail 2011;13:142–7.
3. Mozaffarian D, Benjamin EJ, Go AS, et al. Heart disease and stroke statistics–2015 update: a report from the American Heart Association. Circulation 2015;131:e29–322.
4. Ezekowitz JA, Rowe BH, Dryden DM, et al. Systematic review: implantable cardioverter defibrillators for adults with left ventricular systolic dysfunction. Ann Intern Med 2007;147:251–62.
5. McAlister FA, Ezekowitz J, Hooton N, et al. Cardiac resynchronization therapy for patients with left ventricular systolic dysfunction: a systematic review. JAMA 2007;297:2502–14.
6. Epstein AE, DiMarco JP, Ellenbogen KA, et al. 2012 ACCF/AHA/HRS focused update incorporated into the ACCF/AHA/HRS 2008 guidelines for device-based therapy of cardiac rhythm abnormalities: a report of the American College of Cardiology Foundation/American Heart Association Task Force on Practice Guidelines and the Heart Rhythm Society. J Am Coll Cardiol 2013;61:e6–75.
7. Epstein AE, Dimarco JP, Ellenbogen KA, et al. ACC/AHA/HRS 2008 guidelines for device-based therapy of cardiac rhythm abnormalities. Heart Rhythm 2008;5:e1–62.
8. Bardy GH, Lee KL, Mark DB, et al. Amiodarone or an implantable cardioverter-defibrillator for congestive heart failure. N Engl J Med 2005;352:225–37.
9. Moss AJ, Hall WJ, Cannom DS, et al. Improved survival with an implanted defibrillator in patients with coronary disease at high risk for ventricular arrhythmia. Multicenter Automatic Defibrillator Implantation Trial Investigators. N Engl J Med 1996;335:1933–40.
10. Moss AJ, Zareba W, Hall WJ, et al. Prophylactic implantation of a defibrillator in patients with myocardial infarction and reduced ejection fraction. N Engl J Med 2002;346:877–83.
11. Buxton AE, Lee KL, DiCarlo L, et al. Electrophysiologic testing to identify patients with coronary artery disease who are at risk for sudden death. Multicenter Unsustained Tachycardia Trial Investigators. N Engl J Med 2000;342:1937–45.
12. Cleland JGF, Daubert J-C, Erdmann E, et al. The effect of cardiac resynchronization on morbidity and mortality in heart failure. N Engl J Med 2005;352:1539–49.
13. Bristow MR, Saxon LA, Boehmer J, et al. Cardiac-resynchronization therapy with or without an implantable defibrillator in advanced chronic heart failure. N Engl J Med 2004;350:2140–50.
14. Tang AS, Wells GA, Talajic M, et al. Cardiac-resynchronization therapy for mild-to-moderate heart failure. N Engl J Med 2010;363:2385–95.
15. Moss AJ, Hall WJ, Cannom DS, et al. Cardiac-resynchronization therapy for the prevention of heart-failure events. N Engl J Med 2009;361:1329–38.
16. Barsheshet A, Wang PJ, Moss AJ, et al. Reverse remodeling and the risk of ventricular tachyarrhythmias in the MADIT-CRT (Multicenter Automatic Defibrillator Implantation Trial-Cardiac Resynchronization Therapy). J Am Coll Cardiol 2011;57:2416–23.
17. Adelstein E, Schwartzman D, Bazaz R, et al. Outcomes in pacemaker-dependent patients upgraded from conventional pacemakers to cardiac resynchronization therapy-defibrillators. Heart Rhythm 2014;11:1008–14.
18. Kadish A, Dyer A, Daubert JP, et al. Prophylactic defibrillator implantation in patients with nonischemic dilated cardiomyopathy. N Engl J Med 2004;350:2151–8.
19. Desai AS, Fang JC, Maisel WH, et al. Implantable defibrillators for the prevention of mortality in patients with nonischemic cardiomyopathy: a meta-analysis of randomized controlled trials. JAMA 2004;292:2874–9.

20. Moss AJ, Schuger C, Beck CA, et al. Reduction in inappropriate therapy and mortality through ICD programming. N Engl J Med 2012;367:2275–83.

21. Cleland JG, Daubert JC, Erdmann E, et al. Longer-term effects of cardiac resynchronization therapy on mortality in heart failure [the CArdiac REsynchronization-Heart Failure (CARE-HF) trial extension phase]. Eur Heart J 2006;27:1928–32.

22. Carson P, Anand I, O'Connor C, et al. Mode of death in advanced heart failure: the Comparison of Medical, Pacing, and Defibrillation Therapies in Heart Failure (COMPANION) trial. J Am Coll Cardiol 2005;46:2329–34.

23. Al-Majed NS, McAlister FA, Bakal JA, et al. Meta-analysis: cardiac resynchronization therapy for patients with less symptomatic heart failure. Ann Intern Med 2011;154:401–12.

24. Gold MR, Linde C, Abraham WT, et al. The impact of cardiac resynchronization therapy on the incidence of ventricular arrhythmias in mild heart failure. Heart Rhythm 2011;8:679–84.

25. Ouellet G, Huang DT, Moss AJ, et al. Effect of cardiac resynchronization therapy on the risk of first and recurrent ventricular tachyarrhythmia events in MADIT-CRT. J Am Coll Cardiol 2012;60:1809–16.

26. Shukla G, Chaudhry GM, Orlov M, et al. Potential proarrhythmic effect of biventricular pacing: fact or myth? Heart Rhythm 2005;2:951–6.

27. Boriani G, Ziacchi M, Diemberger I, et al. Cardiac resynchronization therapy: the conundrum of predicting response in the individual patient. J Cardiovasc Med (Hagerstown) 2014;15:269–72.

28. Boriani G, Biffi M, Martignani C, et al. Cardiac resynchronization by pacing: an electrical treatment of heart failure. Int J Cardiol 2004;94:151–61.

29. Bax JJ, Gorcsan J 3rd. Echocardiography and noninvasive imaging in cardiac resynchronization therapy: results of the PROSPECT (Predictors of Response to Cardiac Resynchronization Therapy) study in perspective. J Am Coll Cardiol 2009;53:1933–43.

30. Hsu JC, Solomon SD, Bourgoun M, et al. Predictors of super-response to cardiac resynchronization therapy and associated improvement in clinical outcome: the MADIT-CRT (Multicenter Automatic Defibrillator Implantation Trial with Cardiac Resynchronization Therapy) study. J Am Coll Cardiol 2012;59:2366–73.

31. Barsheshet A, Goldenberg I, Moss AJ, et al. Response to preventive cardiac resynchronization therapy in patients with ischaemic and nonischaemic cardiomyopathy in MADIT-CRT. Eur Heart J 2011;32:1622–30.

32. Ypenburg C, Schalij MJ, Bleeker GB, et al. Impact of viability and scar tissue on response to cardiac resynchronization therapy in ischaemic heart failure patients. Eur Heart J 2007;28:33–41.

33. Bleeker GB, Kaandorp TA, Lamb HJ, et al. Effect of posterolateral scar tissue on clinical and echocardiographic improvement after cardiac resynchronization therapy. Circulation 2006;113:969–76.

34. Bilchick KC, Kuruvilla S, Hamirani YS, et al. Impact of mechanical activation, scar, and electrical timing on cardiac resynchronization therapy response and clinical outcomes. J Am Coll Cardiol 2014;63:1657–66.

35. Chung ES, Leon AR, Tavazzi L, et al. Results of the Predictors of Response to CRT (PROSPECT) trial. Circulation 2008;117:2608–16.

36. Ghio S, Freemantle N, Scelsi L, et al. Long-term left ventricular reverse remodelling with cardiac resynchronization therapy: results from the CARE-HF trial. Eur J Heart Fail 2009;11:480–8.

37. Benjamin EJ, Levy D, Vaziri SM, et al. Independent risk factors for atrial fibrillation in a population-based cohort. The Framingham Heart Study. JAMA 1994;271:840–4.

38. Ruwald AC, Kutyifa V, Ruwald MH, et al. The association between biventricular pacing and cardiac resynchronization therapy-defibrillator efficacy when compared with implantable cardioverter defibrillator on outcomes and reverse remodelling. Eur Heart J 2015;36:440–8.

39. Healey JS, Hohnloser SH, Exner DV, et al. Cardiac resynchronization therapy in patients with permanent atrial fibrillation: results from the Resynchronization for Ambulatory Heart Failure Trial (RAFT). Circ Heart Fail 2012;5:566–70.

40. Noheria A, DeSimone CV, Lachman N, et al. Anatomy of the coronary sinus and epicardial coronary venous system in 620 hearts: an electrophysiology perspective. J Cardiovasc Electrophysiol 2013;24:1–6.

41. Habib A, Lachman N, Christensen KN, et al. The anatomy of the coronary sinus venous system for the cardiac electrophysiologist. Europace 2009;11(Suppl 5):v15–21.

42. van Rees JB, de Bie MK, Thijssen J, et al. Implantation-related complications of implantable cardioverter-defibrillators and cardiac resynchronization therapy devices: a systematic review of randomized clinical trials. J Am Coll Cardiol 2011;58:995–1000.

43. Kutyifa V, Zareba W, McNitt S, et al. Left ventricular lead location and the risk of ventricular arrhythmias in the MADIT-CRT trial. Eur Heart J 2013;34:184–90.

44. Adelstein E, Alam MB, Schwartzman D, et al. Effect of echocardiography-guided left ventricular lead placement for cardiac resynchronization therapy on mortality and risk of defibrillator therapy for ventricular Arrhythmias in Heart Failure Patients (from the Speckle Tracking Assisted Resynchronization Therapy for Electrode Region [STARTER] Trial). Am J Cardiol 2014;113:1518–22.

45. Hlatky MA. Cost effectiveness of cardiac resynchronization therapy. J Am Coll Cardiol 2005;46:2322–4.

46. Feldman AM, de Lissovoy G, Bristow MR, et al. Cost effectiveness of cardiac resynchronization therapy in the Comparison of Medical Therapy, Pacing, and Defibrillation in Heart Failure (COMPANION) trial. J Am Coll Cardiol 2005;46:2311–21.

47. Rozmus G, Daubert JP, Huang DT, et al. Venous thrombosis and stenosis after implantation of pacemakers and defibrillators. J Interv Card Electrophysiol 2005;13:9–19.

48. Da Costa SS, Scalabrini Neto A, Costa R, et al. Incidence and risk factors of upper extremity deep vein lesions after permanent transvenous pacemaker implant: a 6-month follow-up prospective study. Pacing Clin Electrophysiol 2002;25:1301–6.

49. Bracke F, Meijer A, Van Gelder B. Venous occlusion of the access vein in patients referred for lead extraction: influence of patient and lead characteristics. Pacing Clin Electrophysiol 2003;26:1649–52.

50. Antonelli D, Turgeman Y, Kaveh Z, et al. Short-term thrombosis after transvenous permanent pacemaker insertion. Pacing Clin Electrophysiol 1989;12:280–2.

51. Goto Y, Abe T, Sekine S, et al. Long-term thrombosis after transvenous permanent pacemaker implantation. Pacing Clin Electrophysiol 1998;21:1192–5.

52. Zuber M, Huber P, Fricker U, et al. Assessment of the subclavian vein in patients with transvenous pacemaker leads. Pacing Clin Electrophysiol 1998;21:2621–30.

53. Poole JE, Gleva MJ, Mela T, et al. Complication rates associated with pacemaker or implantable cardioverter-defibrillator generator replacements and upgrade procedures: results from the REPLACE registry. Circulation 2010;122:1553–61.

54. Krahn AD, Lee DS, Birnie D, et al. Predictors of short-term complications after implantable cardioverter-defibrillator replacement: results from the Ontario ICD Database. Circ Arrhythm Electrophysiol 2011;4:136–42.

55. Gasparini M. Avoiding unnecessary aggressive ICD programming after MADIT-RIT and ADVANCE III trials. J Am Coll Cardiol 2014;63:189–90.

56. Saeed M, Hanna I, Robotis D, et al. Programming implantable cardioverter-defibrillators in patients with primary prevention indication to prolong time to first shock: results from the PROVIDE study. J Cardiovasc Electrophysiol 2014;25:52–9.

57. Tan VH, Wilton SB, Kuriachan V, et al. Impact of programming strategies aimed at reducing nonessential implantable cardioverter defibrillator therapies on mortality: a systematic review and meta-analysis. Circ Arrhythm Electrophysiol 2014;7:164–70.

58. Brignole M, Auricchio A, Baron-Esquivias G, et al. 2013 ESC guidelines on cardiac pacing and cardiac resynchronization therapy: the task force on cardiac pacing and resynchronization therapy of the European Society of Cardiology (ESC). Developed in collaboration with the European Heart Rhythm Association (EHRA). Eur Heart J 2013;34:2281–329.

59. Epstein AE, Dimarco JP, Ellenbogen KA, et al. ACC/AHA/HRS 2008 guidelines for device-based therapy of cardiac rhythm abnormalities: executive summary. Heart Rhythm 2008;5:934–55.

60. Curtis AB, Worley SJ, Adamson PB, et al. Biventricular pacing for atrioventricular block and systolic dysfunction. N Engl J Med 2013;368:1585–93.

61. Lam SK, Owen A. Combined resynchronisation and implantable defibrillator therapy in left ventricular dysfunction: Bayesian network meta-analysis of randomised controlled trials. BMJ 2007;335:925.

Why We Have to Use Cardiac Resynchronization Therapy– Pacemaker More

Jean-Claude Daubert, MD*, Raphaël Martins, MD, PhD,
Christophe Leclercq, MD, PhD

KEYWORDS

- Cardiac resynchronization therapy • Pacemaker • Chronic heart failure

KEY POINTS

- Cardiac resynchronization therapy (CRT) may use either a pacemaker (CRT-P) or a biventricular implantable cardioverter-defibrillator (CRT-D). Both are electrical treatment modalities that have been validated for the management of chronic heart failure (CHF).
- There is currently no strong scientific evidence indicating that a CRT-D must be offered to all candidates for CRT.
- The preferential choice of CRT-P in the remainder of patients is currently an acceptable one.
- Another direction to explore is downgrading from CRT-D to CRT-P at the time of battery depletion in patients with large reverse remodeling and no ventricular tachycardia and ventricular fibrillation detected.

Supported by extensive clinical evidence, electrical device therapy for heart failure has had impressive development during the last 15 years. Patients with chronic heart failure (CHF) may benefit from implantable electrical cardiac devices with a view to (1) resynchronize the failing discoordinated heart to improve mechanical performance or (2) prevent the risk of arrhythmic death by automatic cardioversion-defibrillation. These 2 therapies can be applied separately with dedicated devices. Cardiac resynchronization therapy (CRT) may use specific pacemakers (CRT-P) or an implantable cardioverter defibrillator (ICD). Or these can be applied together with a combined device, the biventricular implantable cardioverter-defibrillator (CRT-D). Today, the proportion of CRT-D devices among all CRT devices implanted worldwide is about 75%, reaching 90% or more in the United States and in some European countries such as Germany and Italy.[1] By contrast, other European countries are still implanting a significant number

of CRT-P devices: 39% in France, 44% in Sweden, 46% in and Belgium in 2013. Why are there such different practices in highly developed countries with common scientific guidelines and similar or nearly similar levels of health expenditure? The response to this intriguing question remains unclear. This article attempts to answer these important questions for clinical practice: Is the growing use of CRT-D devices supported by solid clinical evidence? Is the risk-benefit and cost-benefit profile of CRT-D better than CRT-P in CHF patients?

DO ALL HEART FAILURE PATIENTS WITH EJECTION FRACTION LESS THAN 35% NEED AN IMPLANTABLE CARDIOVERTER DEFIBRILLATOR?

The widespread use of CRT-D is justified because all patient candidates for CRT are theoretically indicated for an ICD. The use of ICDs for primary prevention in heart failure is based on the high

University of Rennes, Rennes 35000, France
* Corresponding author. rue Saint-Sauveur, Rennes 35000, France.
E-mail address: jcdaubert@orange.fr

cardiacEP.theclinics.com

proportion of sudden death in total mortality in CHF patients with reduced left ventricular ejection fraction (LVEF). Data from large drug trials with events adjudication committees show a range between 35% to 58% in the Metoprolol Randomized Intervention Trial in Congestive Heart Failure (MERIT-HF),[2] which is probably explained by the inclusion of 41% of subjects in New York Heart Association (NYHA) functional class II. As the severity of CHF increases, the proportion of sudden death relative to overall mortality decreases and, conversely, the percentage of deaths attributed to worsening heart failure increases.[2] In MERIT-HF, the relative proportion of sudden death was 84% in NYHA class II subjects, 51% in class III, and 33% in class IV when the total 1-year mortality rate was 6.3%, 10.5%, and 18.6%, respectively. Therefore, the greatest benefit of ICDs is likely to be for patients with mild-to-moderate heart failure. The Sudden Cardiac Death in Heart Failure Trial (SCD-HeFT) is, thus far, the only trial showing a reduction of all-cause mortality by ICD therapy in subjects with mild-to-moderate heart failure and LVEF less than 35%.[3] In that study, which enrolled subjects optimally treated for CHF, ICD therapy was compared with amiodarone or placebo. Although amiodarone conferred no benefit compared with placebo, a significant 23% relative reduction in the risk of overall mortality was observed among the ICD recipients. However, these apparently spectacular results must be interpreted cautiously. The demographic characteristics of the SCD-HeFT population were quite peculiar (see later discussion). In addition, the trial had to include more than 2500 subjects followed up for a median of 45.5 months and be extended for another year to show a statistically significant, albeit modest, absolute risk reduction (ARR) of 7.2% at 5 years. Finally, in agreement with the epidemiologic data mentioned earlier, a subgroup analysis showed that the risk reduction was confined to NYHA class II subjects (hazard ratio [HR] 0.54 [0.40–0.74], probability [P]<.001, ARR 11.9% at 5 years). No treatment benefit was observed among the 30% more severely affected subjects (HR 1.16 [0.84–1.61], P = .30). Finally, the clinical benefit by the ICD was similar in subjects with ischemic cardiomyopathy (HR 0.79 [0.60–1.04]) and nonischemic cardiomyopathy (HR 0.73 [0.50–1.07]). These findings were incorporated in recent guidelines on heart failure[4] with recommendation to implant an ICD in subjects with symptomatic heart failure (NYHA class II-III) and an ejection fraction less than or equal to 35%, despite greater than or equal to 3 months of treatment with optimal pharmacologic therapy, who are expected to survive for greater than 1 year with good functional status, irrespective of the cause. The recommendation is class IA for ischemic and IB for nonischemic due to the wider evidence in ischemic patients.

The Real World and the Individual Patient

Randomized trials are often criticized because they enroll highly selected subjects, unlike those encountered in the real life. This criticism is particularly applicable in the treatment of CHF. Considering the large randomized studies of drugs or devices in CHF conducted in recent times, the mean age of the populations was relatively young, between 60 and 67 years, and the proportion of women was small, between 20% and 32%. The most striking example is the SCD-HeFT, with a population 60.1 years old on average and 23% women.[3] These demographic characteristics are largely different from the real life in which the mean ages are more than 70 years and the proportion of women approaches 50%.[5] It is, therefore, problematic to apply recommendations issued from randomized trials to the general population of patients with CHF. Common sense dictates that these recommendations would have to be applied to similar or identical patient populations as the studies used to validate the clinical indication. In the case of the SCD-HeFT, the treatment should be logically offered to young or relatively young patients without serious comorbidities. However, most patients with moderate to severe CHF are older and have various concomitant disorders.[5]

IS THE CLINICAL SUPERIORITY OF CARDIAC RESYNCHRONIZATION THERAPY–DEFIBRILLATOR COMPARED WITH CARDIAC RESYNCHRONIZATION THERAPY–PACEMAKER CLEARLY ESTABLISHED?

Current clinical evidence is based on the results of randomized controlled trials, principally the Comparison of Medical Therapy, Pacing, and Defibrillation in Heart Failure (COMPANION) trial, a post hoc analysis from REsynchronization reVErses Remodeling in Systolic left vEntricular dysfunction (REVERSE) study in subjects with mild CHF, meta-analyses, or extensive reviews and some large-scale registries.

New York Heart Association Functional Class III-IV

Several randomized trials have been conducted to ascertain the clinical impact of CRT in subjects with moderate-to-severe CHF using CRT-P, CRT-D, or both.[6–12] Meta-analyses have also been published.[13–15] Results, with a remarkable consistency between trials, have shown that, in this subject population, CRT in addition to optimal pharmacologic therapy has a highly favorable and sustained impact on all of the treatment objectives, including (1) improvement in symptoms, quality of life, and exercise capacity; (2) reduction in morbidity related to heart failure with, in particular, a 30% to 52% decrease in the number of hospitalizations for worsening heart failure; and (3) reverse ventricular remodeling. A consistent finding in the randomized trials designed with greater than or equal to 6 months of follow-up has been an up to 15% absolute reduction in left ventricular end-diastolic diameter and an up to 6% increase in LVEF, conferred by CRT. These effects were significantly greater in patients with nonischemic than in patients with ischemic cardiomyopathy. The fourth objective is a positive impact on mortality with a significant reduction in all-cause mortality after 1 to 2 years.

The COMPANION trial examined the effects of CRT-P and CRT-D compared with optimal medical treatment on morbidity and mortality.[10,11] CRT-P and CRT-D were both associated with a 20% reduction in the primary combined endpoint of all-cause mortality and all-cause hospitalization (P<.01). However, only CRT-D, compared with controls, was associated with a significant decrease in total mortality at 1 year (HR: 0.64 [0.48–0.86], P = .003), whereas the 24% relative reduction in mortality associated with CRT-P was marginally significant (HR 0.76 [0.58–1.01], P = .059) (**Fig. 1**). Although the study was powered to answer the question, no head-to-head comparison between CRT-D and CRT-P was planned in the protocol. A post hoc analysis presented 1 year later[15] failed to show any significant incremental survival benefit by CRT-D compared with CRT-P (HR 0.92, P = .33).

The CArdiac REsynchronisation-Heart Failure (CARE-HF) trial enrolled 813 subjects.[12] CRT-P plus standard pharmacologic treatment was compared with pharmacologic treatment alone. At the end of a mean follow-up of 29 months, a relative risk reduction of 37% in the composite endpoint of death and hospitalization for major cardiovascular events (P<.001) and 36% risk for all-cause mortality (ARR 10%; P<.002) were observed. That was the first demonstration that CRT per se could have a major impact on mortality. This effect was mainly attributable to a marked reduction in CHF-related deaths. In the main study, 35% of the deaths in the CRT arm were sudden, very similar to what was observed in the CRT-P arm of the COMPANION trial.[10] However a significant reduction in the risk of sudden cardiac death (HR 0.54, P = .006) could be shown after extending the planned follow-up period to 36 months in the CRT group.[16] Reverse remodeling was evoked as a possible mechanism for this favorable but delayed effect.

In summary, data from COMPANION suggest that CRT-D might reduce the risk of sudden death in NYHA class III-IV heart failure subjects at least in a mid-term perspective. At 1-year follow-up, the incidence of sudden cardiac death was 16% in the CRT-D arm, a 55% relative risk reduction compared with CRT-P. However, there is no evidence that this early benefit is sustained over time and may durably impact total mortality. The results of the post hoc analysis of COMPANION do no support this hypothesis.[15]

In practice, only a new randomized study comparing the 2 treatment modalities might resolve this issue. Based on the results of the CARE-HF trial,[11] and assuming that the combination of CRT and defibrillation back-up could prevent two-thirds of sudden deaths, a study would require 1300 subjects per group and a follow-up

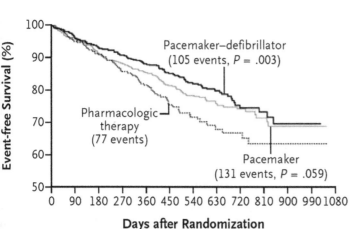

Fig. 1. All-cause mortality in CRT-D subjects, CRT-P subjects, and controls in the COMPANION trial.

period equivalent to that of the CARE-HF trial to have a statistical power of 90% to detect a 5% absolute relative risk reduction of death from any cause with the use of combined therapy compared with CRT alone. Unfortunately, no institution or industry sponsorship was found to promote this study. The issue is still pending, maybe definitely!

New York Heart Association Functional Class I-II

The main treatment goals for patients with asymptomatic or mildly symptomatic left ventricular systolic dysfunction (NYHA class I-II) are different from those set for heart failure patients in class III-IV, consisting primarily of (1) preventing disease progression and (2) reducing cardiac mortality with a special focus on sudden death prevention. Specific endpoints are needed to evaluate these specific objectives. The most relevant are probably (1) a composite of symptoms, morbidity, and mortality[17,18] and (2) reverse remodeling.

In NYHA class I-II patients, the clinical evidence for CRT is principally based on 3 large randomized controlled trials. REVERSE compared CRT-on and CRT-off in subjects implanted either with a CRT-D or a CRT-P.[19] The Multicenter Automatic Defibrillator Implantation Trial With Cardiac Resynchronization Therapy (MADIT-CRT)[20] and RAFT (Resynchronization-Defibrillation for Ambulatory Heart Failure Trial)[21] compared CRT-D and ICD alone in subjects all receiving a defibrillator. The main findings were that (1) CRT reduces significantly the risk of disease progression as assessed by a clinical composite score. This effect was manifest after 2 years in the European cohort of REVERSE.[22,23] In addition, (2) CRT significantly reduces the risk of a combined endpoint of all-cause death or heart failure event. In MADIT-CRT, after a mean follow-up of 2.4 years,[20] the primary endpoint had occurred in 17.2% subjects in the CRT-D group compared with 25.3% in the ICD-only group (HR 0.66, P<.001). The benefit was driven by a 41% reduction in the risk for heart failure events. In RAFT, the subjects were followed for a mean of 40 months.[21] Another primary outcome (3) occurred in 33.2% subjects in the ICD–CRT group and 40.3% in the ICD group (HR 0.75 [0.64–0.87], P<.001). When follow-up is long enough, CRT reduces total mortality. In RAFT,[21] 186 subjects died in the ICD–CRT group compared with 236 in the ICD-only group (HR 0.75 [0.62–0.91], P = .003). Similar observations were made in the posttrial follow-up of MADIT-CRT[22] over a median period of 5.6 years. The cumulative rate of death from any cause among subjects with

typical left bundle-branch block (LBBB) was 18% among subjects randomly assigned to CRT-D compared with 29% among those randomly assigned to defibrillator therapy alone (adjusted HR 0.59 [0.43–0.80], P<.001). The next outcome (4) was that CRT induces large and sustained reverse remodeling. In REVERSE, in which left ventricular end-systolic index (LVESVi) was a powered secondary endpoint,[19,22] a mean reduction of 27.5 plus or minus 31.8 mL/m^2 was observed in the CRT-on group compared with 2.7 plus or minus 25.8 mL/m^2 in the CRT-off group (P<.0001). Reverse remodeling was progressive, with the greatest effect during the first 6 months and further improvements developing over the following 12 months. In MADIT-CRT, a mean increase in LVEF of 11% was observed at 1 year together with a mean 52 mL drop in left ventricular end-diastolic volume.[20] Interestingly, the posttrial follow-up of REVERSE over 5 years[24–26] showed a remarkable stability of left ventricular volumes and ejection fraction over time in the CRT-on subjects (Fig. 2). The final outcome (5) was that in these asymptomatic or slightly-symptomatic subjects CRT did not show any significant effect on symptoms, exercise capacity, and quality-of life-scores.

Cardiac Resynchronization Therapy–Defibrillator Compared with Cardiac Resynchronization Therapy–Pacemaker

A post hoc analysis in REVERSE[27] compared the long-term (5-year) outcomes of subjects who received a CRT-P and those implanted with a CRT-D. The analysis was confined to the 419 subjects who were randomized to active CRT. CRT-P or CRT-D devices were implanted based on national guidelines at the time of enrollment, with 74 subjects receiving CRT-P devices and the remaining 345 subjects receiving CRT-D devices. After 12 months of CRT, changes in the clinical composite score, LVESVi, 6-minute walk time, and quality-of-life indices were similar between CRT-P and CRT-D subjects. However, long-term follow-up showed lower mortality in the CRT-D group (Fig. 3). By multivariable analysis, CRT-D (HR 0.35, P = .003) was an independent predictor of survival. These data suggest that the addition of a defibrillator function to CRT is associated with improved long-term survival compared with CRT pacing alone in NYHA class I-II subjects. One important limitation of this study is the dissimilarity in size between the 2 groups with possible bias in recruitment.

META-ANALYSES

An individual subject meta-analysis of 5 randomized trials assessing the effects of CRT on

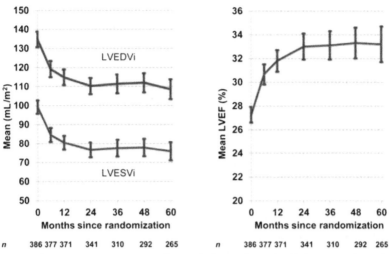

Fig. 2. 5-year posttrial follow-up in REVERSE. Left panel shows change in left ventricular volumes over time. LVEDVi, left ventricular end-diastolic volume index; LVESVi, left ventricular end-systolic index. Right panel shows change in LVEF over time.

morbidity and mortality in a total of 3872 subjects with symptomatic heart failure was recently published by Cleland and colleagues.[25] According to studies, subjects were in NYHA class II (48.5% of the entire population) or in NYHA class III-IV. CRT by CRT-D, or CRT-P or both was compared with optimal medical treatment alone or optimal medical treatment plus an ICD. Overall, CRT was associated with relative risk reduction of 35% in the combined endpoint of all-cause death or heart failure hospitalization (HR 0.65 [0.68–0.74]) and of 34% for all-cause mortality (0.66 [0.37–0.77]). The mortality benefit was particularly marked in NYHA class II subjects (HR 0.62 [0.48–0.80]). Subgroup analysis showed there were no significant

differences in mortality benefit between subjects with CRT-D or ICD alone, or without an ICD. The relative risk reduction was 31% (HR 0.69 [0.56–0.85]) in ICD subjects compared with 37% (0.63 [0.50–0.79]) in subjects with no ICD. In this study, the mean age was similar (65 years) in the different groups.

In a collaborative network analysis on 22 studies and 15,031 subjects, Liang and colleagues[28] showed no significant mortality benefit of CRT-D compared with CRT-P (odds ratio [OR] 0.93 [0.63–1.33]), a result very similar to what was observed in the post hoc analysis of COMPANION.[15] CRT-D was superior to CRT-P in reducing the risk of sudden death (OR 0.39 [0.22–0.65]) but only CRT-P reduced

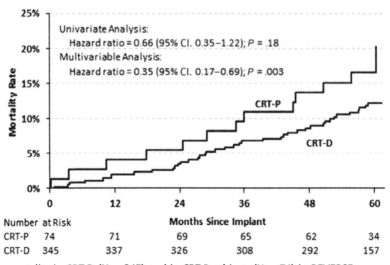

Fig. 3. All-cause mortality in CRT-D (N = 345) and in CRT-P subjects (N = 74) in REVERSE.

significantly the risk of heart failure death (OR 0.64 [0.42–0.90]).

REAL LIFE REGISTRIES COMPARING CARDIAC RESYNCHRONIZATION THERAPY–PACEMAKER AND CARDIAC RESYNCHRONIZATION THERAPY–DEFIBRILLATOR

The European Cardiac Resynchronization Therapy Survey

The European CRT Survey was a joint initiative of the Heart Failure Association (HFA) and the European Heart Rhythm Association of the European Society of Cardiology evaluating the contemporary implantation practice of CRT in Europe.[29] A total of 2438 subjects with successful CRT implantation were enrolled from 141 centers in 13 countries between November 2008 and June 2009. Follow-up (mean 12-months) included symptom severity, cardiovascular hospitalization, and survival. Interestingly, the population included important groups of subjects poorly represented in randomized controlled trials, including very elderly subjects, subjects with previous device implantation, and subjects with atrial fibrillation. Regarding device type, 72% subjects received a CRT-D and 28% received a CRT-P. There were significant differences in baseline characteristics between the 2 groups. In particular, CRT-P subjects were much older (mean age 75 vs 68 years for CRT-D, P<.0001; age >75 years 52% vs 23%, P<.0001) and had a higher prevalence of atrial fibrillation. During follow-up, 207 (10%) subjects died, 346 (16%) had a cardiovascular hospitalization, and 501 (24%) died or had cardiovascular hospitalization. Worse NYHA functional class, atrial fibrillation, ischemic cause, and device type (CRT-P: HR 1.65 [1.11, 2.44], P = .013), but not age, were associated with poorer survival. The 1-year mortality rate was 11% with CRT-P and 8% with CRT-D (**Fig. 4**). Device type did not independently predict cardiovascular hospitalization nor the combined endpoint of death or cardiovascular hospitalization. In summary, CRT-D is associated with a slight survival benefit but major differences in baseline characteristics limit the practical value of this finding.

Budapest Registry

In 2013, Kutyifa and colleagues[30] reported the results of a large Hungarian single-center registry aimed at evaluating all-cause mortality in subjects implanted either with a CRT-D or a CRT-P, stratified by cause. Between 2000 and 2011, 1122 CRT, 693 CRT-P, and 429 CRT-D devices were

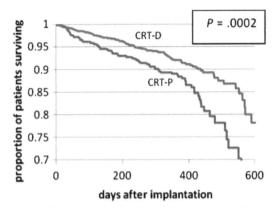

Fig. 4. All-cause mortality in CRT-D and CRT-P subjects in the European CRT registry.

implanted. During the median follow-up of 28 months, 379 subjects died, 250 subjects (36%) with an implanted CRT-P and 129 subjects (30%) with an implanted CRT-D. In the total cohort, there was no evidence of mortality benefit in subjects implanted with a CRT-D compared with a CRT-P (HR 0.98 [0.73–1.32], P = .884). In subjects with ischemic cardiomyopathy, CRT-D treatment was associated with a significant 30% risk reduction in all-cause mortality compared with CRT-P (HR 0.70 [0.51–0.97], P = .03). In non-ischemic subjects, there was no mortality benefit of CRT-D compared with CRT-P (HR 0.98 [0.73–1.32], P = .894; interaction P = .15). As in other studies, CRT-P subjects were older (mean age 66.3 vs 63.9 years) and had less ischemic cause but more atrial fibrillation compared with CRT-D subjects.

The CeRtiTuDe Cohort Study

The CeRtiTuDe Cohort Study was an initiative of the Working Group on Arrhythmia and Cardiac Pacing of the French Society of Cardiology.[31] Based on a large multicenter registry with prospective follow-up (2-year) and specific cause-of-death adjudication, the study objectives were to describe the characteristics of CRT-D and CRT-P subjects in a real-world scenario and to analyze to what extent CRT-P subjects would have additionally benefited from a back-up defibrillator. A total of 1705 consecutive subjects with successful CRT implantation (CRT-P, 535; CRT-D, 1170) were enrolled in 41 centers in France between January 2008 and December 2010. Mean follow-up was 2 years. Preliminary results were presented at the Heart Rhythm Society meeting in 2014. As expected, CRT-P subjects compared with CRT-D were much older (75.9 vs 65.6 years;

$P<.0001$), less often male (69.5 vs 80.8%; $P<.0001$), and had more severe symptoms (NYHA class I-IV 88% vs 80%; $P = .002$), more atrial fibrillation (38.7% vs 22.1%; $P<.0001$), and more severe comorbidities. At 2-year follow-up, 270 subjects died, which is a 77.9 per 1000 annual mortality rate. Mortality rate among CRT-P was twice as high as CRT-D (**Fig. 5**).

By multivariate analysis, CRT type was not an independent predictor of mortality ($P = .07$). By cause-of-death analysis, 95% of the excess mortality among CRT-P subjects was related to an increase in nonsudden death (heart failure death and noncardiovascular death). These findings show that the mortality excess in CRT-P patients compared with CRT-D is mainly related to different baseline patient characteristics and that the addition of an ICD function would probably not have resulted in a survival benefit in this elderly population with comorbidities.

DECREASING NEED OF IMPLANTABLE CARDIOVERTER DEFIBRILLATOR THERAPY AFTER CARDIAC RESYNCHRONIZATION THERAPY

If CRT could be proarrhythmic in specific patients and specific circumstances, the antiarrhythmic properties would predominate. This was shown first by Higgins and colleagues[32] in the VENTAK CHF trial in which 32 subjects with CRT-D devices were randomized 1 month after the implantation for a crossover comparison of 3 months of biventricular pacing and 3 months of inhibited pacing. The primary study endpoint was appropriate therapies. Of the 32 subjects, 13 (41%) received appropriate therapy for ventricular tachycardia (VT) and ventricular fibrillation (VF) at least once in the 6-month monitoring period. Five subjects

(16%) had at least 1 VT/VF episode while programmed to biventricular pacing, whereas 11 (34%) had at least 1 episode while programmed to no pacing ($P<.035$). The significant reduction in VT/VF episodes was attributed to better hemodynamic conditions by CRT.

Recent trials in NYHA class I-II subjects reinforce these findings and show a significant association between reverse remodeling and the reduced risk of VT/VF.

In REVERSE,[33] the time to first appropriately treated VT/VF episode was compared between CRT-on and CRT-off during the randomized period of the trial in the 508 subjects who received a CRT-D. Overall, there were no differences in VT/VF episodes or VT storm between groups. Specifically, in the CRT-on group, the estimated event rate was 18.7% at 2 years, compared with 21.9% in the CRT-off group (HR 1.05, $P = .84$). However, among CR-on subjects, those with reverse remodeling as defined by 6-months LVESVi decrease greater than 15% had a reduced incidence of VT/VF compared with those without remodeling (5.6% vs 16.3%; HR 0.31, $P<.001$) (**Fig. 6**).

In MADIT-CRT,[34,35] the cumulative probability of a first VT/VF episode at 2 years was highest (28%) among low echocardiographic responders to CRT-D defined by a 1-year decrease in LVESVi less than 25%, intermediate among ICD-only subjects (21%), and lowest (12%) among high echocardiographic responders to CRT-D defined by LVESVi decrease greater than or equal to 25% ($P<.001$). Multivariate analysis showed that high responders to CRT-D had a significant 55% reduction in the risk of new VT/VF compared with ICD-only subjects ($P<.001$), whereas the risk of VTA was not significantly different between low responders and ICD-only subjects. Consistently, assessment of echo response as a continuous

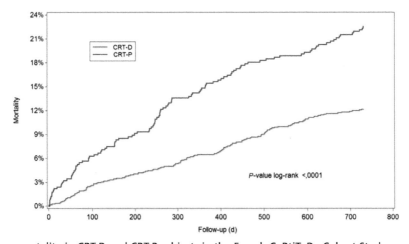

Fig. 5. All-cause mortality in CRT-D and CRT-P subjects in the French CeRtiTuDe Cohort Study.

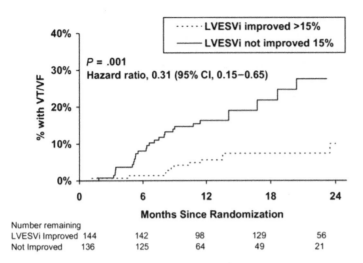

Fig. 6. Risk of new VT/VF in REVERSE according the magnitude of reverse remodeling at 6-months post-CRT. Comparison of subjects with LVESVi reduction greater or less than 15%.

measure showed that incremental 10% reductions in LVESVi were associated with corresponding reductions in the risk of new VT/VF or appropriate shock.

In a subsequent analysis, the MADIT-CRT investigators showed that hyper-responder subjects who achieved LVEF normalization (>50%) at 12 months had very low absolute and relative risk of new VT/VF (**Fig. 7**) and a favorable clinical course during the 2.2-year follow-up.[33] In detail, only 1 subject in this group had new VT/VF after implant, not necessitating shock delivery when there was no significant reduction in the risk of inappropriate shock (13%) compared with subjects with LVEF less than 35% or LVEF 36% to 50% at 12 months. The investigators concluded that these subjects

could be considered for downgrade from CRT-D to CRT-P at the time of battery depletion if no VT/VF has occurred. They account for approximately 10% of the CRT population.

COST AND COST-EFFECTIVENESS OF CARDIAC RESYNCHRONIZATION THERAPY–DEFIBRILLATOR VERSUS CARDIAC RESYNCHRONIZATION THERAPY–PACEMAKER

Cost-effectiveness analyses based on the COMPANION, CARE-HF, and REVERSE data[34–36] indicate that both CRT-P and CRT-D are cost-effective with regard to accepted benchmarks for therapeutic interventions. The 2 therapies are

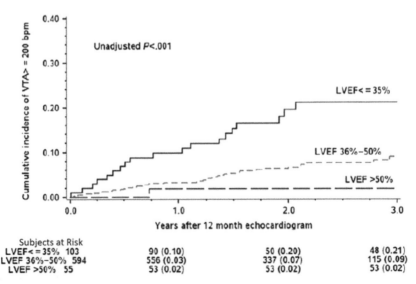

Fig. 7. Risk of new VT/VF episode in MADIT-CRT according to the value of LVEF at 1 year: less than or equal to 35%, 36% to 50%, or greater than 50% (hyper-responders).

cost-effective at the national willingness to pay thresholds of approximately €15000 for CRT-P and €35000 to €50000 for CRT-D per quality-adjusted life year (QALY) gained. The incremental cost to pay per QALY gained is thus 2 to 3 times higher with CRT-D compared with CRT-P. Further analyses[34] showed that overall cost of using a CRT-D strategy compared with a CRT-P strategy is age-sensitive. Overall cost increases progressively with age at the time of implantation. For example, Yao and colleagues[34] calculated an incremental cost of €48800 for a patient implanted at 65 years and of €73300 when implanted at 75 years. CRT-D thus seems less beneficial in older patients.

SAFETY ISSUES AND RISK-BENEFIT PROFILE OF CARDIAC RESYNCHRONIZATION THERAPY–DEFIBRILLATOR VERSUS CARDIAC RESYNCHRONIZATION THERAPY–PACEMAKER

Safety is another important issue to discuss in mildly symptomatic patients with a relatively low mortality risk. There is cumulative evidence that implanting CRT-D devices is associated with a higher perioperative and postoperative risk of major complications compared with CRT-P. Romeyer-Bouchard and colleagues[37] were the first to report an increased risk of infection with CRT-D devices compared with CRT-P. Data were recently reinforced by the results of a large population-based cohort study in all Danish subjects who underwent a cardiovascular implantable electronic device (CIED) procedure from May 2010 to April 2011.[38] The study population consisted of 5918 consecutive subjects implanted with a conventional pacemaker (single- or dual-chamber), an ICD (single- or dual-chamber), a CRT-P, or a CRT-D. Compared with conventional pacemaker, the incremental risk of perioperative or 6-months postoperative complications was 1.5 (0.9–2.3), nonstatistically significant ($P = .11$) for CRT-P and 2.6 (1.9–3.4), $P<.001$, for CRT-D (**Fig. 8**).

By multivariate analysis, CRT-D was the only type of CIED associated with an increased risk of major complications. Notably, the risk of 6-month right ventricular lead complications was twice higher in CRT-D versus CRT-P (2.4% vs 1.2%) and the global rate of right ventricular lead revision was 3 times higher for ICD leads versus pacing leads (3.2 [1.7–5.8], $P<.001$). These data confirm that problems linked to the defibrillation lead remain a real safety issue for CRT-D devices. The relatively poor ICD leads reliability contrasts with the excellent long-term performances of pacing leads, including left ventricular leads. The Kleeman report published in 2007[39] indicated that the overall risk of ICD lead failure was much higher than initially expected (15% at a median follow-up of 2.6 years). It increases progressively over time with an estimated survival rate without lead defect of 85% at 3 years and 60% at 8 years. A trend to an increased risk was observed in subjects with multiple leads, in particular subjects with a biventricular device. Newer lead models are as much affected as older models, as recently illustrated by the Sprint Fidelis and RIATA alerts.[40,41] ICD lead failure may have serious clinical consequences, including life-threatening complications. Most frequent are inappropriate shocks that may severely impair quality of life and compromise patient psychological stability.

WHAT DO THE GUIDELINES SAY?

Based on current scientific evidence, international guidelines give the same level of recommendation for CRT-P and CRT-D use. The 2 treatment modalities are both recommended to reduce morbidity and mortality in patients who are symptomatic (NYHA class II-IV, ambulatory) despite optimal medical therapy, have a reduced ejection fraction (LVEF<35%), the evidence of electrical dyssynchrony by LBBB pattern, and/or QRS width greater than 150 millisecond.[42,43] No clear preference is given to any treatment modality compared with the other.

The strengths and weaknesses of each CRT modality are summarized in **Table 1**.

In practice, it is not ethically wrong to address the issue of priorities in therapeutic objectives

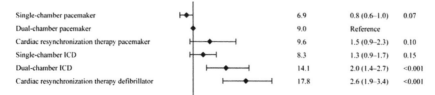

Single-chamber pacemaker		6.9	0.8 (0.6–1.0)	0.07
Dual-chamber pacemaker		9.0	Reference	
Cardiac resynchronization therapy pacemaker		9.6	1.5 (0.9–2.3)	0.10
Single-chamber ICD		8.3	1.3 (0.9–1.7)	0.15
Dual-chamber ICD		14.1	2.0 (1.4–2.7)	<0.001
Cardiac resynchronization therapy defibrillator		17.8	2.6 (1.9–3.4)	<0.001

Fig. 8. Predictors of complications following implantation. (*Adapted from* Kirkfeldt RE, Johansen JB, Nohr EA, et al. Complications after cardiac implantable electronic device implantations: an analysis of a complete, nationwide cohort in Denmark. Eur Heart J 2014;35(18):1191; with permission.)

Table 1
The strengths and weaknesses of each cardiac resynchronization therapy modality

	CRT-D	CRT-P
Mortality reduction	Similar level of evidence CRT-D slightly better	Similar level of evidence CRT-P slightly worse
Complications	Higher	Lower
Costs	Higher	Lower

From Brignole M, Auricchio A, Baron-Esquivias G, et al. 2013 ESC Guidelines on cardiac pacing and cardiac resynchronization therapy: the task force on cardiac pacing and resynchronization therapy of the European Society of Cardiology (ESC). Eur Heart J 2013;34:2313; with permission.

according to different CHF populations. Besides heart failure severity, age and comorbidities, in particular renal insufficiency, remain the stronger predictors of death in CHF.[44] In elderly patients with comorbidities whose longevity remains limited despite all therapeutic efforts, improving quality of life, reducing the rates of hospitalizations for management of CHF, and preserving patient autonomy are probable priorities. Moreover, treatment that lowers mortality and prolongs life with comfortable conditions, which the CRT-P achieves at a modest cost, may be viewed as a beneficial option.

SUMMARY

Both CRT-P and CRT-D are electrical treatment modalities that have been validated for the management of CHF. There is currently no strong scientific evidence indicating that a CRT-D must be offered to all candidates for CRT. Plain common sense should limit the prescription of these costly and complicated devices for patients in need of secondary prevention or for the purpose of primary prevention in younger patients without major comorbidities. The preferential choice of CRT-P in the remainder of patients is currently acceptable. Another direction to explore could be to downgrade from CRT-D to CRT-P at the time of battery depletion in patients with large reverse remodeling and no VT/VF detected.

REFERENCES

1. Eucomed statistics on cardiac rhythm management products, 2005–2013. Available at: www.eucomed. org/medical-technology/fact-figures.
2. MERIT-HF Study Group. Effect of metoprolol CR/XL in chronic heart failure: Metoprolol CR/XL Randomised Intervention Trial in Congestive Heart Failure (MERIT-HF). Lancet 1999;353:2001–7.
3. Bardy G, Lee KL, Mark DB, et al. Amiodarone or an implantable cardioverter-defibrillator for congestive heart failure. N Engl J Med 2005;352: 225–37.
4. McMurray JJ, Adamopoulos S, Anker SD, et al. ESC Guidelines for the diagnosis and treatment of acute and chronic heart failure 2012: The Task Force for the Diagnosis and Treatment of Acute and Chronic Heart Failure 2012 of the European Society of Cardiology. Developed in collaboration with the Heart Failure Association (HFA) of the ESC. Eur Heart J 2012; 33:1787–847.
5. Cleland JG, Swedberg F, Follath F, et al. The Euro-Heart Failure survey programme—a survey on the quality of care among patients with heart failure in Europe. Part 1: patient characteristics and diagnosis. Eur Heart J 2003;24:442–63.
6. Cazeau S, Leclercq C, Lavergne T, et al. Effects of multisite biventricular pacing in patients with heart failure and intraventricular conduction delay. N Engl J Med 2001;344:873–80.
7. Abraham WT, Fisher WG, Smith AL, et al. Cardiac resynchronization in chronic heart failure. N Engl J Med 2002;346:1845–53.
8. Auricchio A, Stellbrink C, Sack S, et al. Long-term clinical effect of hemodynamically optimized cardiac resynchronization therapy in patients with heart failure and ventricular conduction delay. J Am Coll Cardiol 2002;39:2026–33.
9. Young JB, Abraham WT, Smith AL, et al. Combined cardiac resynchronization and implantable cardioversion defibrillation in advanced chronic heart failure: the MIRACLE ICD trial. JAMA 2003;289: 2685–94.
10. Bristow MR, Saxon LA, Boehmer J, et al. Cardiac resynchronization therapy with or without an implantable defibrillator in advanced chronic heart failure. N Engl J Med 2004;350:2140–50.
11. Lindenfeld J, Feldman AM, Saxon L, et al. Effects of cardiac resynchronization therapy with or without a defibrillator on survival and hospitalizations in patients with New York Heart Association in class IV heart failure. Circulation 2007;115:204–12.
12. Cleland JG, Daubert JC, Erdmann E, et al. The effect of cardiac resynchronization therapy on morbidity and mortality in heart failure. N Engl J Med 2005; 352:1539–49.
13. Bradley DJ, Bradley EA, Baughman KL, et al. Cardiac resynchronization and death from progressive heart failure: a meta-analysis of randomized controlled trials. JAMA 2003;289:730–40.
14. McAlister EA, Ezekowitz JA, Wiebe N, et al. Systematic review: cardiac resynchronization in patients with symptomatic heart failure. Ann Intern Med 2004;141:381–9.

15. Bristow M, Saxon L, DeMarco T, et al. What does an ICD add to CRT in advanced heart failure? An analysis of major clinical endpoints in the CRT vs CRT-D groups in the COMPANION study. Circulation 2005; 112. II-673 (Abst).

16. Cleland JGF, Daubert C, Erdmann E, et al. Longer-term effects of cardiac resynchronisation therapy on mortality in heart failure [the CArdiac REsynchronisation-Heart Failure (CARE-HF) trial extension phase]. Eur Heart J 2006;27:1928–32.

17. Packer M. Proposal for a new clinical end point to evaluate the efficacy of drugs and devices in the treatment of chronic heart failure. J Card Fail 2001;7:176–82.

18. Abraham WT, Young JB, Leon AR, et al. Effects of cardiac resynchronization on disease progression in patients with left ventricular dysfunction, an indication for an implantable cardioverter-defibrillator, and mildly symptomatic heart failure. Circulation 2004;110:2864–8.

19. Linde C, Gold MR, Abraham WT, et al. Randomized trial of cardiac resynchronization in mildly symptomatic heart failure patients and in asymptomatic patients with left ventricular dysfunction and previous heart failure symptoms. J Am Coll Cardiol 2008;52: 1834–43.

20. Moss AJ, Hall WJ, Cannom DS, et al. Cardiac-resynchronization therapy for the prevention of heart-failure events. N Engl J Med 2009;361:1329–38.

21. Tang AS, Wells GA, Talajic M, et al. Cardiac-resynchronization therapy for mild-to-moderate heart failure. N Engl J Med 2010;363:2385–95.

22. Linde C, Gold MR, Abraham WT, et al. Long-term impact of cardiac resynchronization therapy in mild heart failure: five-year results from the REsynchronization reVErses Remodeling in Systolic left vEntricular dysfunction (REVERSE) study. Eur Heart J 2013; 34:2592–9.

23. Goldenberg I, Kutyifa V, Klein HU, et al. Survival with cardiac-resynchronization therapy in mild heart failure. N Engl J Med 2014;370:1694–701.

24. Gold MR, Daubert C, Abraham W, et al. Implantable defibrillators improve survival in mildly symptomatic heart failure patients receiving cardiac resynchronization therapy: analysis of the long-term follow-up of REVERSE. Circ Arrhythm Electrophysiol 2013;6: 1163–8.

25. Cleland JG, Abraham WT, Linde C, et al. An individual patient meta-analysis of five randomized trials assessing the effects of cardiac resynchronization therapy on morbidity and mortality in patients with symptomatic heart failure. Eur Heart J 2013;34: 3547–56.

26. Bogale N, Priori S, Cleland JG, et al. The European CRT Survey: 1 year (9-15 months) follow-up results. Eur J Heart Fail 2012;14:61–73.

27. Kutyifa V, Geller L, Bogyi P, et al. Effect of cardiac resynchronization therapy with implantable cardioverter defibrillator versus cardiac resynchronization therapy with pacemaker on mortality in heart failure patients: results of a high-volume, single-centre experience. Eur J Heart Fail 2014;16:1323–30.

28. Higgins SL, Hummel JD, Niazi IK, et al. Cardiac resynchronization therapy for the treatment of heart failure in patients with intraventricular conduction delay and malignant ventricular tachyarrhythmias. J Am Coll Cardiol 2003;42:1454–9.

29. Gold MR, Linde C, Abraham WT, et al. The impact of cardiac resynchronization therapy on the incidence of ventricular arrhythmias in mild heart failure. Heart Rhythm 2011;8:679–84.

30. Gold MR, Daubert C, Abraham WT, et al. The impact of reverse remodeling on long term survival in mildly symptomatic heart failure patients receiving cardiac resynchronization therapy: results from the REVERSE study. Heart Rhythm 2015;12: 524–30.

31. Marijon E, Leclercq C, Narayanan C, et al. Causes-of-death analysis of patients with cardiac resynchronization therapy: an analysis of the CeRtiTuDe cohort study. Eur Heart J 2015. [Epub ahead of print].

32. Ouellet G, Huang DT, Moss AJ, et al. Effect of cardiac resynchronization therapy on the risk of first and recurrent ventricular tachyarrhythmic events in MADIT-CRT. J Am Coll Cardiol 2012; 60:1809–16.

33. Ruwald MH, Solomon S, Foster E, et al. Left ventricular ejection fraction normalization in cardiac resynchronization therapy and risk of ventricular arrhythmias and clinical outcomes. Results from the Multicenter Automatic Defibrillator Implantation Trial With Cardiac Resynchronization Therapy (MADIT-CRT) trial. Circulation 2014;130: 2278–86.

34. Yao G, Freemantle N, Calvert MJ, et al. The long-term cost-effectiveness of cardiac resynchronisation therapy with or without an implantable cardioverter-defibrillator. Eur Heart J 2006;22:48–51.

35. Linde C, Mealing S, Hawkins N, et al. Cost-effectiveness of cardiac resynchronisation therapy in patients with asymptomatic to mild heart failure: insights from the European cohort of the REVERSE study. Eur Heart J 2010;32:1631–8.

36. Feldman AM, de Lissovoy G, Bristow MR, et al. Cost effectiveness of cardiac resynchronisation therapy in the comparison of medical therapy, pacing and defibrillation (COMPANION) trial. J Am Coll Cardiol 2005;46:2311–21.

37. Romeyer-Bouchard C, Da Costa A, Dauphinot V, et al. Prevalence and risk factors related to infections of cardiac resynchronization therapy devices. Eur Heart J 2010;31:203–10.

38. Kirkfeldt RE, Johansen JB, Nohr EA, et al. Complications after cardiac implantable electronic

device implantations: an analysis of a complete, nationwide cohort in Denmark. Eur Heart J 2014; 35:1186–94.

39. Kleeman T, Becker T, Doenges K, et al. Annual rate of transvenous defibrillation lead defects in implantable cardioverter-defibrillators over a period of >10 years. Circulation 2007;115:2474–80.

40. Maisel WH. Semper fidelis-consumer protection for patients with implanted medical devices. N Engl J Med 2008;358(10):985–7.

41. Hauser RG, Abdelhadi R, McGriff D, et al. Deaths caused by the failure of Riata and Riata ST implantable cardioverter-defibrillator. Heart Rhythm 2012;9: 1227–35.

42. Brignole M, Auricchio A, Baron-Esquivias G, et al. 2013 ESC Guidelines on cardiac pacing and cardiac resynchronization therapy: the Task Force on cardiac pacing and resynchronization therapy of the European Society of Cardiology (ESC). Eur Heart J 2013;34:2281–329.

43. Tracy CM, Epstein AE, Darbar D, et al. 2012 ACCF/ AHA/HRS focused update incorporated into the ACCF/AHA/HRS 2008 guidelines for device-based therapy of cardiac rhythm abnormalities: a report of the American College of Cardiology Foundation/ American Heart Association Task Force on Practice Guidelines and the Heart Rhythm Society. J Am Coll Cardiol 2012;60:1298–313.

44. Barlera S, Tavazzi L, Franzosi MG, et al. Predictors of mortality in 6975 patients with chronic heart failure in the GISSI-HF trial: proposal for a nomogram. Circ Heart Fail 2013;6:31–9.

Cardiac Resynchronization Therapy in Women

Maria Rosa Costanzo, MD, FESC

KEYWORDS

- Cardiac resynchronization therapy • Left bundle branch block • Women • Heart failure

KEY POINTS

- Women are underrepresented in all cardiac resynchronization (CRT) studies, in which they are typically less than 30% of the population.
- Most of the available data show that CRT produces a greater clinical benefit in women than in men.
- In several studies, women have left bundle branch block (LBBB) more frequently than men.
- Women have true LBBB at QRS durations shorter than those of men with LBBB.
- Although plausible, it is unknown whether sex differences in cardiac remodeling influence the response to CRT.

INTRODUCTION

Cardiac resynchronization therapy (CRT) has been studied for 2 decades, and trials conducted over this period of time have first shown that CRT enhances functional capacity, then that this improvement is due to augmentation of left ventricular (LV) systolic function, reduction in LV volumes and mitral regurgitation, and finally that this beneficial reverse myocardial remodeling achieved with CRT is associated with improved survival and fewer events in patients with heart failure (HF) with mild to severe disease.[1–5]

Studies of CRT and clinical experience have also shown that variable percentages of patients fail to improve with CRT (nonresponders), whereas some CRT recipients experience near normalization of their LV systolic function (super-responders). This diversity of responses has driven the performance of numerous studies and analyses aimed at the identification of predictors of outcomes after CRT.[6–8]

Female sex is one of the factors that has repeatedly emerged as a predictor of CRT benefit.[9,10]

However, the interpretation of the data regarding sex-specific CRT effects is hindered by many important facts: (1) There are no prospective, randomized controlled clinical trials (RCTs) specifically comparing CRT responses in male versus female patients with HF. (2) The sources of information currently available include observational retrospective studies, databases, registries, and post hoc analyses of RCT and meta-analyses. (3) Regardless of the data source, women are underrepresented in both RTCs and observational studies in which female patients are typically only 30% or less of subjects.[11,12] There are several potential causes for the low proportion of women undergoing CRT (**Box 1**). Despite the limitations inherent to all the analyses on the effects of CRT in women, sufficient and important information can be gathered from the available literature to (1) summarize the findings up to date, (2) identify

Dr M.R. Costanzo receives reimbursement for travel and consulting honoraria from St. Jude Medical. The Advocate Heart Institute receives research grants from St. Jude Medical.
Advocate Heart Institute, Edward Heart Hospital, 4th Floor, 801 South Washington Street, Naperville, IL 60566, USA
E-mail address: mariarosa.Costanzo@advocatehealth.com

Card Electrophysiol Clin 7 (2015) 721–734
http://dx.doi.org/10.1016/j.ccep.2015.08.018
1877-9182/15/$ – see front matter © 2015 Elsevier Inc. All rights reserved.

the gaps in our knowledge, and (3) shed light on
which studies should be performed to confirm or
refute the belief that women and men have differential responses to CRT.

OBSERVATIONAL STUDIES

The key findings and limitations of observational
studies evaluating gender differences in response
to CRT are summarized in **Boxes 2 and 3**.

In a retrospective study of 550 patients (22%
women, 69% New York Heart Association
[NYHA] III, 31% NYHA IV) undergoing CRT at a
single center between 2000 and 2009, female
sex predicted a 48% lower mortality from

cardiovascular (CV) death ($P = .0051$) and all-
cause mortality ($P = .0022$), a 44% decrease in
the combined end point CV death/HF hospitalizations ($P = .0036$), and a 33% reduction in death
from any cause/hospitalizations for major adverse
CV events ($P = .0214$).[10] Compared with men,
women had a 45% lower pump failure mortality
rate ($P = .0330$) but similar frequency of sudden
cardiac death. A decrease in LV end diastolic volume (LVEDD) by 15% or greater occurred more
often in female than male patients (62% vs 44%,
respectively, $P = .0051$). The rate of response to
CRT, defined as improvement by 1 or greater
NYHA class, 25% or greater in 6-minute walking
distance, or a composite clinical score (which
included these two variables plus survival free
from HF hospitalizations for ≥ 1 year after implantation) was 78% and similar for both sexes. By
multivariable analysis, the association between female sex and lower morbidity and mortality was independent of age, LV ejection fraction (LVEF),
atrial rhythm, HF cause, QRS duration, CRT device
type, NYHA functional class, and decrease in
LVEDD (adjusted hazard ratio [HR]: 0.48,
$P = .0086$).[10] Although these findings suggest
that the factors responsible for the better outcomes may be intrinsic to female sex, they do
not uncover their precise nature. In addition, the
study provides data only on QRS duration but
not on its configuration, making it impossible to
determine if the greater benefit of CRT in women
is due to a higher frequency of true left bundle
branch block (LBBB), an electrocardiographic
feature that underlies true dyssynchronous conduction and, therefore, predicts greater benefit
from CRT.[11–17]

Results in sharp contrast with the aforementioned study emerged from another retrospective
cohort analysis of 728 consecutive patients

(22.8% women) undergoing CRT between 2002 and 2008.[18] At baseline women were younger (66 vs 69 years; P<.001), had higher rates of nonischemic cardiomyopathy (68% vs 36%; P<.001) and LBBB despite similar QRS duration (63% vs 42%; P<.001), lower rates of atrial fibrillation (AF) (20% vs 32%; P = .050), and smaller LVEDD (64 mm vs 66 mm; [P = .03]). Both female and male patients had significantly improved clinical and echocardiographic parameters after CRT, but women had greater improvement in NYHA functional class (−0.79 vs × 0.56; P = .009). In unadjusted analyses, women were at a lower risk of death than men after CRT (HR = 0.51; 95% confidence interval [CI] = 0.35–0.75; P<.001). However, by multivariate analysis, age at CRT placement, HF cause, NYHA functional class, and lead location were independent predictors of survival, whereas female sex was not.[18] These results suggest that nonischemic HF cause and other clinical variables, rather than factors intrinsic to female sex, drive the superior CRT outcomes in women.[19,20] In addition to its retrospective nature, the interpretation of these results is limited by the fact that an improvement in NYHA functional class by only 0.5 or greater was sufficient to define subjects as CRT responders.[18]

Contrasting findings were reported in another retrospective analysis of 619 (19% women) predominantly NYHA class III patients who underwent CRT implant between 1998 and 2008; were followed for an average of 3.6 years; and had a 1-, 5-, and 10-year survival of 91%, 63%, and 39%, respectively.[21] Of 12 variables included in the multivariate analysis, female sex was the *only* independent predictor of all-cause mortality (HR = 0.44; 95% CI = 0.21–0.90; P = .025). The secondary end point of combined all-cause mortality or HF hospitalization did not differ between sexes. There was a trend toward a higher rate of device-related complications in women than in men (13% vs 8%; P = .079). This study has important limitations typical of many observational analyses. These limitations include (1) the absence of information on QRS configuration (LBBB vs other conduction abnormalities), (2) failure to index LV volumes to body surface area, and (3) the inclusion of 96 (15%) patients receiving off-label CRT implantation (42 individuals with LVEF >35% and 54 patients with QRS duration <120 milliseconds). Nevertheless, in this study, sex was independently associated with improved survival after CRT even after adjustment for variables known to predict outcomes in patients with HF, including age, NYHA class, LVEF, mean arterial pressure, ischemic HF cause, renal dysfunction, hyponatremia, anemia, and diabetes.[22] In contrast to other studies in which AF occurs more frequently in men than in women, in this study, AF occurred at similar rates in both sexes and did not increase the risk of poorer outcomes.[10,11,18]

In 693 patients from 2 international centers, patients were grouped as nonresponders/modest (395), moderate (186), or super-responders (112) to CRT, according to an absolute postimplant change in LVEF of 5% or less, 6% to 15%, and greater than 15%, respectively.[23] Compared with the other 2 groups, super-responders were more likely to be female and to have nonischemic cardiomyopathy, lower creatinine, and lower pulmonary artery systolic pressure. Super-responders also had lower baseline LVEF than nonresponders/modest responders (23% vs 26%; P = .05). Improvement in NYHA functional class and LVEDD was greatest in super-responders. By Kaplan-Meier analysis, these patients achieved better survival compared with both nonresponders/modest responders (P<.001) and moderate responders (P = .049). Together with nonischemic HF cause, female sex was associated with a 2-fold increase in the odds of super-response to CRT after adjustment for age, QRS duration, and time from implant to LVEF measurement.[23] Enthusiasm for the findings of this analysis is tempered by (1) the tertiary care nature of the 2 centers in which patients' characteristics may not reflect those of community-dwelling individuals; (2) the definition of super-response, which may explain why more than 50% of the subjects were classified as nonresponders; and (3) the variable times at which pre- and post-CRT LVEF were measured, which makes it difficult to estimate the tempo of reverse remodeling and its association with changes in symptoms.

One study of 212 NYHA class III and IV patients undergoing CRT at a single institution between 1998 and 2008 deserves special mention because it included only patients with true LBBB (QRS ≥120 milliseconds, monophasic QS or rS in V_1, monophasic R wave in V_6) and with nonischemic HF cause.[24] Furthermore, nearly 50% of the subjects were women. Additional unique aspects of this study are that 2 key features of CRT response were examined separately: probability and magnitude of CRT effect. First, the investigators tested whether the response to CRT differs above and below a cut point of QRS length of 150 milliseconds. Second, the relationship of QRS duration to the probability of response was examined across the continuum of the entire QRS duration range. The influence of sex on CRT response was also assessed using QRS duration as both a categorical and a continuous variable. The response to CRT was defined as an increase in LVEF of 5% or greater from baseline to the follow-up echocardiogram, which was done at least 3 months after CRT implant.[24]

Rates of CRT response were greater in women than in men (84% vs 58%; *P*<.001). Women had higher response rates than men at both a QRS duration less than 150 milliseconds (86% vs 36%; *P*<.001) and at a QRS length of 150 milliseconds or greater (83% vs 69%; *P* = .05). These findings indicate that, although the female CRT response was high regardless of QRS length, the male CRT response was significantly higher only at longer QRS durations (*P* = .001). Sex-specific differences were even more striking when the QRS length was analyzed as a continuous variable. Curve profiles differed significantly, with the widest sex disparity found at QRS lengths between 130 and 160 milliseconds. In women, the QRS length-CRT response relationship was nonlinear and a remarkably high probability (≈90%) of CRT response was maintained at QRS durations between approximately 130 and 175 milliseconds. Men, in contrast, exhibited low response rates for QRS lengths less than 140 milliseconds, followed by a progressive improvement in response to CRT with increasing QRS lengths.[24] These findings suggest that, for any given QRS duration, women may have relatively greater electrical dyssynchrony and, thus,

derive greater CRT benefit. This phenomenon is not entirely explained by the fact that normal QRS duration values are 5 to 10 milliseconds shorter in women than in men because even a frameshift of 10 milliseconds would not superimpose the sex curves, which, in this study, followed entirely different trajectories (**Fig. 1**). Thus, any single QRS duration value has different implications in women versus men.[9,25] This point is particularly relevant for midrange QRS values for which CRT prescription is controversial, as reflected by differing recommendations in US versus European practice guidelines. Specifically, indiscriminate adoption of 150-millisecond QRS duration as the threshold for CRT prescription, although correct in men, could deny a life-saving therapy to a large contingent of appropriate female candidates.[17,26–28]

ANALYSES FROM DATABASES

The results of the aforementioned study are corroborated by the analysis of approximately 145,000 US Medicare recipients undergoing CRT-defibrillator (CRT-D) between 2002 and 2008 and followed up for up to 90 months.[11] After controlling for comorbidities, the presence of LBBB was associated with significantly lower all-cause mortality in women than in men (26% vs

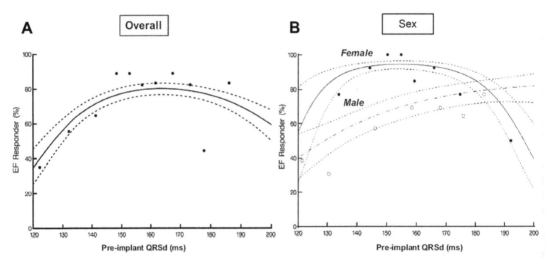

Fig. 1. Probability of CRT response according to QRS duration (QRSd). Parametric model: multivariable logistic regression shown with the corresponding 68% confidence limits (comparable with ± standard deviation). The decile points representing mean percentage of responders according the deciles QRSd are given a crude verification model fit. (*A*) Overall. Closed symbols represent decile points based on the equal number of patients (17 or 18 patients). (*B*) Sex-specific plot based on a patient with baseline LVEDD 6 cm, baseline LEVF 20%, and 2 years from implant to follow-up echocardiography. Each decile point represents an average of approximately 10 patients (*closed symbols women; open symbols men*). Shapes were confirmed by nonparametric modeling. (*From* Varma N, Manne M, Nguyen D, et al. Probability and magnitude of response to cardiac resynchronization therapy according to QRS duration and gender in non-ischemic cardiomyopathy and LBBB. Heart Rhythm 2014;11:1144; with permission.)

15%; $P<.001$). Similar differences occurred in the end point of HF hospitalization or death. Based on these findings, it is possible to conclude that among Medicare beneficiaries receiving CRT-D, LBBB predicts better outcomes in women than in men (**Fig. 2**). One possible explanation for this sex disparity in response to CRT-D is that men may have more false-positive LBBB diagnoses than women. Indeed one study comparing CRT outcomes between patients who met strict LBBB criteria versus those who only met conventional LBBB criteria showed that those meeting the more rigorous LBBB criteria had better echocardiographic responses and longer event-free survival, independent of QRS duration.[29] In fact, recent studies have suggested that use of conventional LBBB criteria misdiagnose up to 30% of patients and that this erroneous classification occurs more frequently in men than in women.[30] Therefore, it is possible that LBBB predicts better outcome in women because, among those diagnosed with LBBB, women more frequently exhibit true dyssynchronous LV activation and are, thus, more likely to benefit from CRT.[11]

Another analysis aimed at assessing mortality by sex in 31,892 CRT-D recipients enrolled in the National Cardiovascular Data Registry between 2006 and 2009 and followed for a median of 2.9 years also showed that, among patients with LBBB, women had a 21% lower mortality risk than men ($P<.001$).[11] Comparison of outcomes in patients with LBBB and a QRS duration of 140 to 149 milliseconds versus those with LBBB and QRS duration of 120 to 129 milliseconds showed that, among individuals with the longer QRS length, the mortality risk decreased by 27% in women and only by 18% in men. When mortality was evaluated in patients with LBBB by 10-millisecond increments in QRS duration, the survival benefit from CRT was extended to shorter QRS durations in women than in men. Importantly, in the non-LBBB population, the mortality risk was similar between sexes regardless of QRS duration[11] (**Fig. 3**). These findings confirm the hypothesis that only with true LBBB the LV lateral wall is activated approximately 100 milliseconds later than the interventricular septum due to the impairment of electrical propagation in the rapidly conducting His-Purkinje system.[13–17] With LBBB, CRT reduces this delay, thereby improving cardiac output and mechanical efficiency.[11] In patients with prolonged QRS duration but without LBBB, LV activation through the His-Purkinje system may not be impaired. These facts may explain the greater CRT benefit in women with LBBB and QRS durations shorter than 150 milliseconds compared with that of men with similar QRS durations but with conduction abnormalities that do not meet the criteria for LBBB[30] (**Fig. 4**).

The key findings of analyses evaluating sex differences in response to CRT in large databases are summarized in **Box 4**.

ANALYSES FROM REGISTRIES

Data from a 2-centers registry of 334 patients with consecutive HF (19.7% women) who underwent CRT showed that, compared with men, women had significantly greater reductions in LV volumes at the 6- and 12-month follow-up ($P<.05$ and $<.001$, respectively) and a significantly higher LVEF (41% vs 34%; $P<.01$) at 1 year.[31] Multiple regression analysis, including sex, age, HF cause, NYHA functional class, QRS duration, baseline left ventricular end-diastolic volume index (LVEDVi), left ventricular end-systolic volume index (LVESVi), LVEF, and use of angiotensin-converting enzyme inhibitors/angiotensin receptor blockers and beta-blockers, revealed that female sex remains independently associated with greater reduction in LVESVi (**Fig. 5**). At the 12-month follow-up, the proportion of responders (defined in terms of LESVi reduction by at least 10%) was higher in women than in men (76.1% vs 59.3%, $P<.05$). Cumulative survival at 1 year was 88% and similar in men and women. Several aspects of this registry analysis deserve mention: (1) Of the 2 participating centers, one was a university hospital and the other a community hospital, which reduces the selection bias associated with the inclusion of only one type of institution. (2) Most patients (94% of men and 96% of women) had LBBB, a factor that eliminates the influence of nonspecific conduction abnormalities on the results of the analysis. (3) At 1 month after CRT implant, *all* patients underwent optimization of atrioventricular (AV) delay, defined as the interval associated with the longest filling time and the best myocardial performance index, eliminating the influence of suboptimal AV delay on CRT response. (4) The multivariable analysis adjusted for the use of antineurohormonal medications, which are themselves associated with reverse remodeling in patients with HF. (5) This analysis is one of the few analyses in which LV volumes were indexed to body surface areas (BSA), a factor that is essential for a meaningful comparison of echocardiographic CRT response between men and women, because females have smaller BSA than men. Because of the unique characteristics of this analysis, it is possible to suggest sex-based differences in physiologic LV remodeling may determine the sex differences in CRT response.[32–40]

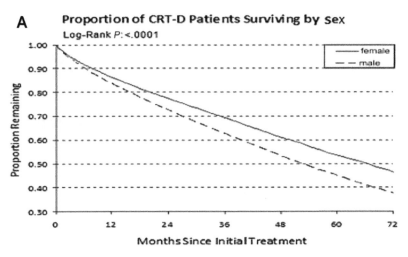

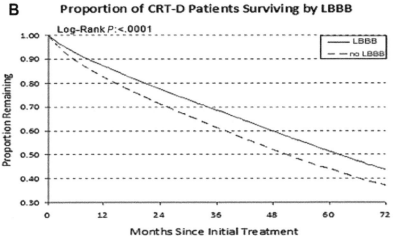

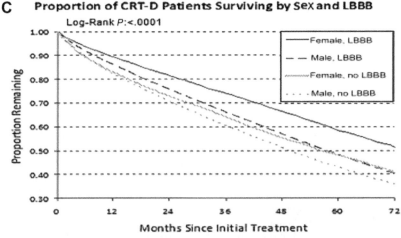

Fig. 2. Kaplan-Meier plots of survival. Results are stratified according to sex (*A*), LBBB (*B*), or both (*C*). Women had better survival than men, and patients with LBBB had better survival than non-LBBB patients. (*From* Loring Z, Canos DA, Selzman K, et al. Left bundle branch block predicts better survival in women than men receiving cardiac resynchronization therapy. JACC Heart Fail 2013;1:240; with permission.)

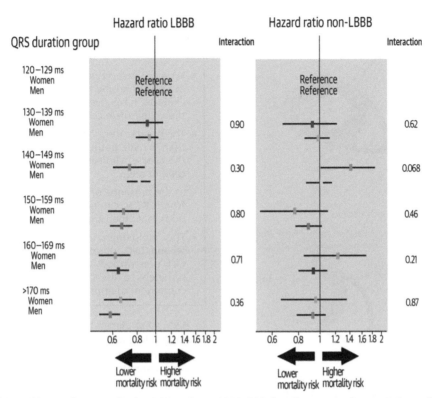

Fig. 3. Multivariable HRs for mortality in LBBB and non-LBBB QRS duration groups by sex. Points reflect HRs for all-cause mortality in LBBB (*left*) and non-LBBB (*right*) in 10 milliseconds. QRS duration groups for men and women. Lines indicate 95% confidence bounds. Sex-by-treatment interaction probability values are reported for every QRS duration category. (*From* Zusterzeel R, Curtis JP, Canos DA, et al. Sex-specific mortality risk by QRS morphology and duration in patients receiving CRT. J Am Coll Cardiol 2014;64:891; with permission.)

In contrast, data from 6994 patients enrolled in the Registry to Improve the Use of Evidence-Based Heart Failure Therapies in the Outpatient Setting (IMPROVE-HF), which analyzed the vital status at 24 months by device status and sex, showed that, after adjustment for baseline patient and practice characteristics, sex was not an independent predictor of CRT outcomes and both sexes exhibited a similar and significant clinical improvement after CRT.[41] Based on their findings, the investigators concluded that device therapies should be offered to all eligible patients with HF, without modification of selection criteria based on sex. The results of this analysis, however, should be interpreted cautiously for the reasons outlined in **Box 5**.

POST HOC ANALYSES OF RANDOMIZED CONTROLLED CLINICAL TRIALS

Earlier CRT trials including the Multicenter InSync Randomized Clinical Evaluation (MIRACLE), the Comparison of Medical Therapy, Pacing and Defibrillation in Heart Failure (COMPANION), and

Cardiac Resynchronization–Heart Failure (CARE-HF), all of which enrolled patients with NYHA functional class III and IV HF, yielded conflicting results on whether women derive greater benefit from CRT than men.[1–3] Although MIRACLE showed a signal for greater CRT benefit in female subjects, the COMPANION and CARE-HF trials revealed no sex-related differences in survival after CRT. None of the aforementioned trials, however, conducted analyses specifically aimed at investigating which factors may be responsible for sex differences in CRT responses and outcomes. The first RCT to do so was the Multicenter Automatic Defibrillator Implantation Trial With Cardiac Resynchronization Therapy (MADIT-CRT) trial, which enrolled patients with milder HF (NYHA functional class I and II).[9] In this study, compared with the 1367 (75%) male patients, the 453 (25%) female patients were more likely to have a nonischemic HF cause (76% vs 36%; P<.001) and LBBB (87% vs 65%; P<.01). Compared with women receiving only ICD therapy, those undergoing CRT-D had a significant 69% reduction in death or HF (P<.001) and a 70% reduction in HF alone

A Normal Conduction

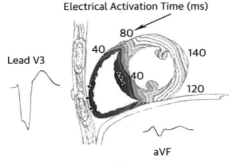

Electrical Activation Time (ms)

B Left Bundle Branch Block

Electrical Activation Time (ms)

Fig. 4. Electrical activation of the ventricle in normal conduction and LBBB. Sagittal view of ventricles in normal conduction (*A*) and LBBB (*B*). Activation starts at the small arrows and spreads in a wave front with each line representing successive 10 milliseconds. The delay between activation of the interventricular septum and free wall is only approximately 40 milliseconds in normal conduction but approximately 100 milliseconds in LBBB. (*From* Strauss DG, Selvester RH, Lima JA, et al. ECG quantification of myocardial scar in cardiomyopathy patients with or without conduction defects: correlation with cardiac magnetic resonance and arrhythmogenesis. Circ Arrhythm Electrophysiol 2008;1(5):327–36; with permission.)

(*P*<.001). In the total population, female CRT-D recipients had a significant 72% reduction in all-cause mortality (*P* = .02), which did not occur in similarly treated men (HR: 1.05; *P* = .83). In women, mortality was further reduced by 82% and 78%, respectively, when QRS duration was 150 milliseconds or greater and LBBB was present. These outcomes did not occur in men. Importantly, sex-by-treatment interactions for mortality reduction were significant at *P*<.05 for death or HF, HF only, and all-cause mortality. Furthermore, the better outcomes observed after CRT-D in women were also associated with consistently greater echocardiographic evidence of reverse cardiac remodeling in female compared with male subjects. These findings are strengthened by the fact that LV volumes were indexed

to BSA, thus eliminating the confounding factor of potentially greater BSA in male than female patients. Two issues pertaining to the MADIT-CRT analysis cannot be ignored: (1) Women had an overall higher likelihood of all device-related adverse events than men (10.5% vs 7.9%; *P* = .001;). (2) Men had higher rates of renal dysfunction, ischemic HF cause, and included a lower percentage of patients taking beta-blockers, all factors that predict a poor prognosis in patients with HF.[9]

In the European cohort of the Resynchronization Reverses Remodeling in Systolic Left Ventricular Dysfunction (REVERSE) trial involving 162 patients (20% female) with NYHA class I and II HF, LVEF of 0.35, or less and QRS of 120 milliseconds or greater, the clinical composite end point of worsened HF was reduced to a similar degree with CRT therapy in women and men.[42] The REVERSE trial, however, had higher LVEF and less prolonged QRS duration criteria for enrollment than the MADIT-CRT study; the power to identify sex differences in outcomes was limited by the trial's small sample size.[5,9]

Additional insights into the differential sex effects of CRT were provided by an analysis of the SMART-AV (SmartDelay determined AV Optimization: A Comparison of AV Optimization Methods Used in Cardiac Resynchronization Therapy) trial, which randomized 980 CRT candidates (32% women) to either optimized electrogram-based AV delays automatically programmed by the CRT device (SmartDelay, Boston Scientific Marlborough, MA), AV delay optimized according to the iterative echocardiography method, or a fixed empirical AV delay of 120 milliseconds.[43] All

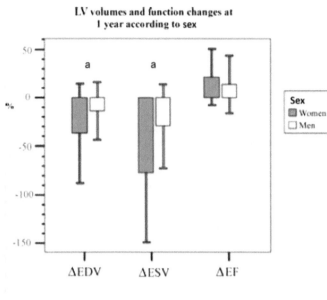

LV volumes and function changes at 1 year according to sex

Sex
▨ Women
☐ Men

ΔEDV   ΔESV   ΔEF

Fig. 5. Changes in LV volume and LVEF from baseline to 12 months. Compared with men, women show significantly greater LVEDV and LVESV reduction without significant difference in LVEF improvement from before to after CRT. LV volumes were indexed to body surface area; [a] P<.01 between men and women. ΔEDV, change in LV end-diastolic volume; ΔESV, change in LV end-systolic volume. (*From* Lilli A, Ricciardi G, Porciani MC, et al. Cardiac resynchronization therapy: gender related differences in left ventricular reverse remodeling. Pacing Clin Electrophysiol 2007;30(11):1352; with permission.)

patients were followed for 6 months. After adjustments for baseline differences, compared with women assigned to a fixed AV interval and to the entire male cohort, female subjects undergoing AV optimization exhibited significantly greater LV volumes reductions, changes that were entirely concentrated in women with NICM. Interestingly, in these patients, AV optimization significantly shortened the sensed AV delay setting from 120 milliseconds to a median programmed AV delay of 100 milliseconds regardless of AV optimization method. In women, but not in men, AV optimization incrementally increased the magnitude of LV

Box 5
The IMPROVE-HF Registry: reasons for caution regarding the conclusions that CRT benefits do not differ by sex

- There was underrepresentation of women, which constituted only 30% of the sample size.
- The average QRS duration was only 134 milliseconds in men and 128 milliseconds in women.
- Information on QRS duration was unavailable for one-third of the population.
- There was no information on whether QRS duration was prolonged because of LBBB or other conduction abnormalities.
- The data provided was inadequate to support the conclusion that the effects of CRT do not differ between sexes.

---

volumes reduction when compared with an empirical AV interval setting. In addition, regardless of inclusion or exclusion of patients with AF/flutter, the mean biventricular pacing percentages were greater for women than for men (99% vs 98%; $P = .003$ and 99% vs 98%; $P = .011$, respectively). The reasons for why the effects of AV optimization in women were more pronounced remain unclear but may be due to inherent differences in atrial geometry and/or PR intervals between men and women.[44] As a group, first-degree AV block was more prevalent in men than in women. Hence, shorter baseline PR intervals in women could have competed with biventricular pacing if the programmed AV interval was inappropriately programmed. Therefore, AV delay optimization may have potentially reduced the number of women with suboptimal resynchronization because of shorter PR intervals promoting intrinsic ventricular activation. The impact of the findings of this analysis on our understanding of potentially greater CRT effects in women than in men is somewhat diminished by the lack of evaluation of outcomes, such as mortality and HF events, absence on information regarding the ventricular ectopy burden, and the short follow-up time (6 months). Similar findings of greater biventricular pacing in women than in men (96% vs 94%; $P<.0004$) were also observed after 2 years of follow-up in the Management of Atrial Fibrillation Suppression in AF-HF Comorbidity Therapy (MASCOT) study, which enrolled NYHA class III/IV patients with a class I CRT indication and examined the effects of an AF suppression algorithm in CRT recipients. In addition, after adjustment for CV history, women had lower all-cause mortality (P = .0007), less cardiac death (P = .04), and fewer HF hospitalizations (P = .01).[45] It should be noted, however, that the MASCOT study was not powered to detect differences in mortality between the two groups assigned to have the AF suppression algorithm either on or off. Furthermore, the study outcomes may have been influenced by significant differences in the percentages of men and woemn receiving CRT-D or CRT-P (CRT-D: men 61% vs women 35% and CRT-P: men 38% vs women 65%; P<.0001). Although women had a greater reduction in LVEDD than did men (−8.2 mm ±11.1 mm vs −1.1 mm ±22.1 mm; P<.02), this finding is inconclusive because LV volumes were not indexed to BSA. Although both sexes improved similarly in NYHA class, women reported greater improvement than men in quality-of-life score (−21.1 ±26.5 vs −16.2 ±22.1, respectively; P<.0001). The reasons why quality of life improved to a greater extent in women than in men, although NYHA improved similarly in the 2 sexes, remain unclear.

META-ANALYSES

A unique meta-analysis was recently conducted by the US Food and Drug Administration (FDA) using pooled data from 3 randomized controlled trials, MADIT-CRT, the Resynchronization-Defibrillation for Ambulatory Heart Failure Trial (RAFT), and REVERSE.[4,5,9,46,47] The restriction to these 3 trials is because the inclusion criteria for the FDA analysis required that the study be a randomized clinical trial comparing CRT-D versus implantable cardioverter defibrillator (ICD) primarily in patients with mild HF (NYHA class II), that it report HF and mortality outcomes, and that individual patient data from the study be available to the FDA as a part of a premarket approval application. The analysis included 4076 patients, 22% of whom were women. The primary and secondary end points of the analysis were time to HF event or death and death alone, respectively. Given the different duration of the 3 trials, follow-up for this analysis was censored at 3 years. In addition to confirming that women benefited from CRT-D more than men, the key finding of this analysis is that the main sex differences occurred in patients with LBBB and a QRS of 130 to 149 milliseconds (**Fig. 6**). In this group, women had a 76% reduction in HF or death (absolute CRT-D to ICD difference, 23%; HR = 0.24, [95% CI, 0.11–0.53]; P<.001) and a 76% reduction in death alone (absolute difference 9%; HR, 0.24, [95%CI, 0.06–0.89]; P = .03), while at the same QRS durations there was no significant

benefit in men for either the primary (P = .38) or secondary end point (P = .60). Importantly, neither women nor men with conventionally diagnosed LBBB benefited from CRT-D at QRS less than 130 milliseconds, but both sexes with LBBB had improved outcomes at QRS durations of 150 milliseconds or greater. These findings are critically important because recent professional guidelines restrict the class I indication for CRT-D to patients with LBBB and QRS of 150 milliseconds or greater and give only a class IIa indication for CRT-D to patients with LBBB and a QRS of 120 to 149 milliseconds. Because women are less likely to receive CRT-D than men are, the present findings argue for the development of sex-specific CRT-D indications.[28] Specifically, based on the results of the FDA meta-analysis, women with LBBB and QRS duration of 120 to 149 milliseconds may deserve advancement to a class I CRT-D indication. However, the FDA meta-analysis summarized earlier only included patients with mild HF; therefore, its findings cannot be extrapolated to patients with more severe HF. This gap has been partially filled by a recent meta-analysis of 27,547 individuals (24.1% women) with mild to severe HF enrolled in 45 controlled and observational studies performed between 2004 and 2014, which were selected by having reported sex-stratified relative risk estimates for all-cause mortality.[48] Even with inclusion of studies conducted on patients with NYHA class III and IV HF, female patients had better outcomes after CRT compared with male patients, with a significant 33% reduction in the risk of death from any cause (HR = 0.67; 95% CI = 0.61–0.74; P<.001), 20% reduction in death or HF hospitalization (HR = 0.80; 95% CI = 0.71–0.90; P<.001), 41% reduction in cardiac death (HR = 0.59; 95% CI = 0.42–0.84; P<.001), as well as a 41% reduction in ventricular arrhythmias or sudden cardiac death (HR = 0.59; 95% CI = 0.49–0.70; P<.001).[48] These more favorable responses to CRT in women were consistently associated with greater echocardiographic evidence of reverse cardiac remodeling than in men. A novel and interesting dimension of this meta-analysis is the finding that the sex-based difference in response to CRT seemed to be more evident in the European cohort than in the American cohort (HR = 0.57; 95% CI = 0.50–0.65 for the European studies vs an HR = 0.70; 95% CI = 0.58–0.80 in the American studies P = .04).[48] The reasons for these geographic differences in CRT response are unknown and deserve further evaluation.

Although significant heterogeneity was observed among the 45 available studies

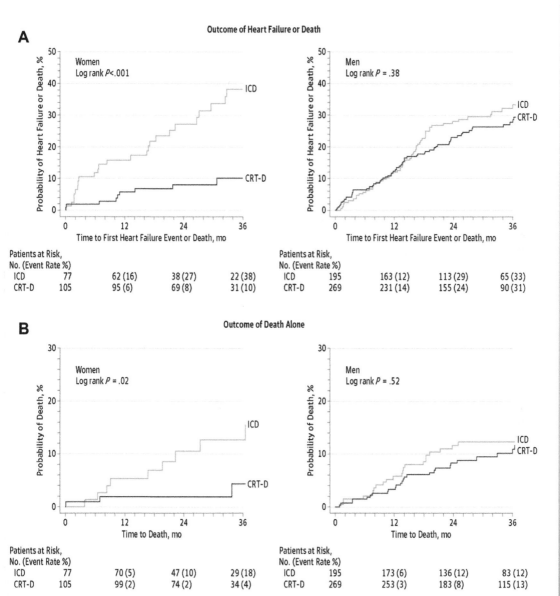

Fig. 6. Kaplan-Meier estimates of heart failure or death (*A*) and death alone (*B*) in LBBB and QRS of 130 to 149 milliseconds stratified by sex. (*From* Zusterzeel R, Selzman KA, Sanders WE, et al. Cardiac resynchronization therapy in women. US Food and DRUG Administration meta-analysis of patient-level data. JAMA Intern Med 2014;174:1345; with permission.)

(I^2 = 29.49%; 95% CI = 0%–51.36%; P = .03), little of it was explained by study design, percentage of women, sample size, number of events, duration of follow-up, average LVEF, whether risk profiles were adjusted, or whether patients with AF were enrolled.

SUMMARY

The beneficial effects of CRT on functional capacity, quality of life, reverse cardiac remodeling, and survival have been conclusively demonstrated in

multiple RCTs. Despite the ubiquitous underrepresentation of women in these trials, as well as in investigations from observational studies, databases, registries, and meta-analyses, most of the data show that CRT produces a greater clinical benefit in women than in men. In some, but not in all, studies female sex remains a predictor of greater response for CRT after adjustment for HF cause, functional limitation, concomitant AF, device type, background medical therapy, and various comorbidities, including diabetes mellitus, renal impairment, and pulmonary arterial hypertension. More difficult is to understand the role of LBBB in influencing sex responses to CRT. In several studies, women have LBBB more frequently than men. In some analyses, female sex remains an independent predictor of response to CRT even after adjusting for QRS configuration, whereas in others it is the presence of LBBB and not sex that is the factor that determines the CRT benefit. One study has shown that LBBB is often misdiagnosed unless stringent electrocardiographic criteria are used and that an erroneous diagnosis of LBBB is made more often in men than in women.[29,30] A frequent and important observation is that women have true LBBB at QRS durations shorter than those of men with LBBB.[11,24,29,46] This phenomenon is not entirely explained by the fact that normal QRS duration values are 5 to 10 milliseconds shorter in women than in men because the trajectories of CRT response by sex are not superimposable. In women, the relationship between QRS duration and CRT response seems to be nonlinear, with remarkably high CRT response rates (90%) being maintained over a wide range of QRS lengths (130–175 milliseconds).[24] In contrast, men exhibit a low CRT response rate at QRS lengths less than 140 milliseconds followed by a progressive increase. Thus, individual QRS durations have different connotations in women versus men. This point is especially relevant for midrange QRS values for which CRT prescription remains controversial. Specifically, the use of a QRS duration of 150 milliseconds as the threshold for recommending CRT, although appropriate in men, could deny a life-saving therapy to many women likely to benefit from CRT.[24,28]

Many elegant studies have shown profound sex differences in myocardial remodeling in response to aging, arterial hypertension, aortic stenosis, myocardial infarction, and HF: compared with men, women generally exhibit greater concentric cardiac hypertrophy and less chamber dilatation and myocyte loss.[32–40] If and how these sex differences in cardiac remodeling influence the response to CRT is unknown, and they should be the focus of future laboratory and clinical investigation.

REFERENCES

1. Abraham WT, Fisher WG, Smith AL, et al, MIRACLE Study Group, Multicenter InSync Randomized Clinical Evaluation. Cardiac resynchronization in chronic heart failure. N Engl J Med 2002;346:1845–53.
2. Bristow MR, Saxon LA, Boehmer J, et al, Comparison of Medical Therapy, Pacing and Defibrillation in Heart Failure (COMPANION) Investigators. Cardiac resynchronization therapy with or without an implantable defibrillator in advanced heart failure. N Engl J Med 2004;350:2140–50.
3. Cleland JG, Daubert JC, Erdmann E, et al, Cardiac Resynchronization-Heart Failure (CARE-HF) Study Investigators. The effect of cardiac resynchronization on morbidity and mortality in heart failure. N Engl J Med 2005;352:1539–49.
4. Moss AJ, Hall WJ, Cannom DS, et al, MADIT-CRT Trial Investigators. Cardiac-resynchronization therapy for the prevention of heart failure events. N Engl J Med 2009;361:1329–38.
5. Linde C, Abraham WT, Gold MR, et al, REVERSE (REsynchronization reVErses Remodeling in Systolic left vEntricular dysfunction) Study Group. Randomized trial of cardiac resynchronization in mildly symptomatic heart failure patients and in asymptomatic patients with left ventricular dysfunction and previous heart failure symptoms. J Am Coll Cardiol 2008;52:1834–43.
6. Leclercq C, Gras D, Le Helloco A, et al. Hemodynamic importance of preserving the normal sequence of ventricular activation in permanent cardiac pacing. Am Heart J 1995;129:1133–41.
7. Hsu JC, Solomon SD, Bourgoun M, et al. Predictors of super-response to cardiac resynchronization therapy and associated improvement in clinical outcome: the MADITCRT (Multicenter Automatic Defibrillator Implantation Trial with Cardiac Resynchronization Therapy) study. J Am Coll Cardiol 2012;59:2366–73.
8. Castellant P, Fatemi M, Bertault-Valls V, et al. Cardiac resynchronization therapy: "nonresponders" and "hyperresponders". Heart Rhythm 2008;5:193–7.
9. Arshad A, Moss AJ, Foster E, et al, MADIT-CRT Executive Committee. Cardiac resynchronization therapy is more effective in women than in men: the MADIT-CRT (Multicenter Automatic Defibrillator Implantation Trial with Cardiac Resynchronization Therapy) trial. J Am Coll Cardiol 2011;57:813–20.
10. Leyva F, Foley PW, Chalil S, et al. Female gender is associated with a better outcome after cardiac resynchronization therapy. Pacing Clin Electrophysiol 2011;34:82–8.
11. Loring Z, Canos DA, Selzman K, et al. Left bundle branch block predicts better survival in women than men receiving cardiac resynchronization therapy. JACC Heart Fail 2013;1:237–44.
12. Sipahi I, Chou JC, Hyden M, et al. Effect of QRS morphology on clinical event reduction with cardiac resynchronization therapy: meta-analysis of randomized controlled trials. Am Heart J 2012;163:260–7.e3.
13. Bilchick KC, Kamath S, DiMarco JP, et al. Bundle-branch block morphology and other predictors of outcome after cardiac resynchronization therapy in Medicare patients. Circulation 2010;122:2022–30.

14. Peterson PN, Greiner MA, Qualls LG, et al. QRS duration, bundle-branch block morphology, and outcomes among older patients with heart failure receiving cardiac resynchronization therapy. JAMA 2013;310:617–26.

15. Rickard J, Bassiouny M, Cronin EM, et al. Predictors of response to cardiac resynchronization therapy in patients with a non-left bundle branch block morphology. Am J Cardiol 2011;108:1576–80.

16. Rickard J, Kumbhani DJ, Gorodeski EZ, et al. Cardiac resynchronization therapy in non-left bundle branch block morphologies. Pacing Clin Electrophysiol 2010;33:590–5.

17. Zareba W, Klein H, Cygankiewicz I, et al, MADIT-CRT Investigators. Effectiveness of cardiac resynchronization therapy by QRS morphology in the Multicenter Automatic Defibrillator Implantation Trial-Cardiac Resynchronization Therapy (MADIT-CRT). Circulation 2011;123:1061–72.

18. Xu YZ, Friedman PA, Webster T, et al. Cardiac resynchronization therapy: do women benefit more than men? J Cardiovasc Electrophysiol 2012;23:172–8.

19. Bleeker GB, Schalij MJ, Boersma E, et al. Does a gender difference in response to cardiac resynchronization therapy exist? Pacing Clin Electrophysiol 2005;28:1271–5.

20. van Campen CM, Visser FC, van der Weerdt AP, et al. FDG PET as a predictor of response to resynchronisation therapy in patients with ischaemic cardiomyopathy. Eur J Nucl Med Mol Imaging 2007;34:309–15.

21. Zabarovskaja S, Gadler F, Braunschweig F, et al. Women have better long-term prognosis than men after cardiac resynchronization therapy. Europace 2012;14:1148–55.

22. Lund LH, Mancini D. Heart failure in women. Med Clin North AM 2004;88:1321–45.

23. Killu AM, Grupper A, Friedman PA, et al. Predictors of outcomes of "super-response" to cardiac resynchronization therapy. J Card Fail 2014;20:379–86.

24. Varma N, Manne M, Nguyen D, et al. Probability and magnitude of response to cardiac resynchronization therapy according to QRS duration and gender in non-ischemic cardiomyopathy and LBBB. Heart Rhythm 2014;11:1139–47.

25. Macfarlane P, Oosterom A, Pahlm O, et al. Normal limits in comprehensive electrocardiology. 2nd edition. London: Springer; 2010. Appendix 1: Adult Normal Limits ISBN:978-1-84882-045-6 (Print); 978-1-84882-046-3 (Online).

26. Stavrakis S, Lazzara R, Thadani U. The benefit of CRT and QRS duration: a meta-analysis. J Cardiovasc Electrophysiol 2012;23:163–8.

27. Dupont M, Rickard J, Baranowski B, et al. Differential response to CRT and clinical outcomes according to QRS morphology and QRS duration. J Am Coll Cardiol 2012;60:592–8.

28. Tracy CM, Epstein AE, Darbar D, et al. 2012ACCF/AHA/HRS focused update of the 2008 guidelines for device-based therapy of cardiac rhythm abnormalities: a report of the ACC/AHA task force on practice guidelines and the Heart Rhythm Society. Circulation 2012;126:1784–800.

29. Mascioli G, Padeletti L, Sassone B, et al. Electrocardiographic criteria of true left bundle branch block; a simple sign to predict a better clinical and instrumental response to CRT. Pacing Clin Electrophysiol 2012;35:927–33.

30. Strauss DG, Selvester RH, Wagner GS. Defining left bundle branch block in the era of cardiac resynchronization therapy. Am J Cardiol 2011;107:927–34.

31. Lilli A, Ricciardi G, Porciani MC, et al. Cardiac resynchronization therapy: gender related differences in left ventricular reverse remodeling. PACE 2007;30:1349–55.

32. Olivetti G, Giordano G, Corradi D, et al. Gender differences and aging: effects on the human heart. J Am Coll Cardiol 1995;26:1068–79.

33. Carroll JD, Carroll EP, Feldman T, et al. Sex-associated differences in left ventricular function in aortic stenosis of the elderly. Circulation 1992;86:1099–107.

34. Kostkiewicz M, Tracz W, Olszowska M, et al. Left ventricular geometry and function in patients with aortic stenosis: gender differences. Int J Cardiol 1999;71:57–61.

35. Bella JN, Palmieri V, Wachtell K, et al. Sex-related difference in regression of left ventricular hypertrophy with antihypertensive treatment: the LIFE study. J Hum Hypertens 2004;18:411–6.

36. Gerdts E, Zabalgoitia M, Bjornstad H, et al. Gender differences in systolic left ventricular function in hypertensive patients with electrocardiographic left ventricular hypertrophy (the LIFE study). Am J Cardiol 2001;87:980–3.

37. Tamura T, Said S, Gerdes AM. Gender-related differences in myocyte remodeling in progression to heart failure. Hypertension 1999;33:676–80.

38. Luchner A, Brockel U, Muscholl M, et al. Gender-specific differences of cardiac remodeling in subjects with left ventricular dysfunction: a population-based study. Cardiovasc Res 2002;53:720–7.

39. Crebbe DL, Dipla K, Ambati S, et al. Gender differences in postinfarction hypertrophy in end-stage failing hearts. J Am Coll Cardiol 2003;41:300–6.

40. Guerra S, Leri A, Wang X, et al. Myocyte death in the failing human heart is gender dependent. Circ Res 1999;85:856–66.

41. Wilcox JE, Fonarow GC, Zhang Y, et al. Clinical effectiveness of cardiac resynchronization and implantable cardioverter-defibrillator therapy in men and women with heart failure; findings from IMPROVE-HF. Circ Heart Fail 2014;7:146–53.

42. Daubert C, Gold MR, Abraham WT, et al. Prevention of disease progression by cardiac resynchronization therapy in patients with asymptomatic or mildly symptomatic left ventricular dysfunction: insights from the European cohort of the REVERSE (Resynchronization Reverses Remodeling in Systolic Left Ventricular Dysfunction) trial. J Am Coll Cardiol 2009;54:1837–46.

43. Cheng A, Gold M, Waggoner AD, et al. Potential mechanisms underlying the effect of gender on response to cardiac resynchronization therapy: insights from the SMART-AV multicenter trial. Heart Rhythm 2012;9(5):736–41.

44. D'Andrea A, Scarafile R, Riegler L, et al. Right atrial size and deformation in patients with dilated cardiomyopathy undergoing cardiac resynchronization therapy. Eur J Heart Fail 2009;11:1169–77.

45. Schubert A, Muto C, Maounis T, et al. Gender-related safety and efficacy of cardiac resynchronization therapy. Clin Cardiol 2013;36:683–90.

46. Zusterzeel R, Selzman KA, Sanders WE, et al. Cardiac resynchronization therapy in women. US Food and DRUG Administration meta-analysis of patient-level data. JAMA Intern Med 2014;174: 1340–8.

47. Tang AS, Wells GA, Talajic M, et al, Resynchronization-Defibrillation for Ambulatory Heart Failure Trial Investigators. Cardiac resynchronization therapy for mild-to-moderate heart failure. N Engl J Med 2010;363:2385–95.

48. Cheng YJ, Zhang J, Li WJ, et al. More favorable response to cardiac resynchronization therapy in women than in men. Circ Arrhythm Electrophysiol 2014;7:807–15.

How to Improve CRT Benefit on Atrial Fibrillation Patients

Atrial Fibrillation During Cardiac Resynchronization Therapy

Mariëlle Kloosterman, BSc, Alexander H. Maass, MD, PhD, Michiel Rienstra, MD, PhD, Isabelle C. Van Gelder, MD, PhD*

KEYWORDS

- Implantation • Biventricular pacing • Heart failure • Atrioventricular junction ablation

KEY POINTS

- Atrial fibrillation (AF) has a high prevalence (20%–40%) among patients with heart failure (HF) receiving cardiac resynchronization therapy (CRT).
- Randomized data on success of CRT in patients with AF are sparse and in part come from patients undergoing atrioventricular junction (AVJ) ablation for untreatable AF rather than from patients with HF and AF.
- Every effort should be made to assess success of biventricular (BiV) pacing.

INTRODUCTION

More than 2 decades of research has established CRT as one of the most exciting advancements in HF treatment. CRT improves left ventricular (LV) function by restoring intraventricular, interventricular, and atrioventricular dyssynchrony thereby conferring symptomatic relief and survival benefits to most recipients.[1–5] CRT has an established role as an efficacious and safe device-based, nonpharmacologic approach for patients with HF, impaired LV function (left ventricular ejection fraction [LVEF] ≤35%), electrical dyssynchrony (QRS duration ≥120 ms), sinus rhythm, and optimal medical therapy. However, optimal CRT use in patients with HF and AF, an important subgroup of patients, remains uncertain.

AF and HF can be characterized as the twin epidemics of modern cardiovascular medicine. AF is the most common arrhythmia in patients with HF, with the prevalence of AF in patients with HF ranging from 10% to 15% in New York Heart Association (NYHA) class II to up to 50% in NYHA class IV[6] and with the incidence of new-onset atrial tachyarrhythmias (ATs) and AF ranging from 20% to 40% according to CRT device diagnostics.[7] The latest European Society of Cardiology (ESC) guidelines and American College of Cardiology Foundation/American Heart Association/Heart Rhythm Society (ACCF/AHA/HRS) guidelines consider patients with permanent AF as eligible to receive CRT (class II A, level of evidence B) (**Table 1**).[8,9] However, guidelines about heart rate control during AF, that is, drug therapy, or ablation in the heterogeneous group of patients with AF undergoing CRT, and recommendations about nonpermanent AF, are missing.

This review gives an overview of the barriers during CRT and the current literature (**Table 2**) on the effect of CRT in patients with AF. These barriers include the occurrence of new or recurrent

Disclosures: Dr I.C. Van Gelder reports receiving grant support for the institution from Medtronic, Biotronik, and St. Jude Medical. Dr A.H. Maass reports receiving lecture fees from Biotronik, Boston Scientific, Medtronic, Sorin, and St. Jude Medical.
Department of Cardiology, Thoraxcenter, University Medical Center Groningen, PO Box 30.001, 9700 RB Groningen, The Netherlands
* Corresponding author.
E-mail address: i.c.van.gelder@umcg.nl

cardiacEP.theclinics.com

Table 1
Clinical practice recommendations to CRT in patients with permanent atrial fibrillation issued by the European Society of Cardiology in collaboration with the European Heart Rhythm Association

Recommendations	Class	Level
Patients with HF, wide QRS, and reduced LVEF		
CRT should be considered in patients with chronic HF, intrinsic QRS ≥120 ms, and LVEF ≤35% who remain in NYHA functional class III and ambulatory IV despite adequate medical treatment, provided that a BiV pacing as close to 100% as possible can be achieved	IIa	B
AV junction ablation should be added in case of incomplete BiV pacing	IIa	B
Patients with uncontrolled heart rate who are candidates for AV junction ablation		
CRT should be considered in patients with reduced LVEF who are candidates for AV junction ablation for rate control	IIa	B

Abbreviations: AV, atrioventricular; BiV, biventricular; CRT, cardiac resynchronization therapy; HF, heart failure; LVEF, left ventricular ejection fraction; NYHA, New York Heart Association.

From European Society of Cardiology (ESC), European Heart Rhythm Association (EHRA), Brignole M, et al. 2013 ESC guidelines on cardiac pacing and cardiac resynchronization therapy. Europace 2013;15(8):1097; with permission of Oxford University Press (UK) (c) European Society of Cardiology, www.escardio.org.

AF and other ATs that hamper CRT response due to the inability to continuously pace the ventricles. Finally, the role of AVJ ablation is discussed.

DETRIMENTAL EFFECT OF ATRIAL FIBRILLATION ON RESPONSE TO CARDIAC RESYNCHRONIZATION THERAPY

AF and ATs have a high prevalence in real-world patients with CRT. In recent CRT trials, the cumulative incidence of new-onset AF/ATs ranged between 20% and 40% according to device interrogations[10–15] (**Table 3**).

The incidence of new-onset AT/AF is important because it can be associated with less response to CRT and more cardiac adverse events during long-term follow-up. Buck and colleagues[16]

showed that in 114 consecutive patients of whom 56 (49%) had (prior) AF (23 AF present at implantation of CRT and 33 a prior history of AF) and 58 who had no history of AF, new-onset AF occurred in 14 (24%) patients during a median follow-up of 18 months. New-onset AF was associated with a lower response (4 [29%] responders versus 10 [71%] nonresponders, $P = .02$), with response being defined as a decrease in LV end-systolic volume greater than or equal to 10%.

Episodes with AT/AF are regularly recurring phenomena. During a median follow-up of 13 months, AT/AF episodes of greater than 10 min occurred in 361 (30%) of 1193 patients.[17] Device-detected AT/AF lead to a higher risk of all-cause mortality (ACM) or HF hospitalizations (hazard ratio [HR], 2.16; $P = .032$) (**Fig. 1**). These AT/AF episodes can also lead to uncontrolled ventricular rates. During a median follow-up of 18 months, 443 of 1404 patients with HF experienced episodes of AF, being uncontrolled in 34% (**Fig. 2**).[14] Suboptimal CRT delivery with BiV pacing less than 95% was significantly and inversely correlated to ventricular heart rate, decreasing by 7% for each 10-beats-per-minute increase in ventricular rate. Uncontrolled ventricular rate was associated with HF hospitalizations and ACM (HR, 1.69; 95% confidence interval [CI], 1.01–2.83; $P = .046$).

A large retrospective, cross-sectional analysis of 80,768 patients, using the Medtronic Discovery Link database, showed that BiV pacing less than 98% was observed in 40.7% of patients.[18] Among those with suboptimal pacing, AT/AF was the most common reason for loss of BiV pacing, with the contribution of AT/AF to the loss of CRT increasing with lesser percentages of BiV pacing (**Fig. 3**). Comparably, in another retrospective, observational analysis of the Discovery Link database including only patients with an atrial lead for AF diagnostics and device programming with the intent of achieving continuous BiV pacing, 8686 (8%) of 54,019 patients included had persistent or permanent AF. Nearly half (47%) of the patients with persistent AF had less than 90% BiV pacing during AF. Relative to patients with high BiV pacing, patients with moderate (90%–98%) BiV pacing had a 20% increase in mortality rate (HR, 1.20; 95% CI, 1.15–1.26; $P<.001$), and the patients who received low (<90%) BiV pacing had a 32% increase in mortality rate (HR, 1.32, 95% CI, 1.23–1.41; $P<.001$).

Hayes and colleagues[19] observed that patients with AF were able to experience only similar survival rates as patients in sinus rhythm if the ventricular heart rate could be successfully suppressed and the BiV pacing rates exceeded 98.5%.

But how can the effective percentage of BiV pacing be assessed? There is often discrepancy

Table 2
Overview studies

Trial Name	Year	Study Design	Treatment	Underlying Rhythm	No. of Patients	Follow-up Duration (mo)	Mean Age (y)	Male Sex (%)	AVJ Ablation (%)	NYHA Class (%) II	III	IV	Mean LVEF (%)	Mean QRS (ms)	Soft End Points	Hard End Points
ICD vs CRT-D																
RAFT[26]	2012	RCT	ICD vs CRT-ICD	Perm. AF	115 114	40	72 70	85 90	0.4	75 69	— —	— —	23 22	151 153	No difference in 6MWD or QoL score	No difference in ACM or HF hospitalization
MADIT-CRT Substudy, Ruwald et al[27]	2015	RCT	ICD vs CRT-ICD ≤90% BiV 91%–96% BiV ≥97% BiV	—	520 80 134 485	37	64 66 67 63	70 72 71 67	—	88 90 87 89	— — — —	— — — —	29 29 29 29	164 160 161 164	—	Risk of ACM reduced by 52% in BiV ≥97% (HR, 0.48, P<.016), compared with patients with ICD. No difference if ≤90% BiV pacing
MADIT-CRT Substudy, Ruwald et al[28]	2014	RCT	ICD or CRT-D	No history AT/AF History AT/AF	1101 (668 CRT-D) 140 (51 CRT-D)	37	64 67	68 81	—	59 37	— —	— —	29 28	162 168	—	CRT-D associated with 57% risk reduction of HF and ACM compared with ICD only in patients with in-trial AT (HR, 0.43, 95% CI, 0.19–0.99, P = .047) and in-trial AF (HR, 0.30; 95% CI, 0.10–0.87, P = .027)
BiV pacing vs RV pacing																
MUSTIC-AF[29]	2002	Crossover	3 mo BiV pacing and 3 mo RV pacing	Perm. AF	43	6	65	81	63	—	100	—	26	209	Effective BiV improved 6MWD with 32 m (Δ9.3%, P = .05) and peak VO$_2$ with 1.7 mL/kg/min (Δ13%, P = .04) compared with VVIR	—

(continued on next page)

Table 2
(continued)

Trial Name	Year	Study Design	Treatment	Underlying Rhythm	No. of Patients	Follow-up Duration (mo)	Mean Age (y)	Male Sex (%)	AVJ Ablation (%)	NYHA Class (%) II	III	IV	Mean LVEF (%)	Mean QRS (ms)	Soft End Points	Hard End Points
PAVE[30]	2005	RCT	RV pacing	AF	81	24	67	64	100	46	29	—	45	—	Increase in 6MWD (+31% vs +24%, P = .04) and LVEF (46% vs 41%, P = .03) in BiV pacing compared with RV pacing	—
			BiV pacing	AF	103	21	70	63	100	54	33	—	47	—		
Brignole et al[31]	2011	Prosp.	RV pacing	AF	89	20	72	73	100	—	53	37			—	Composite end point of HF death, HF hospitalization or worsening HF occurred significantly less often in CRT; HR, 0.37, 95% CI, 0.12–0.5, P = .001
			BiV pacing	AF	97		72	67	100	—	45	38				
AF vs sinus rhythm																
Molhoek et al[33]	2004	Prosp.	CRT	SR	30	25	68	80	0	—	—	—	23	180	Both groups improved in NYHA, QoL, and 6MWD. SR more often improved in NYHA class (80% vs 64%, P<.05)	CM between SR and AF not different (10% vs 23%, P = .07)
				Perm. AF	30	19	63	90	57	—	—	—	20	205		
Delnoy et al[34]	2006	Prosp.	CRT	SR	167	23	72	68	0	19	64	15	22	171	Changes in NYHA class, 6MWD, QoL, and LVEF were similar	No difference in survival in SR (10.2%) vs AF (7.3%, P = .34)
				Pers. or Perm. AF	96		73	75	22	22	63	14	25	171		

Study	Year	Design	Therapy	Group	N	FU (mo)								Echocardiographic/functional outcome	Comments
SPARE[36]	2008	Retrosp.	CRT	SR	344	12	67	76	0	—	73	25		166	Improvement in QoL, 6MWD, and left ventricular reverse remodeling comparable	HF death at 12 mo higher in AF (17/126; 13.5%) than SR (14/344; 4.1%; P<.001). Perm AF independent predictor for HF death (HR, 5.4; 95% CI, 1.9–15.1)
				AF	126		69	81	15	—	89	26		170		
Effect of AVJ ablation															
Gasparini et al[37]	2006	Prosp.	CRT	SR	511	25	63	77	0	—	90	26		165	AF + AVJ group only showed improvement of LVEF (P<.001), LVESV (P<.001), and exercise capacity (P<.001)	—
				AF + drugs	48		64	83	0	—	100	25		172		
				AF + AVJ	114		67	87	100	—	96	27		162		
Gasparini et al[38]	2008	Prosp.	CRT	SR	1042	34	63	75	0	6	79	15	24	170	—	Patients with AF similar adjusted HR for ACM and CM (HR, 0.9; 95% CI, 0.57–1.42, P = .64) and (HR, 0.64; 95% CI, 0.66–1.66, P = .99) as SR In AF + AVJ significant improved overall survival compared with AF + drugs (HR, 0.26; 95% CI, 0.09–0.73, P = .010) for ACM (HR, 0.31; 95% CI, 0.10–0.99, P = .048) for CM and (HR, 0.15; 95% CI, 0.03–0.70, P = .016) for HF death
				AF + drugs	25		66	78	0	3	81	16	25	168		
				AF + AVJ	118		67	86	100	5	78	17	27	155		

(continued on next page)

Table 2
(continued)

Trial Name	Year	Study Design	Treatment + Underlying Rhythm — Treatment	Treatment + Underlying Rhythm — Underlying Rhythm	No. of Patients	Follow-up Duration (mo)	Mean Age (y)	Male Sex (%)	AVJ Ablation (%)	NYHA Class (%) II	NYHA Class (%) III	NYHA Class (%) IV	Mean LVEF (%)	Mean QRS (ms)	Outcome — Soft End Points	Outcome — Hard End Points
CERTIFY[39]	2013	Prosp.	CRT	SR	6046	37	66	78	0	—	74	26	—	158	—	Long-term survival in AF + AVJ similar to SR (P = NS). ACM (HR, 1.52; 95% CI, 1.26–1.82, P = .52) and CM (HR, 0.88; 95% CI, 0.66–1.17, P = .39) higher for AF + drugs, both compared SR and AF + AVJ groups (both P<.001)
				AF + drugs	895		70	85	0	—	83	26	—	155		
				AF + AVJ	443		68	84	100	—	85	27	—	159		
Dong et al[40]	2010	Prosp.	CRT-D	Medical therapy only	109	9	72	87	0	—	—	—	23	175	Improvement in NYHA class higher in +AVJ ablation than drugs group (−0.7 ± 0.8 vs −0.4 ± 0.8, P = .04)	AVJ ablation independently associated with survival benefit from ACM (HR, 0.13; 95% CI, 0.03–0.58, P = .007) and from combined ACM, heart transplant, and left ventricular assist device (HR, 0.19; 95% CI, 0.06–0.62, P = .006)
				AVJ ablation	45		68	84	100	—	—	—	26	161		

Abbreviations: 6MWD, 6-minute walking distance; ACM, all-cause mortality; BiV, biventricular; CERTIFY, Cardiac Resynchronization Therapy in Atrial Fibrillation Patients Multinational Registry; CM, cardiac mortality; ICD, implantable cardioverter defibrillator; LVESV, left ventricular end-systolic volume; MADIT-CRT, Multicenter Automatic Defibrillator Implantation Trial-Cardiac Resynchronization Therapy; PAVE, Left Ventricular-Based Cardiac Stimulation Post AV Nodal Ablation Evaluation; Perm., permanent; Pers., persistent; Prosp., prospective; QoL, quality of life; RAFT, Resynchronization for Ambulatory Heart Failure Trial; Retrosp., retrospective; RV, right ventricular; SPARE, Spanish Atrial Fibrillation and Resynchronization study; SR, sinus rhythm.

Data from Refs.[26–40]

Table 3
The incidence of new or recurrent AT/AF based on device diagnostics

Study	Year	Mean LVEF (%)	Patients (%) with New or Recurrent AF/AT Based on Device Diagnostics
Leclerq et al[10]	2010	25	21
Borleffs et al[11]	2009	23	25
Marijon et al[12]	2010	25	27
Caldwell et al[13]	2009	25	27
Boriani et al[14]	2011	27	32
Puglisi et al[15]	2008	27	42

Data from Refs.[10–15]

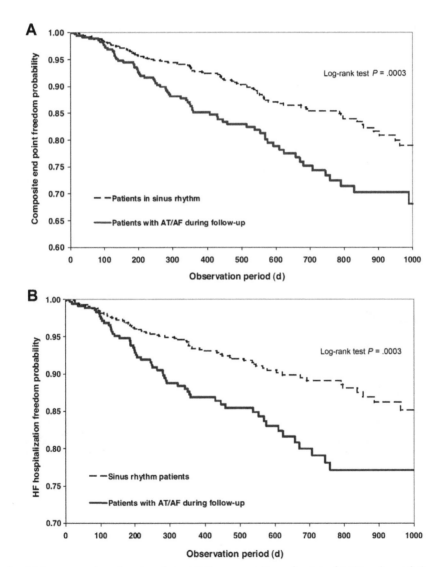

Fig. 1. Kaplan-Meier curves show freedom from (A) the composite end point of ACM or heart failure (HF) hospitalization or (B) HF hospitalization for patients with atrial tachycardia or atrial fibrillation (AT/AF) (red lines) versus patients without AT/AF (black lines) during follow-up. (From Santini M, Gasparini M, Landolina M, et al. Device-detected atrial tachyarrhythmias predict adverse outcome in real-world patients with implantable biventricular defibrillators. J Am Coll Cardiol 2011;57(2):171; with permission of Elsevier.)

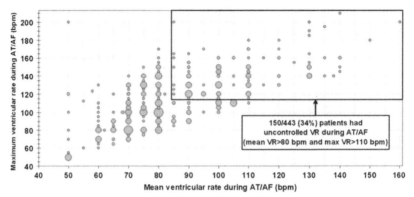

Fig. 2. Maximum ventricular rate (VR) during atrial fibrillation as a function of mean VR during atrial fibrillation. Each point represents 1 patient; in case multiple patients have same VR values, the dimension of the point represents the number of patients with equal data. The black box outlines the patients with uncontrolled VR (mean VR >80 beats per minute [bpm] and maximum VR >110 bpm). (*From* Boriani G, Gasparini M, Landolina M, et al. Incidence and clinical relevance of uncontrolled ventricular rate during atrial fibrillation in heart failure patients treated with cardiac resynchronization therapy. Eur J Heart Fail 2011;13(8):871; with permission of John Wiley & Sons.)

between the percentage of BiV pacing that is recorded by the device and the actual true BiV capture.[20] Often during AF, BiV pacing is artificially high because of invalid counting of fusion and pseudo–fusion complexes. One way to assess effective BiV pacing is by performing an exercise test. Loss of BiV pacing may become apparent as it can be easily detected on the electrocardiograms (ECGs). Maass and colleagues[21] showed

the importance of exercise tests to guarantee better response to CRT. Their retrospective study involved 114 consecutive patients. At moderate exercise, defined as 25% of the maximal exercise tolerance, that is, comparable to daily life exercise, nonresponders frequently exceeded the upper rate of the device (13 [22%] vs 2 [3%], *P*<.0001). The influence of heart rate exceeding the upper rate of the device was restricted to patients with

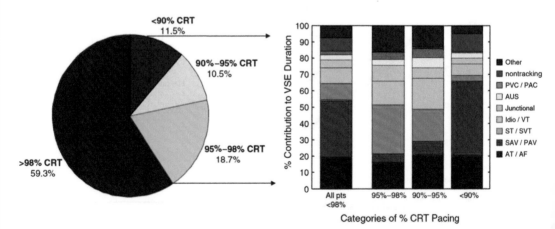

Fig. 3. (*Left*) The percentage of biventricular cardiac resynchronization therapy (CRT) pacing for 80,768 patients. (*Right*) The reasons for ventricular sensing episodes (VSEs) plotted according to the severity of CRT pacing loss. AUS, atrial undersensing with appropriate ventricular sensing; Idio/VT, idioventricular rhythm, ventricular tachyarrhythmia, or ventricular oversensing; PAC, premature atrial contraction; pts, patients; PVC, premature ventricular contraction; ST/SVT, sinus tachycardia or supraventricular tachycardia that exceeded the upper tracking rate; sensed atrioventricular (SAV)/paced atrioventricular (PAV) interval: intrinsic AV conduction was faster than the programmed sensed or paced AV delays; atrial tachycardia (AT)/atrial fibrillation (AF): 10 or more consistent beats without CRT that occurred during AT/AF. (*From* Cheng A, Landman SR, Stadler RW. Reasons for loss of cardiac resynchronization therapy pacing: insights from 32 844 patients. Circ Arrhythm Electrophysiol 2012;5(5):886; with permission of Wolters Kluwer Health, Inc.)

AF. The percentage of BiV pacing recorded by the device was marginally but significantly lower in patients in whom the heart rate exceeded the sensor rate of the device during minimal exercise (99% [60–100] vs 98% [37–100], P = .003). These patients exceeding the upper rate at moderate exercise probably also more frequently exceed the upper rate during their daily activities. Close examination of exercise tests and subsequent adequate reprogramming of the device, increasing rate controlling drug dosages, or performing AVJ ablation may prevent this problem.

Device diagnostics and programming are essential to define AF burden and maintain BiV pacing. The Clinical Effect of Heart Failure Management via Home Monitoring with a Focus on Atrial Fibrillation (EFFECT) study (ClinicalTrials.gov Identifier: NCT00811382) will assess whether management of AF as well as the early optimization of CRT via home monitoring decreases mortality and morbidity compared with conventional treatment in subjects with a standard indication for CRT with implantable cardioverter defibrillator (ICD) backup and AF.

Another important consequence of AF may be inappropriate shocks. Appropriate shocks have been described to occur more often in patients with AF.[22–24] In a large observational cohort including 106,513 patients receiving dual-chamber ICD or CRT devices, a total of 22,062 patients (21%) received shocks. AF with rapid ventricular rate was present in 11% of all patients. In the 43,962 patients with CRT-D, a higher proportion of patients with AF with rapid ventricular rate (37%) received shocks compared with patients with AF without rapid ventricular rate (20%) or those without AF (14%) (P<.001).[25]

In a single-center retrospective study following 223 patients receiving a CRT-D without a history of AF, 55 (25%) developed AF during a follow-up of 33 ± 16 months. The average AF burden was 6.7%. Patients who developed AF more often experienced appropriate (27% vs 16%, P<.05) as well as inappropriate shocks (31% vs 6%, P<.001). They were also more often hospitalized (36% vs 18%, P<.005).[11]

STUDIES INVESTIGATING THE BENEFICIAL EFFECT OF CARDIAC RESYNCHRONIZATION THERAPY IN THE PRESENCE OF ATRIAL FIBRILLATION

A substudy from the Resynchronization for Ambulatory Heart Failure Trial (RAFT) is the only randomized study to compare CRT with intrinsic conduction, rather than right ventricular (RV) pacing, in patients with permanent AF and HF. Of the 1798 patients enrolled in the RAFT study, 229 patients had permanent AF at baseline and were randomized to either an ICD or an ICD + CRT.[26] Only 1 patient received an AVJ ablation. Patients with permanent AF, who were otherwise CRT candidates, appeared to gain minimal benefit from CRT-ICD compared with a standard ICD because no difference in total mortality rates between the 2 groups was found (see **Table 2**). However, there was a trend for fewer HF hospitalizations in the ICD + CRT group (HR, 0.58; 95% CI, 0.38–1.01; P = .052). This was a prespecified subanalysis of the RAFT trial that was not powered to rule out moderate-sized treatment effects. Also, suboptimal pacing (<95%) occurred in two-thirds of patients.

In a substudy from the Multicenter Automatic Defibrillator Implantation Trial-Cardiac Resynchronization Therapy (MADIT-CRT) including 1219 patients with a left bundle branch block, the association between BiV pacing and CRT efficacy, when compared with ICD, on outcome was studied.[27] During a median follow-up of 3.1 years, the risk of death was reduced by 52% in patients with CRT-D with BiV pacing greater than or equal to 97% when compared with patients with ICD, again highlighting the importance of assessment of efficacious BiV pacing. Another substudy of MADIT-CRT[28] analyzed the benefit of CRT-D in patients with AT/AF. The percentage of patients who received BiV pacing greater than or equal to 92% was not different between patients with in-trial AT/AF (87.5%) and patients without in-trial AT/AF (90.2%; P = .43) The benefit of CRT-D was not attenuated because of in-trial AT/AF, CRT-D was associated with a 57% risk reduction of ACM compared with ICD only in patients with in-trial AT, and similar results were found among patients who had in-trial AF.

The Multisite Stimulation in Cardiomyopathies (MUSTIC)-AF trial[29] was the first to evaluate CRT in 59 patients with both permanent AF and a need for ventricular pacing using a single, blind, crossover design. Patients were monitored during two 3-month treatment periods of conventional VVIR (single-chamber ventricular demand pacing) versus BiV pacing. The study had a high dropout rate (42%); only 37 patients completed both crossover phases. Effective BiV pacing (defined as >75%) improved 6-minute walking distance (6MWD) and peak oxygen uptake (V_{O2}).

The Left Ventricular-Based Cardiac Stimulation Post AV Nodal Ablation Evaluation (PAVE) study[30] compared chronic BiV pacing with RV pacing in patients undergoing AVJ ablation for management of AF with rapid ventricular heart rate, thus not in the setting of severe HF. In patients with BiV pacing, 6MWD improved significantly when compared with right-ventricular pacing. (+31% vs +24%, P = .04) In addition, LVEF was significantly greater (46 vs 41%, P = .03). These effects seemed most beneficial in patients with impaired systolic function or symptomatic HF.

The group from Brignole reported similar findings.[31] They examined whether CRT was superior to conventional RV pacing in reducing HF events in patients with severely symptomatic permanent AF undergoing AVJ ablation. A total of 186 patients were followed up for a median duration of 20 months. The composite end point of cardiac mortality (CM), HF hospitalization or worsening HF, occurred significantly less often in the CRT group.

In a follow-up study of the MUSTIC trial,[32] 33 patients with AF and 42 patients in sinus rhythm were followed longitudinally at 9 and 12 months. At the 9- and 12-month follow-up, all patients in sinus rhythm and 88% of patients in the AF group were programmed to BiV pacing. Patients with AF, of whom 63% had undergone a previous AVJ ablation, were able to experience results comparable with those in sinus rhythm. Compared with baseline they had increased 6MWD (55 m, P = .004), improved quality of life (QoL) with a reduction of 14 points in the Minnesota score (P = .002), an improved NYHA class by 0.8 (P = .0001), and improved LVEF (+4%) after CRT.

In a small study, Molhoek and colleagues[33] compared the effect of CRT in 30 patients in sinus rhythm with 30 patients with permanent AF. In 28 patients (15 with sinus rhythm and 13 with AF), a conventional indication existed for an ICD. These patients received a combined device. NYHA class, QoL, and 6MWD improved significantly in the 2 groups after 6 months. There was no difference in clinical improvement between patients with AF with (57%) and without AVJ ablation. However, in patients with AF with no AVJ ablation, the percentage of ventricular pacing was significantly lower (82% vs 100%, P<.05).

Delnoy and colleagues[34] studied the usefulness of CRT in 96 patients with HF and AF versus 167 patients with HF and sinus rhythm. About 21% of patients with AF had an AVJ ablation at baseline. NYHA class, 6MWD, QoL scores, and LVEF improved significantly after 3 and 12 months in both groups, and changes were similar. ACM rates were comparable.

The Cardiac Resynchronisation in Heart Failure (CARE-HF) trial[5] was a multicenter, randomized trial that compared the effect of standard pharmacologic therapy alone with that of a combination of standard therapy and CRT. Mean follow-up duration was 29.4 months. A retrospective analysis of the CARE-HF trial focused on the effect of new-onset AF on the outcome and efficacy of CRT. The incidence of AF was assessed by adverse event reporting and by ECG during follow-up, not by continuous monitoring as is performed by the device nowadays. AF was documented in 124 of 813 (15%) patients, 66 in the CRT group and 58 in the medical therapy only group. In the entire study group, development of AF was associated with an increased rate of ACM or unplanned hospitalization for a major cardiovascular event (HR, 2.00; 95% CI, 1.58–2.54; P<.0001). New-onset AF, however, was not independently associated with an increased risk of ACM (HR, 1.17; 95% CI, 0.82–1.67; P = .37). The effect of CRT was not modified by new episodes of AF (P value for interaction, .74).[35]

In the Spanish Atrial Fibrillation and Resynchronization (SPARE) study,[36] the benefits and mortality in patients with AF or sinus rhythm undergoing CRT were compared. The cumulative percentage of ventricular pacing in the AF group was 94% ± 8% at 12 months. AF was reported as an independent risk factor for mortality from HF after CRT implantation, despite similar functional improvement and remodeling as those in sinus rhythm.

The most important contributions to this field came from studies by Gasparini and colleagues.[37] They studied the role of AVJ ablation in patients with permanent AF and HF during CRT. The decision whether to perform AVJ ablation or not depended on the percentage of BiV pacing, based on device interrogation at 2 months follow-up, whereby 85% or less BiV pacing was the cutoff value for performing an AVJ ablation. During long-term follow-up, up to 4 years, patients with permanent AF showed large and sustained improvements of LV function and functional capacity, similar to patients in sinus rhythm. However, this occurred only in the group of patients with AF that underwent AVJ ablation.

Data from 2008, including 1285 consecutive patients of whom 243 had AF (49% AVJ ablation) and 1042 sinus rhythm, showed that between patients with sinus rhythm and AF, adjusted HRs were similar for ACM and CM. However, AVJ ablation significantly improved overall survival compared with optimal medical rate control therapy alone.[38]

The Cardiac Resynchronization Therapy in Atrial Fibrillation Patients Multinational Registry (CERTIFY)[39] confirmed these findings. During a median follow-up of 37 months, outcome of patients with permanent AF undergoing CRT combined with either AVJ ablation (n = 443) or rate-slowing drugs (n = 895) was compared with that of patients in sinus rhythm (n = 6046). Long-term survival after CRT among patients with AF + AVJ ablation is similar to that observed among patients in sinus rhythm. Mortality is higher for patients with AF treated with rate-slowing drugs only (**Fig. 4**).

Dong and colleagues[40] followed up 154 patients with AF of whom 45 (29%) received AVJ ablation, whereas the other 109 patients (71%) received optimal rate controlling therapy during CRT. The survival benefit was significantly higher (+19.5%, P = .008) for the group receiving AVJ ablation.

THE ROLE OF ATRIOVENTRICULAR JUNCTION ABLATION

If pharmacologic rate control proves ineffective, AVJ ablation can be performed. The procedure eliminates native atrioventricular (AV) conduction and ensures a high percentage of BiV pacing. There is a growing amount of evidence that investigates the effect of the ablate-and-pace strategy in patients undergoing CRT. Many important studies have already been mentioned. A systematic review of Ganesan and colleagues[41] supports that AVJ ablation is associated with a substantial reduction in ACM, primarily by reducing cardiovascular mortality, as well as with improvements in NYHA class when compared with medical therapy only in 768 patients with AF who received CRT. But careful institution of rate control drugs has not been properly investigated. However, there are studies that argue in favor of the use of medication alone, alleging that sufficiently high degrees of ventricular capture and thus BiV pacing can be achieved without AVJ ablation.[42,43] Two other points should also be kept in mind. First, the CRT studies that have investigated the role of AVJ node ablation have been biased in terms of patient selection. Patients receiving AVJ ablation have been patients with symptomatic permanent AF. The necessity of AVJ ablation for patients with paroxysmal or persistent AF is unclear. Second, AVJ ablation is associated with a number of disadvantages, including pacemaker dependency, which puts the patients in a vulnerable position, especially in case of lead or device failure. Results from the REPLACE study,[44] the first prospective, multicenter study of complications related to pacemaker, ICD, and CRT generator changes, report a major complication rate of 4.0% in patients who had a generator replacement without a plan to add a transvenous lead. The overall 6-month complication rate in patients receiving generator replacement combined with a plan to add 1 or more transvenous leads is substantial with 15.3%, with the highest risks occurring in patients who had an upgrade to or a revised CRT device (18.7%; 95% CI, 15.1–22.6). This knowledge should be weighed when deciding about AVJ ablation.

RECOMMENDATIONS

Current data demonstrate that a favorable effect of CRT can be achieved in patients with AF, and the authors are confident that patients with AF can achieve similar benefits from CRT as patients in sinus rhythm. However, this requires careful and attentive management (**Fig. 5**). The incidence of AT/AF episodes during CRT is high, and therefore careful analysis of device diagnostics, standard 12-lead ECGs, and Holter recordings is mandatory to assess underlying rhythm in all patients receiving CRT. In case of AF, the goal is to achieve BiV pacing as close to 100% as possible. Exercise tests may help determine the effective percentage of BiV pacing.

The following points should be kept in mind:

- Be aware of the development of AF in every patient receiving CRT.
- The first option is to restore sinus rhythm. Prophylaxis with amiodarone or even an atrial ablation may be necessary.
- Even if a rhythm control strategy is adopted, β-blockers should be instituted to prevent rapid conduction of AF during a recurrence.
- Exercise tests may help to assess continuous BiV pacing during (moderate) exercise since

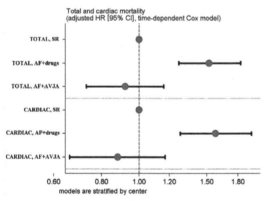

Fig. 4. Hazard ratio (HR) for total mortality and cardiac mortality after CRT comparing patients with sinus rhythm (SR) with patients with permanent AF, respectively, with or without atrioventricular junction ablation (AVJA). The sinus rhythm group was the reference. (*From* Gasparini M, Leclercq C, Lunati M, et al. Cardiac resynchronization therapy in patients with atrial fibrillation: the CERTIFY study (Cardiac Resynchronization Therapy in Atrial Fibrillation Patients Multinational Registry). JACC Heart Fail 2013;1(6):505; with permission of Elsevier.)

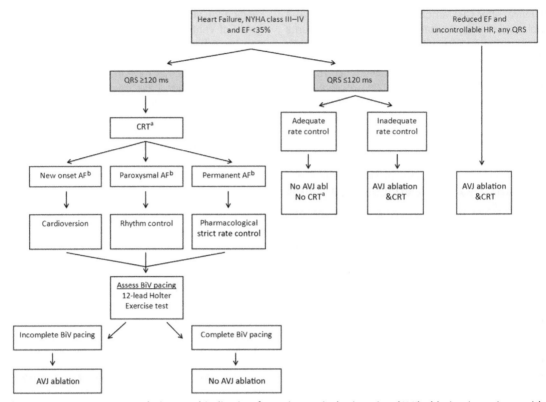

Fig. 5. Treatment recommendations and indication for atrioventricular junction (AVJ) ablation in patients with atrial fibrillation (AF). EF, ejection fraction; HR, heart rate. [a] Consider ICD according to guidelines, [b] determine indication for anticoagulation therapy. (*Adapted from* European Society of Cardiology (ESC), European Heart Rhythm Association (EHRA), Brignole M, et al. 2013 ESC guidelines on cardiac pacing and cardiac resynchronization therapy: the Task Force on cardiac pacing and resynchronization therapy of the European Society of Cardiology (ESC). Developed in collaboration with the European Heart Rhythm Association (EHRA). Europace 2013;15(8):1096; with permission of Oxford University Press (UK) (c) European Society of Cardiology, www.escardio.org).

device counters often mention inappropriate percentages.

- If AF becomes more permanent, every effort should be made to guarantee optimal BiV pacing. Either with drugs or, when this become ineffective, with an AVJ ablation.
- After an AVJ ablation, patients become pacemaker dependent, which may cause problematic situations once complications occur, for example, at the moment of replacement.

SUMMARY

Does it matter for CRT success if the atria are fibrillating? Patients with AF are able to experience significant advantages of CRT as long as effective BiV pacing is achieved. However, BiV pacing cannot be effective unless AV conduction is sufficiently suppressed. Exercise tests, device diagnostics, and programming are essential to define AF burden and assess effective BiV pacing; this is especially important considering that around

20% to 40% of patients in sinus rhythm at baseline experience episodes of AT/AF during follow-up. Patients with device-detected AT/AF are at risk of cardiac deterioration and have a worse prognosis. Combining an active clinical approach with remote monitoring may prevent hemodynamic deterioration and allows tailored diagnostic and therapeutic strategies for the heterogeneous group of patients with AF receiving CRT. Efforts dedicated toward establishing tailored treatment will help to adequately manage AF issues in patients with HF who are treated with CRT. If possible, medical rhythm control should be the preferred strategy. However, in case of nonresponse and in case of any doubt on continuous pacing, AVJ ablation should be performed.

REFERENCES

1. Abraham WT, Fisher WG, Smith AL, et al. Cardiac resynchronization in chronic heart failure. N Engl J Med 2002;346(24):1845–53.

2. Auricchio A, Stellbrink C, Sack S, et al. Long-term clinical effect of hemodynamically optimized cardiac resynchronization therapy in patients with heart failure and ventricular conduction delay. J Am Coll Cardiol 2002;39(12):2026–33.

3. Bristow MR, Saxon LA, Boehmer J, et al. Cardiac-resynchronization therapy with or without an implantable defibrillator in advanced chronic heart failure. N Engl J Med 2004;350(21):2140–50.

4. Cazeau S, Leclercq C, Lavergne T, et al. Effects of multisite biventricular pacing in patients with heart failure and intraventricular conduction delay. N Engl J Med 2001;344(12):873–80.

5. Cleland JG, Daubert JC, Erdmann E, et al. The effect of cardiac resynchronization on morbidity and mortality in heart failure. N Engl J Med 2005;352(15):1539–49.

6. Maisel WH, Stevenson LW. Atrial fibrillation in heart failure: epidemiology, pathophysiology, and rationale for therapy. Am J Cardiol 2003;91(6A):2D–8D.

7. Upadhyay GA, Steinberg JS. Managing atrial fibrillation in the CRT patient: controversy or consensus? Heart Rhythm 2012;9(8 Suppl I):S51–9.

8. European Society of Cardiology (ESC), European Heart Rhythm Association (EHRA), Brignole M, Auricchio A, et al. 2013 ESC guidelines on cardiac pacing and cardiac resynchronization therapy: the Task Force on cardiac pacing and resynchronization therapy of the European Society of Cardiology (ESC). Developed in collaboration with the European Heart Rhythm Association (EHRA). Europace 2013; 15(8):1070–118.

9. Epstein AE, DiMarco JP, Ellenbogen KA, et al. 2012 ACCF/AHA/HRS focused update incorporated into the ACCF/AHA/HRS 2008 guidelines for device-based therapy of cardiac rhythm abnormalities: a report of the American College of Cardiology Foundation/American Heart Association Task Force on PRACTICE Guidelines and the Heart Rhythm Society. J Am Coll Cardiol 2013;61(3):e6–75.

10. Leclercq C, Padeletti L, Cihak R, et al. Incidence of paroxysmal atrial tachycardias in patients treated with cardiac resynchronization therapy and continuously monitored by device diagnostics. Europace 2010;12(1):71–7.

11. Borleffs CJ, Ypenburg C, van Bommel RJ, et al. Clinical importance of new-onset atrial fibrillation after cardiac resynchronization therapy. Heart Rhythm 2009;6(3):305–10.

12. Marijon E, Jacob S, Mouton E, et al. Frequency of atrial tachyarrhythmias in patients treated by cardiac resynchronization (from the prospective, multicenter Mona Lisa study). Am J Cardiol 2010;106(5):688–93.

13. Caldwell JC, Contractor H, Petkar S, et al. Atrial fibrillation is under-recognized in chronic heart failure: insights from a heart failure cohort treated with cardiac resynchronization therapy. Europace 2009; 11(10):1295–300.

14. Boriani G, Gasparini M, Landolina M, et al. Incidence and clinical relevance of uncontrolled ventricular rate during atrial fibrillation in heart failure patients treated with cardiac resynchronization therapy. Eur J Heart Fail 2011;13(8):868–76.

15. Puglisi A, Gasparini M, Lunati M, et al. Persistent atrial fibrillation worsens heart rate variability, activity and heart rate, as shown by a continuous monitoring by implantable biventricular pacemakers in heart failure patients. J Cardiovasc Electrophysiol 2008; 19(7):693–701.

16. Buck S, Rienstra M, Maass AH, et al. Cardiac resynchronization therapy in patients with heart failure and atrial fibrillation: importance of new-onset atrial fibrillation and total atrial conduction time. Europace 2008;10(5):558–65.

17. Santini M, Gasparini M, Landolina M, et al. Device-detected atrial tachyarrhythmias predict adverse outcome in real-world patients with implantable biventricular defibrillators. J Am Coll Cardiol 2011; 57(2):167–72.

18. Cheng A, Landman SR, Stadler RW. Reasons for loss of cardiac resynchronization therapy pacing: insights from 32 844 patients. Circ Arrhythm Electrophysiol 2012;5(5):884–8.

19. Hayes DL, Boehmer JP, Day JD, et al. Cardiac resynchronization therapy and the relationship of percent biventricular pacing to symptoms and survival. Heart Rhythm 2011;8(9):1469–75.

20. Kamath GS, Cotiga D, Koneru JN, et al. The utility of 12-lead Holter monitoring in patients with permanent atrial fibrillation for the identification of nonresponders after cardiac resynchronization therapy. J Am Coll Cardiol 2009;53(12):1050–5.

21. Maass AH, Buck S, Nieuwland W, et al. Importance of heart rate during exercise for response to cardiac resynchronization therapy. J Cardiovasc Electrophysiol 2009;20(7):773–80.

22. Poole JE, Johnson GW, Hellkamp AS, et al. Prognostic importance of defibrillator shocks in patients with heart failure. N Engl J Med 2008;359(10): 1009–17.

23. Daubert JP, Zareba W, Cannom DS, et al. Inappropriate implantable cardioverter-defibrillator shocks in MADIT II: frequency, mechanisms, predictors, and survival impact. J Am Coll Cardiol 2008; 51(14):1357–65.

24. van Rees JB, Borleffs CJ, de Bie MK, et al. Inappropriate implantable cardioverter-defibrillator shocks: incidence, predictors, and impact on mortality. J Am Coll Cardiol 2011;57(5):556–62.

25. Fischer A, Ousdigian KT, Johnson JW, et al. The impact of atrial fibrillation with rapid ventricular rates and device programming on shocks in 106,513 ICD and CRT-D patients. Heart Rhythm 2012;9(1):24–31.

26. Healey JS, Hohnloser SH, Exner DV, et al. Cardiac resynchronization therapy in patients with permanent

atrial fibrillation: results from the resynchronization for ambulatory heart failure trial (RAFT). Circ Heart Fail 2012;5(5):566–70.

27. Ruwald AC, Kutyifa V, Ruwald MH, et al. The association between biventricular pacing and cardiac resynchronization therapy-defibrillator efficacy when compared with implantable cardioverter defibrillator on outcomes and reverse remodelling. Eur Heart J 2015;36(7):440–8.

28. Ruwald AC, Pietrasik G, Goldenberg I, et al. The effect of intermittent atrial tachyarrhythmia on heart failure or death in cardiac resynchronization therapy with defibrillator versus implantable cardioverter-defibrillator patients: a MADIT-CRT substudy (Multicenter Automatic Defibrillator Implantation Trial with Cardiac Resynchronization Therapy). J Am Coll Cardiol 2014;63(12):1190–7.

29. Leclercq C, Walker S, Linde C, et al. Comparative effects of permanent biventricular and right-univentricular pacing in heart failure patients with chronic atrial fibrillation. Eur Heart J 2002;23(22): 1780–7.

30. Doshi RN, Daoud EG, Fellows C, et al. Left ventricular-based cardiac stimulation post AV nodal ablation evaluation (the PAVE study). J Cardiovasc Electrophysiol 2005;16(11):1160–5.

31. Brignole M, Botto G, Mont L, et al. Cardiac resynchronization therapy in patients undergoing atrioventricular junction ablation for permanent atrial fibrillation: a randomized trial. Eur Heart J 2011; 32(19):2420–9.

32. Linde C, Leclercq C, Rex S, et al. Long-term benefits of biventricular pacing in congestive heart failure: results from the multisite stimulation in cardiomyopathy (MUSTIC) study. J Am Coll Cardiol 2002;40(1): 111–8.

33. Molhoek SG, Bax JJ, Bleeker GB, et al. Comparison of response to cardiac resynchronization therapy in patients with sinus rhythm versus chronic atrial fibrillation. Am J Cardiol 2004;94(12):1506–9.

34. Delnoy PP, Ottervanger JP, Luttikhuis HO, et al. Comparison of usefulness of cardiac resynchronization therapy in patients with atrial fibrillation and heart failure versus patients with sinus rhythm and heart failure. Am J Cardiol 2007;99(9):1252–7.

35. Hoppe UC, Casares JM, Eiskjaer H, et al. Effect of cardiac resynchronization on the incidence of atrial fibrillation in patients with severe heart failure. Circulation 2006;114(1):18–25.

36. Tolosana JM, Hernandez Madrid A, Brugada J, et al. Comparison of benefits and mortality in cardiac resynchronization therapy in patients with atrial fibrillation versus patients in sinus rhythm (results of the Spanish Atrial Fibrillation and Resynchronization [SPARE] study). Am J Cardiol 2008; 102(4):444–9.

37. Gasparini M, Auricchio A, Regoli F, et al. Four-year efficacy of cardiac resynchronization therapy on exercise tolerance and disease progression: the importance of performing atrioventricular junction ablation in patients with atrial fibrillation. J Am Coll Cardiol 2006;48(4):734–43.

38. Gasparini M, Auricchio A, Metra M, et al. Long-term survival in patients undergoing cardiac resynchronization therapy: the importance of performing atrio-ventricular junction ablation in patients with permanent atrial fibrillation. Eur Heart J 2008; 29(13):1644–52.

39. Gasparini M, Leclercq C, Lunati M, et al. Cardiac resynchronization therapy in patients with atrial fibrillation: the CERTIFY study (Cardiac Resynchronization Therapy in Atrial Fibrillation Patients Multinational Registry). JACC Heart Fail 2013;1(6):500–7.

40. Dong K, Shen WK, Powell BD, et al. Atrioventricular nodal ablation predicts survival benefit in patients with atrial fibrillation receiving cardiac resynchronization therapy. Heart Rhythm 2010;7(9):1240–5.

41. Ganesan AN, Brooks AG, Roberts-Thomson KC, et al. Role of AV nodal ablation in cardiac resynchronization in patients with coexistent atrial fibrillation and heart failure a systematic review. J Am Coll Cardiol 2012;59(8):719–26.

42. Khadjooi K, Foley PW, Chalil S, et al. Long-term effects of cardiac resynchronisation therapy in patients with atrial fibrillation. Heart 2008;94(7):879–83.

43. Schutte F, Ludorff G, Grove R, et al. Atrioventricular node ablation is not a prerequisite for cardiac resynchronization therapy in patients with chronic atrial fibrillation. Cardiol J 2009;16(3):246–9.

44. Poole JE, Gleva MJ, Mela T, et al. Complication rates associated with pacemaker or implantable cardioverter-defibrillator generator replacements and upgrade procedures: results from the REPLACE registry. Circulation 2010;122(16):1553–61.

Atrioventricular Node Ablation

Maurizio Gasparini, MD

KEYWORDS

- Cardiac resynchronization therapy • Atrial fibrillation • Atrioventricular junction ablation

KEY POINTS

- Every effort should be made in all patients receiving cardiac resynchronization therapy (CRT) to approach 100% biventricular (BIV) pacing by a correct device programming, a correct pharmacologic regimen, and atrioventricular (AV) nodal ablation in permanent atrial fibrillation (AF) patients.
- Currently, atrioventricular junction (AVJ) ablation should always be considered a fundamental step in a combined strategy to obtain the best results of CRT in the heart failure (HF) population affected by permanent AF.
- AF in patients with HF may have a significant negative impact on the clinical benefit conveyed by CRT, if not appropriately managed.

WHAT ARE THE INTERACTIONS BETWEEN ATRIAL FIBRILLATION AND HEART FAILURE (ATRIAL FIBRILLATION BEGETS HEART FAILURE AND VICE VERSA)?

The prevalence of AF ranges from approximately 5% in patients with asymptomatic cardiac dysfunction to more than 50% of those with severe symptomatic HF.[1–9] In some patients, the onset of HF and AF coincide, whereas the onset of AF in patients with preexisting HF indicates a poor prognosis. Patients who develop HF as a consequence of AF (approximately 75% of those admitted when these 2 conditions coexist) have a better outcome than those who develop AF after the onset of HF.

AF and HF are believed to directly predispose to each other. They form a sinister synergy, and management of AF in the setting of HF is challenging. Even more problematic is the management of AF patients undergoing CRT.

A distinction has to be made between the 3 forms of AF, namely paroxysmal, persistent, and permanent, the last one being frequent in the advanced phases of HF.

WHAT ARE THE TOOLS TO TREAT ATRIAL FIBRILLATION IN HEART FAILURE?

Paroxysmal AF may be controlled by antiarrhythmic drugs, even if limited by their negative chronotropic effect, much dreaded in left ventricular (LV) dysfunction.

Persistent AF may need repeated cardioversion.

Paroxysmal and persistent AF, at least in an initial stage of AF, may be successfully treated with AF ablation (ie, pulmonary veins isolation). Treating AF substrate in the context of a cardiomyopathy, however, may achieve poor results in advanced HF, because during AF in failing hearts, there is a heterogeneous distribution of fibrosis that likely influences dynamic pattern of AF activation and signal complexity.

Permanent AF requires a satisfying rate control and this is more true in HF.

MEDICAL THERAPY FOR RATE CONTROL IN PERMANENT ATRIAL FIBRILLATION

The aim of the rate-control strategy is to lower heart rate (to allow better diastolic filling and stroke

The author has no conflict of interest.
EP and Pacing Unit, Humanitas Research Hospital, 20089 Rozzano-Milano, Italy
E-mail address: maurizio.gasparini@humanitas.it

Card Electrophysiol Clin 7 (2015) 749–754
http://dx.doi.org/10.1016/j.ccep.2015.08.006

volume increase in hearts with conserved Frank-Starling mechanism). Moreover, heart rate regularization further reinforces favorable effects on diastolic function.

Rate-control drugs considered effective in HF patients with depressed LV function include digoxin, amiodarone, dronedarone, and β-blockers.

Different randomized trials, however, have suggested caution in the use of digoxin and amiodarone in patients with HF due to increased morbidity and mortality.[10]

WHAT ARE THE INTERACTIONS BETWEEN ATRIAL FIBRILLATION AND *CARDIAC RESYNCHRONIZATION THERAPY*?

AF poses several challenges to adequately deliver CRT because fast atrial rhythm conducted to the ventricles may easily override BIV pacing.

An intrinsic, intermediate-to-high, irregular spontaneous AF rhythm reduces the percentage of effectively BIV-paced captured beats (BVP%), because there are phases of competing AF rhythm that cause spontaneous, fusion (hybrid between paced and intrinsic QRS morphologies), or pseudofusion (pacing artifacts delivered but intrinsic QRS morphology not altered) beats, not hemodynamically effective as pure BIV beats (**Fig. 1**).

This phenomenon suggests that the global effective CRT dose may be markedly reduced compared with atrial-synchronous rhythm with a short AV interval (as is achieved during sinus rhythm [SR]). Moreover, in AF patients, during exertion, spontaneous ventricular rate tends to override BIV pacing rates, determining a further reduction of paced beats precisely when patients are most in need of having BIV capture, thus greatly limiting functional capacity.

From a clinical standpoint, it is important to identify symptoms, such as palpitations, and, more importantly, worsening effort dyspnea, which may suggest that the resynchronization effect is reduced because of the interference of underlying AF. Retrieving relevant information (BVP%, duration, numbers of mode switches episodes, and so forth) through device control may complement clinical data; this kind of information is important and is currently easily achieved with home monitoring systems.

Some device-derived features may be helpful to improve rate control and thus improve CRT delivery. These algorithms try to maximize BIV% by stimulating in a BIV mode a native beat or by achieving BIV capture by a higher mean heart rate. They are only partially helpful, however, and not as efficacious as a complete BIV pacing modality.

The recourse to rate-control drugs and/or activation of device-based algorithms is reasonable as a first-line approach when AF/AT burden is low/intermediate.

Findings derived from different large observational cohort studies on the effects of CRT in patients with permanent AF have yielded contrasting results. It is worth emphasizing, however, that when the survival curves of the HF patients with AF treated with a combined device-based/drug regimen are compared, all-cause mortality remains remarkably high, amounting to more than 14% per year in both separate cohorts of nonablated patients (**Fig. 2**).

It follows, therefore, that in HF patients treated with CRT who present with permanent AF or frequent persistent or paroxysmal episodes, the pursuit of an aggressive treatment strategy, such as AVJ ablation, may be warranted.

Atrioventricular Junction Ablation for Optimizing Cardiac Resynchronization Therapy in Permanent Atrial Fibrillation

AVJ ablation is commonly performed in patients with symptomatic, drug-refractory, fast, permanent AF as part of the conventional ablate and pace strategy and has been shown to confer symptomatic relief. AVJ ablation in individuals with AF treated with CRT has initially mainly been confined to selected patients in whom high-rate

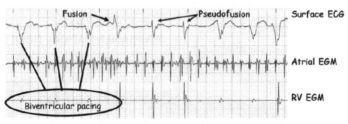

Fig. 1. In a patient with AF and HF treated with CRT, spontaneous irregular intrinsic beats alternate with fusion and pseudofusion beats, thus markedly reducing effective CRT. As shown in the figure, this may occur even during normal rate AF. (RV, right ventricle; EGM, intracavitary electrogram. *From* Gasparini M, Regoli F, Galimberti P, et al. Cardiac resynchronization therapy in heart failure patients with atrial fibrillation. Europace 2009;11(Suppl 5):v82–6; with permission.)

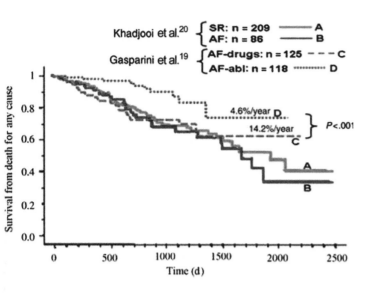

Fig. 2. Comparison of Kaplan-Meier analysis for freedom from death for any cause between HF patients treated with drugs or with ablated AV node (abl). (*From* Gasparini M, Regoli F, Galimberti P, et al. Cardiac resynchronization therapy in heart failure patients with atrial fibrillation. Europace 2009;11(Suppl 5):v82–6; with permission.)

AF or atrial tachycardia (AT) jeopardizes satisfactory BIV stimulation, and, in CRT–implantable cardioverter-defibrillator (ICD) recipients, determines inappropriate ICD interventions. The problem of inappropriate ICD therapies during AF, constituting approximately 30% of all ICD interventions,[11] is that it has an important negative impact on hospitalization rate and quality of life in patients and may be completely resolved after AVJ ablation. In the context of CRT in HF patients with concomitant AF, however, a growing body of evidence has demonstrated that AVJ ablation may be useful to optimize CRT delivery by eliminating the deleterious hemodynamic effects of underlying AF.

In 2006, 1 large observational prospective investigation[12] specifically evaluated the effects of AVJ ablation on CRT delivery using a predefined protocol. This study showed that only AF patients who underwent AVJ ablation showed significant improvements in LV ejection fraction, LV end-systolic volume, and exercise capacity. Furthermore, a significantly higher proportion of responders (response defined as a ≥10% reduction in LV end-systolic volume) were observed in the AVJ ablation group (68%) compared with the nonablated group (18%) at 12 months. As later observed by the same group[13] in a more extensive observational multicenter study, CRT combined with AVJ ablation conferred a significant reduction of deaths for any cause compared with CRT alone, particularly by reducing HF. From this evidence, AVJ ablation was included in European Guidelines.

In 2011 a metanalysis by Wilton and colleagues[14] stated that AVJ ablation may improve CRT outcomes in patients with AF. In 2012, an elegant meta-analysis by Ganesan and colleagues[15] included 6 studies and specifically compared CRT-AF patient outcomes according to AVJ ablation. Patients without AVJ ablation had higher all-cause (relative risk [RR] 0.42) and cardiovascular (RR 0.44) mortality.

A succeeding subanalysis of patients with AF enrolled in the Resynchronization/Defibrillation for Ambulatory Heart Failure Trial (RAFT)[16] showed, however, that, although CRT did reduce HF hospitalization (40% risk reduction), it had no influence on cardiovascular death (hazard ratio [HR] 0.97; 95% CI, 0.55–1.71; P = .91).[16] The conclusion drawn by Healey and colleagues,[16] even if formally absolutely correct, may be misleading. In the authors' opinion, these conclusions do not adequately take into account that AVJ ablation has been performed in only 1 RAFT patient. Probably a more correct final message is simply that patients with AF, who are otherwise CRT candidates, not undergoing AVJ ablation do not reach effective BIV stimulation and, as a consequence, gain a minimal benefit from CRT-with a defibrillator compared with standard ICD.

Definitive data on this topic, in particular strong endpoints of mortality showing clear benefits by AVJ ablation in CRT, have been recently provided by a large multicenter observational study, the Cardiac Resynchronization Therapy in Atrial Fibrillation Patients Multinational Registry (CERTIFY) study.[17] This article reports data of a large cohort of patients (more than 7000) with a significantly long follow-up. The clinical outcome of CRT in patients with HF and permanent AF undergoing CRT in combination with either AVJ ablation (n = 443) or rate-slowing drugs (n = 895) were compared with patients in SR (n = 6046). Over a median follow-up of 37 months (230,000 patient years), total mortality (6.8 vs 6.1), cardiac mortality (4.2 vs 4.0), and HF mortality (3.4 vs 3.5 per 100 person year) (all P = not significant) were similar in patients with AF plus AVJ ablation and patients in SR. In contrast, the AF plus drugs group had a higher total, cardiac, and HF mortality than the SR and the AF plus AVJ ablation groups (11.3, 8.1, and 7.4, respectively; $P<.001$). On multivariable analysis, AF plus AVJ ablation patients displayed values of total (HR 0.93), cardiac (HR 0.88), and HF mortality (HR 0.82) that were similar to those of to the SR group, independent of known confounders. The AF plus drugs group, however, presented higher total (HR 1.52), cardiac (HR 1.57), and HF mortality (HR 1.58) than both the SR and AF plus AVJ ablation groups (both $P<.001$). The study concluded that long-term survival after CRT in patients with AF plus AVJ ablation is similar to that observed in patients in SR whereas mortality is higher in AF patients treated with rate-slowing drugs.

Last but not least, AVJ ablation has been also demonstrated by a multicenter longitudinal study[18] to be the most powerful predictor of SR resumption (SRR) in permanent AF patients treated with CRT. SRR occurs in a significant percentage (10%) of permanent AF patients after CRT by positively affecting atrial electrophysiology (especially by lessening the stretch and change in local and systemic hormonal states). Other factors predicting SRR included smaller left atrial dimension, smaller LV dimension, and shorter QRS after CRT. SRR was usually within 6 months of implantation but observed even after 4 years. The coexistence of 3 predictors versus 0 to 2 predictors increases the likelihood of SRR by 3.5-fold, whereas the presence of all 4 factors improves the probability by a factor of 5.7. Critically, the subgroup of those who resumed SR went on to have a superb prognosis and a much lower death rate than those who remained in AF (0 vs 18 per 100 person-years).

The issue of pacemaker dependency may represent a major problem in indicating AVJ ablation on a large scale. It must be stated, however, that CRT, through BIV pacing, offers dual pacing back-up. In addition, more novel device features (available with home monitoring) instantly detect any alteration in lead parameter. Effective failure of capture, therefore, seems unlikely.

THE IMPORTANCE OF MAXIMIZED BIVENTRICULAR PACING

There is a great need to design randomized controlled trials with strong endpoints,[19] even though such designs may be difficult to implement for ethical and financial reasons, to definitively validate the need of AVJ ablation in this context. The need of AVJ ablation concept, however, has grown parallel to the concept that the highest BIV pacing percentage must be reached in CRT. After the retrospective analysis of Koplan and colleagues[20] showing that the greatest magnitude of benefit was observed with greater than 92% BIV pacing, an elegant work of Hayes and colleagues[21] of more than 30,000 patients followed up by home monitoring showed that mortality was inversely correlated to the percentage of BIV pacing both in SR or paced atrial rhythm and even in AF. The greatest magnitude mortality reduction was observed with a BIV pacing cutoff greater than 98%. AF patients with a BIV pacing percentage greater than 98.5% had a survival rate equivalent to that of their counterparts in normal SR. On the contrary, AF patients with a BIV pacing percentage less than 98.5% showed a significantly higher mortality with respect to SR patients.

A recent article Ousdigian and coauthors[22] assessed the impact of AF on BIV pacing (BIVP%), looking for a possible correlation between BIVP% and all-cause mortality on a wide population accounting for 54,019 patients with a follow-up of 2.3 ± 1.2 years.

A proportion as high as two-thirds of patients with permanent (daily mean AF burden $\geq$23 hours accounting for 69%) and persistent ($\geq$1 day with AF $\geq$6 hours 62%) AF did not achieve high BIVP% (>98%). Relative to no/little AF, patients with AF had increased mortality after adjusting for age, gender, BIVP%, and shocks (permanent: HR 1.28 [1.19–1.38], $P<.001$; and persistent: HR 1.51 [1.41–1.61], $P<.001$). Relative to patients with BIVP% greater than 98%, patients with reduced BIVP% had increased mortality after adjusting for age, gender, AF, and shocks (90%–98%: HR 1.20, $P<.001$ and <90%: HR 1.32, $P<.001$). High BIVP% was associated with the greatest mortality improvement in permanent AF among the AF classifications.

All those data strongly indicate that physicians should always aim for a BIV% of 100% and in AF patients AVJ ablation may be the best (sometimes the only) tool for this scope.

SUMMARY

AF in patients with HF may have a significant negative impact on the clinical benefit conveyed by CRT, if not appropriately managed. Careful overall evaluation is mandatory to precisely define the degree of AT/AF burden to articulate tailored diagnostic and therapeutic strategies. Based on recent observational extensive data, in patients presenting intermediate or elevated AT/AF burden, AVJ ablation may represent a fundamental tool to achieve full CRT delivery, thus conferring marked improvements in global cardiac function, and, by extension, in survival.

REFERENCES

1. Cazeau S, Leclercq C, Lavergne T, et al. Effects of multisite biventricular pacing in patients with heart failure and intraventricular conduction delay. N Engl J Med 2001;344(12):873–80.
2. Abraham WT, Fisher WG, Smith AL, et al. Cardiac resynchronization in chronic heart failure. N Engl J Med 2002;346(24):1845–53.
3. Auricchio A, Stellbrink C, Sack S, et al. Long-term clinical effect of hemodynamically optimized cardiac resynchronization therapy in patients with heart failure and ventricular conduction delay. J Am Coll Cardiol 2002;39(12):2026–33.
4. Bristow MR, Saxon LA, Boehmer J, et al. Cardiac-resynchronization therapy with or without an implantable defibrillator in advanced chronic heart failure. N Engl J Med 2004;350(21):2140–50.
5. Cleland JGF, Daubert JC, Erdmann E, et al. The effect of cardiac resynchronization on morbidity and mortality in heart failure. N Engl J Med 2005; 352(15):1539–49.
6. Auricchio A, Metra M, Gasparini M, et al. Long-term survival of patients with heart failure and ventricular conduction delay treated with cardiac resynchronization therapy. Am J Cardiol 2007;99(2):232–8.
7. Swedberg K, Cleland JGF, Dargie H, et al. Guidelines for the diagnosis and treatment of chronic heart failure: executive summary (update 2005): the task force for the diagnosis and treatment of chronic heart failure of the European Society of Cardiology. Eur Heart J 2005;26(11):1115–40.
8. Vardas PE, Auricchio A, Blanc JJ, et al. Guidelines for cardiac pacing and cardiac resynchronization therapy: the task force for cardiac pacing and cardiac resynchronization therapy of the European Society of Cardiology. Developed in Collaboration with the European Heart Rhythm Association. Eur Heart J 2007;28(18):2256–95.
9. Epstein AE, DiMarco JP, Ellenbogen KA, et al. ACC/AHA/HRS 2008 guidelines for device-based therapy of cardiac rhythm abnormalities: a report of the American College of Cardiology/American Heart Association Task Force on Practice Guidelines (Writing Committee to Revise the ACC/AHA/NASPE 2002 Guideline update for implantation of cardiac pacemakers and antiarrhythmia devices): developed in Collaboration with the American Association for Thoracic Surgery and Society of Thoracic Surgeons. Circulation 2008;117(21):e350–408.
10. Bardy GH, Lee KL, Mark DB, et al. Amiodarone or an implantable cardioverter-defibrillator for congestive heart failure. N Engl J Med 2005;352(3):225–37.
11. Sweeney MO, Wathen MS, Volosin K, et al. Appropriate and inappropriate ventricular therapies, quality of life, and mortality among primary and secondary prevention implantable cardioverter defibrillator patients: results from the pacing fast VT reduces shock therapies (PainFREE Rx II) trial. Circulation 2005; 111(22):2898–905.
12. Gasparini M, Auricchio A, Regoli F, et al. Four-year efficacy of cardiac resynchronization therapy on exercise tolerance and disease progression: the importance of performing atrioventricular junction ablation in patients with atrial fibrillation. J Am Coll Cardiol 2006;48(4):734–43.
13. Gasparini M, Auricchio A, Metra M, et al. Long-term survival in patients undergoing cardiac resynchronization therapy: the importance of performing atrio-ventricular junction ablation in patients with permanent atrial fibrillation. Eur Heart J 2008; 29(13):1644–52.
14. Wilton SB, Leung AA, Ghali WA, et al. Outcomes of cardiac resynchronization therapy in patients with versus those without atrial fibrillation: a systematic review and meta-analysis. Heart Rhythm 2011;8(7):1088–94.
15. Ganesan AN, Brooks AG, Roberts-Thomson KC, et al. Role of AV nodal ablation in cardiac resynchronization in patients with coexistent atrial fibrillation and heart failure a systematic review. J Am Coll Cardiol 2012;59(8):719–26.
16. Healey JS, Hohnloser SH, Exner DV. Cardiac resynchronization therapy in patients with permanent atrial fibrillation: results from the Resynchronization for Ambulatory Heart Failure Trial (RAFT). Circ Heart Fail 2012;5:566–70.
17. Gasparini M, Leclercq C, Lunati M, et al. Cardiac resynchronization therapy in patients with atrial fibrillation: the CERTIFY study (Cardiac resynchronization therapy in atrial fibrillation patients multinational registry). JACC Heart Fail 2013;1(6):500–7.
18. Gasparini M, Steinberg JS, Arshad A, et al. Resumption of sinus rhythm in patients with heart failure and permanent atrial fibrillation undergoing cardiac resynchronization therapy: a longitudinal observational study. Eur Heart J 2010; 31(8):976–83.
19. Steinberg JS. Desperately seeking a randomized clinical trial of resynchronizationtherapy for patients with heart failure and atrial fibrillation. J Am Coll Cardiol 2006;48(4):744–6.

20. Koplan BA, Kaplan AJ, Weiner S, et al. Heart failure decompensation and all-cause mortality in relation to percent biventricular pacing in patients with heart failure: is a goal of 100% biventricular pacing necessary? J Am Coll Cardiol 2009;53(4):355–60.

21. Hayes DL, Boehmer JP, Day JD, et al. Cardiac resynchronization therapy and the relationship of percent biventricular pacing to symptoms and survival. Heart Rhythm 2011;8(9):1469–75.

22. Ousdigian KT, Borek PP, Koehler JL, et al. The epidemic of inadequate biventricular pacing in patients with persistent or permanent atrial fibrillation and its association with mortality. Circ Arrhythm Electrophysiol 2014;7(3):370–6.

How to Improve Cardiac Resynchronization Therapy Benefit in Atrial Fibrillation Patients
Pulmonary Vein Isolation (and Beyond)

Carola Gianni, MD[a,b], Luigi Di Biase, MD, PhD, FHRS[a,c,d,e],
Sanghamitra Mohanty, MD, MS[a], Yalçın Gökoğlan, MD[a],
Mahmut Fatih Güneş, MD[a], Amin Al-Ahmad, MD, FHRS, CCDS[a],
J. David Burkhardt, MD, FHRS[a], Andrea Natale, MD, FESC, FHRS[a,f,g,h,i,j],*

KEYWORDS

- Catheter ablation • Atrial fibrillation • Heart failure • Cardiac resynchronization therapy
- Pulmonary vein ablation • Triggers

KEY POINTS

- Cardiac resynchronization therapy (CRT) is not as effective in heart failure (HF) patients with atrial fibrillation (AF) undergoing CRT for inadequate biventricular capture and loss of atrioventricular (AV) synchrony.
- Catheter ablation of AF can improve CRT benefit by restoring both interventricular and AV synchrony, but no study has specifically addressed this issue.
- Regardless of CRT, many clinical trials have shown that catheter ablation of AF is a safe and effective strategy to achieve rhythm control in patients with HF.
- PVI-alone is not enough in patients with HF and an ablation strategy targeting non-PV triggers and the substrate is necessary.

INTRODUCTION

Atrial fibrillation (AF) and heart failure (HF) often coexist, and when they do clinical outcomes worsen. Although cardiac resynchronization therapy (CRT) is an important treatment for symptomatic HF patients in sinus rhythm (SR) with low left ventricular ejection fraction (LVEF) and ventricular dyssynchrony, its role is still not well defined in patients with AF.

Disclosures: The authors have nothing to disclose and no conflict relevant to the subject matter or materials discussed in this article.
[a] Texas Cardiac Arrhythmia Institute, St. David's Medical Center, 3000 North IH-35, Suite 700, Austin, TX 78705, USA; [b] Department of Clinical Sciences and Community Health, University of Milan, Milan, Italy; [c] Arrhythmia Services, Department of Medicine, Montefiore Medical Center, Albert Einstein College of Medicine, Bronx, NY, USA; [d] Department of Biomedical Engineering, University of Texas, Austin, TX, USA; [e] Department of Cardiology, University of Foggia, Foggia, Italy; [f] MetroHealth Medical Center, Case Western Reserve University School of Medicine, Cleveland, OH, USA; [g] Division of Cardiology, Stanford University, Stanford, CA, USA; [h] Electrophysiology and Arrhythmia Services, California Pacific Medical Center, San Francisco, CA, USA; [i] Division of Cardiovascular Diseases, Scripps Clinic, La Jolla, CA, USA; [j] Dell Medical School, University of Texas, Austin, TX, USA
* Corresponding author. Texas Cardiac Arrhythmia Institute, St. David's Medical Center, 3000 North IH-35, Suite 700, Austin, TX 78705.
E-mail address: dr.natale@gmail.com

Card Electrophysiol Clin 7 (2015) 755–764
http://dx.doi.org/10.1016/j.ccep.2015.08.007
1877-9182/15/$ – see front matter © 2015 Elsevier Inc. All rights reserved.

CRT is not as effective in patients with AF undergoing CRT for two main reasons: loss of atrioventricular (AV) synchrony and inadequate biventricular capture. The latter can be addressed either with pharmacologic therapy to slow ventricular response or with AV node ablation (AVNA) to achieve near 100% biventricular pacing. Both can be restored with strategies that aim to achieve rhythm control, namely antiarrhythmic drugs (AADs) or catheter ablation.

This article discusses the role and techniques of catheter ablation of AF in patients with HF, and its possible application in CRT recipients.

ATRIAL FIBRILLATION AND HEART FAILURE

AF and HF are the two current epidemics of cardiovascular disease and they often coexist.[1,2] The prevalence of AF in patients with HF increases with HF severity, from 10% to 20% in patients with mild to moderate HF to more than 50% in patients with severe HF.[2–5] Inversely, the lifetime prevalence of HF in AF has been estimated at 40%.[3] Coexistence of HF and AF is associated with an increased risk for hospitalization, stroke, and mortality, with a four- to eight-fold increase versus a two-fold increase in AF alone.[2,6,7]

The pathophysiologic relationship between AF and HF is not completely understood.[8] On one hand, it can be attributed to shared risk factors, such as age, diabetes, hypertension, obesity, sleep apnea, valvular or structural heart disease, and coronary artery disease. On the other hand, a vicious cycle where AF begets HF and HF begets AF also plays an important role. Indeed, AF facilitates the development and progression of HF reducing cardiac output by means of heart rate elevation and irregularity and loss of atrial function and AV synchrony.[9–13] Conversely, HF can facilitate the development and progression of AF via atrial dilatation and fibrosis secondary to elevated left ventricular filling pressures, functional valvular regurgitation, and volume retention mediated by activation of the renin-angiotensin-aldosterone system.[11,12]

ATRIAL FIBRILLATION AND CARDIAC RESYNCHRONIZATION THERAPY

It has been estimated that 20% to 25% of those eligible for CRT have AF; despite this, almost all the landmark randomized controlled clinical trials on CRT have excluded patients with pre-existing AF.[3,14,15] Thus, current guidelines are cautious when it comes to CRT in patients with AF and symptomatic systolic dysfunction (Class IIa, Level of Evidence C).[16]

CRT is not as effective in patients with AF: the high intrinsic ventricular rate reduces biventricular capture, thus precluding optimal ventricular synchronization, and loss of atrial systole makes AV optimization impossible.[17] To improve CRT benefit in AF rate and rhythm control strategies are important: the former addresses ventricular desynchronization, whereas the latter can potentially restore interventricular and AV synchrony.

AVNA has emerged as an important adjunctive therapy for CRT recipients with AF. Observational studies have shown that, compared with AV nodal blocking drugs, AVNA increases LVEF, exercise tolerance, and survival.[18] AVNA restores ventricular synchrony but does not address AV optimization, for which a strategy to obtain rhythm control is warranted.

As in patients with normal systolic function, it has been shown that rhythm control with AADs is not superior to rate control in reducing mortality in patients with HF.[19] The lack of benefit from AADs reflects their poor efficacy in maintaining SR, along with their negative inotropic and proarrhythmic effects. Catheter ablation offers an opportunity to achieve and maintain SR without the downsides of AADs.

STUDIES ON ATRIAL FIBRILLATION ABLATION IN PATIENTS WITH HEART FAILURE

Multiple observational studies suggest that catheter ablation for AF is as effective in maintaining SR in patients with HF as it is in those without (**Table 1**).[20–31] The most important difference is a higher risk of recurrence, with more repeat procedures required to achieve comparable AF-free survival in the HF population.[32] Moreover, catheter ablation improves prognostic markers, including left ventricular function (LVEF), exercise capacity, and quality of life (QoL) in HF patients with AF (**Figs. 1** and **2**). The population enrolled in these studies is heterogeneous, and comprises patients with different HF etiologies and AF types. Interestingly, some patients showed normalization of LVEF after AF ablation, with better results seen in patients with a more rapid ventricular response and/or nonischemic cardiomyopathy, suggesting the presence of a reversible AF-induced cardiomyopathy. Indeed, in this subpopulation, effective and sustained maintenance of SR seems to be curative.[33]

To date, five randomized controlled trials have evaluated the role of catheter ablation for rhythm control in patients with HF (**Table 2**).[34–38] Four of them compared AF ablation with rate control, either pharmacologic or through AVNA, and one compared ablation with rhythm control. In the

PABA-CHF trial, patients with mild to moderate HF were randomized either to AF ablation (N = 41) or to AVNA and CRT (N = 40).[34] After 6 months, 71% of the patients in the ablation group were free from AF off AADs and showed superior improvements in LVEF (35% vs 28%; $P<.001$), exercise tolerance (340 vs 297 m at the 6-ft walking test; $P<.001$), and QoL (60 vs 82 on the questionnaire score; $P<.001$). Subsequently, a study conducted MacDonald and colleagues[35] could not demonstrate any statistically significant difference between AF ablation (N = 22) and pharmacologic rate control (N = 19) in terms of LVEF improvement, exercise tolerance, or QoL. However, these results should be interpreted with caution, because the study was likely underpowered with a low success rate in the ablation group (50%).

In contrast, two more recent trials, ARC-HF and CAMTAF, showed a significant improvement in exercise capacity and QoL with AF ablation compared with pharmacologic rate control.[36,37] The CAMTAF trial also showed improvement in LVEF with AF ablation, whereas in the ARC-HF the difference between groups was not significant. Lastly, in the recently presented AATAC-HF, a trial that compared AF ablation with rhythm control in HF patients with persistent AF and a dual-chamber device (implantable cardioverter-defibrillator or CRT-D), ablation was superior to amiodarone in achieving freedom from atrial tachycardia (AT)/AF after 24 months of follow-up (70% vs 34%; log-rank $P<.0001$).[38] Again, LVEF significantly improved and, more interestingly, this was the first study to show a positive effect in both hospitalization (31 vs 57%; $P<.001$) and mortality (8% vs 18%; $P = .037$) rates.

An important observation is that, despite the complex risk profile of this cohort, studies have shown that complication rates in patients with HF undergoing AF ablation are not different from that of patients with a structurally normal heart.[39] Peculiar complications associated with ablation in this cohort, namely device malfunction and exacerbation of HF, can be prevented with adequate planning. Device malfunction is rare, and most commonly secondary to lead dislodgment.[40,41] Recently implanted leads (<6 months) are more prone to dislodgement, thus delaying the procedure can help preventing this complication. In addition, careful manipulation of intracardiac catheters and sheaths is important. More specifically, atrial lead dislodgement occurs when positioning the transseptal sheath in the right atrium before left atrial access, and can be avoided ensuring the sheath is posterior to the lead in the right anterior oblique view. Exacerbation of HF secondary to fluid overload can be minimized with additional preprocedural and postprocedural diuresis and with the use of low-flow open irrigated catheters.[42]

Finally, meta-analyses have confirmed the essence of catheter ablation in this cohort. In a meta-analysis of seven studies including 1851 patients, 64% to 96% of patients with HF were free from AT/AF after a mean of 1.4 procedures.[32] Compared with patients with normal LVEF, there were no differences in complications rates (3.5% vs 2.5%). In a more recent meta-analysis of 26 studies and 1838 patients, success rates were lower (54%–67%) with a slightly higher incidence of complications (4.8%).[43] Interestingly, both studies showed that after ablation patients with HF experienced a similarly significant improvement of LVEF improvement (11% and 13%).[32,43] This effect was confirmed in another meta-analysis of nine studies involving 354 patients that specifically assessed the change in LVEF in which a similar 11% improvement after catheter ablation was reported.[44]

No studies to date have specifically addressed the role of catheter ablation of AF in CRT recipients, so it is still unclear if these therapies offer additive benefits. One can postulate that catheter ablation of AF can improve CRT response by controlling the ventricular rate/regularity and by affecting atrial function, thus promoting adequate interventricular and AV synchrony. More definitive data about the role of AF ablation may come from clinical trials that are enrolling device recipients with AF to be randomized to either catheter ablation or conventional medical therapy. To our knowledge, there are three trials with these characteristics: two ongoing, CASTLE-HF (NCT00643188) and AMICA (NCT0652522); and one yet to be published, AATAC-HF.[38] By studying the subset of patients with ventricular dyssynchrony, one might be able to elucidate the incremental benefit of atrial rhythm control in AF patients with CRT.

ABLATION APPROACH

Pulmonary vein (PV) isolation remains the cornerstone of every AF ablation procedure, but by itself it is not enough in patients with HF. AF patients with HF demonstrate more pronounced atrial remodeling compared with AF patients without HF, leading to electrophysiologic and structural changes that predispose to the development of other triggers and make the atria the perfect substrate for AF to sustain.[12] This may account for the higher prevalence of nonparoxysmal AF in this cohort and a more aggressive ablation

Table 1
Published observational studies on AF ablation in patients with HF

First Author, Country, Year	Study Design	Patients with HF (N)	Age (y)	LVEF (%)	NYHA Class	PAF (%)	Ablation Strategy	Follow-Up (mo)	Redo Rate	Complication Rate	Success Rate	LVEF Change	Exercise Capacity	QoL
Chen, USA, 2004[20]	R	94	57 ± 8	36 ± 8%	2.7 ± 0.5	42%	PVI	14 ± 5	22%	4%	99% (96% off AAD)	+5% (NS)	NA	↑
Hsu, France, 2004[21]	P	58	56 ± 10	35 ± 7%	2.3 ± 0.5	9%	PVI, LA roof, MI	12 ± 7	50%	3%	78% (69% off AAD)	+21%	↑	↑
Tondo, Italy, 2006[22]	P	40	57 ± 10	33 ± 2%	2.8 ± 0.1	25%	PVI, MI, CTI	14 ± 2	33%	13%	87% (49% off AAD)	+14%	↑	↑
Gentlesk, USA, 2007[23]	P	67	54 ± 9	42 ± 9%	NA	70%	Triggers (PVs and non-PV)	20 ± 9	NA	NA	86% (58% off AAD)	+14%	NA	NA
Efremidis, Greece, 2008[24]	P	13	55 ± 22	35% (35–40)	2.0 ± 0.7	0%	PVI, MI, CTI	9 ± 7	NA	0%	62%	+20%	NA	NA
Lutomsky, Germany, 2008[25]	P	18	56 ± 11	41 ± 7% (CMRI)	NA	100%	PVI	5 ± 1	NA	NA	50% off AAD	+11%	NA	NA
De Potter, Spain, 2010[26]	R	36	52 ± 10	41 ± 8%	NA	39%	PVI, PW, MI	14 ± 14	31%	8%	70%[a]	+10%	NA	NA

Choi, USA, 2010[27]	R	15	56 ± 11	37 ± 6%	1.7 ± 0.8	67%	PVI ± LA roof, MI (redo)	16 ± 13	33%	7%	73% off AAD	+13%	NA	NA
Cha, USA, 2011[28]	P	111	55 (49–61)	35% (30–40)	NA	28%	PVI/WACA, non-PV triggers ± LA roof, MI (non-PAF)	12 >60	20%	4%	76 >33% (62 >26% off AAD)	+21%	NA	↑
Anselmino, Italy, 2013[29]	R	196	61 ± 10	40 ± 8%	2.1 ± 0.7	22%	PVI ± LA roof, MI, CFAE (non-PAF, redo)	46 (16–64)	30%	11%	62%	+10%	↑	↑
Nedios, Germany, 2014[30]	R	69	60 ± 9	33 ± 6%	2.4 ± 0.5	36%	PVI ± PW, MI (non-PAF)	28 ± 11	46%	1%	65%	+15%	NA	NA
Lobo, Brazil, 2015[31]	R	31	60 ± 11	45 ± 6%	2.2 ± 0.6	7%	PVI, SVC isolation, CTI, AF nests, triggers	20 ± 17	26%	0%	77%	+14%	↑	NA

Abbreviations: AAD, antiarrhythmic drugs; AF, atrial fibrillation; CFAE, complex fractionated electrograms; CMRI, cardiac MRI; CTI, cavotricuspid isthmus; LA, left atrium; LVEF, left ventricular ejection fraction; MI, mitral isthmus; NA, not available; NS, nonsignificant; NYHA, New York Heart Association; P, prospective; PAF, paroxysmal atrial fibrillation; PV, pulmonary vein; PVI, pulmonary vein isolation; PW, posterior wall; QoL, quality of life; R, retrospective; SVC, superior vena cava; WACA, wide atrial circumferential ablation.

[a] AAD regimen nonspecified.

Data from Refs.[20–31]

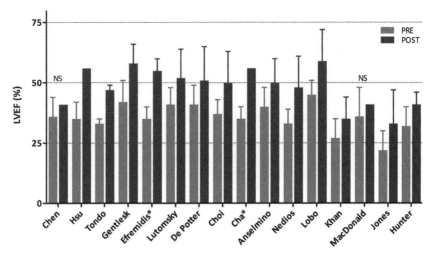

Fig. 1. Mean LVEF at baseline (PRE) and at the end of follow-up (POST) of published studies on AF ablation in patients with HF. NS, nonsignificant. *Columns* and *error bars* display mean and standard deviation, except for asterisks, median and interquartile range.

strategy, addressing other targets, such as non-PV triggers or the substrate, is necessary.

Our experience is that addressing non-PV triggers, even empirically, leads to better outcomes

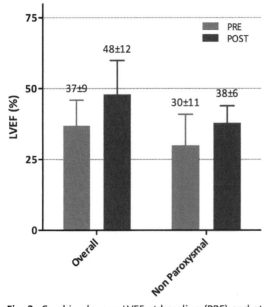

Fig. 2. Combined mean LVEF at baseline (PRE) and at the end of follow-up (POST) of published studies on AF ablation in patients with HF. On the *left*, studies with paroxysmal and nonparoxysmal AF patients; on the *right*, studies with only nonparoxysmal AF patients. Only studies with normally distributed data were included in the analysis; data are expressed as mean and standard deviation.

in this population, as compared with ablation of complex fractionated atrial electrograms or left linear lesions (mitral isthmus, roof line).[45] Non-PV triggers are particularly prevalent in patients with more persistent AF, enlarged left atrium, and underlying heart disease.[46,47] Remodeled atria can harbor non-PV triggers by means of fibrosis, intracellular calcium overload, and activation of atrial stretch-activated ion channels.[48–50] Because HF is generally a progressive disease, continuing atrial remodeling with subsequent emergence of non-PV triggers may well account for the higher risk of AF recurrence after ablation in patients with HF.

Our ablation approach in patients with AF and HF consists of formal PV isolation, confirmed by a circular mapping catheter, followed by ablation of the entire posterior wall down to the coronary sinus and to the left side of the septum, anterior to the right PVs. After this extensive ablation, if AF does not terminate, we perform external cardioversion and when the patient is in stable SR, we proceed with high-dose isoproterenol infusion (20–30 µg/minute) for 10 to 15 minutes to elicit non-PV triggers and look for PV reconnection. If any consistent ectopic atrial activity and/or AT start, we map and ablate it with elimination of those arrhythmias as an end point. Most commonly, the sites of non-PV triggers are the coronary sinus, left atrial appendage, and superior vena cava and the ablation end point is complete isolation of these structures, again confirmed by absent activity as recorded by the circular mapping catheter.

Table 2
Published randomized clinical trials on AF ablation in patients with HF

First Author, Country, Year	Intervention	Patients with HF (N)	Age (y)	LVEF (%)	NYHA Class	PAF (%)	Ablation Strategy	Follow-Up (mo)	Redo Rate	Complication Rate	Success Rate	LVEF Change	Exercise Capacity	QoL
Khan, USA, 2008[34] PABA-CHF	RFA vs AVNA + CRT	41	60 ± 8	27 ± 8%	NA	49%	PVI, LA lines, CFAE	6	20%	8%	88% (71% off AAD)	+8%	↑	↑
MacDonald, UK, 2011[35]	RFA vs rate control	22	62 ± 7	36 ± 12% (CMRI)	2.9 ± 0.3	0%	PVI, LA roof, CFAE ± CTI	10 ± 3	27%	15%	50%[a]	+5% (NS)	=	=
Jones, UK, 2013[36] ARC-HF	RFA vs rate control	26	64 ± 10	22 ± 8% (RNVG)	2.5 ± 0.5	0%	PVI, LA roof, MI, CFAE, CTI	12	19%	15%	88% (84% off AAD)	+11%	↑	↑
Hunter, UK, 2014[37] CAMTAF	RFA vs rate control	26	55 ± 12	32 ± 8%	2.6 ± 0.5	0%	WACA, CFAE, LA roof, MI ± CTI	12	54%	8%	73% off AAD	+9%	↑	↑
Di Biase, USA, 2015[38] AATAC-HF	RFA vs rhythm control	102	NA	NA	NA	0%	PVI ± PW, non-PV triggers	24	NA	NA	70% off AAD	NA	NA	NA

Abbreviations: AAD, antiarrhythmic drugs; AF, atrial fibrillation; CFAE, complex fractionated electrograms; CMRI, cardiac MRI; CRT, cardiac resynchronization therapy; CTI, cavotricuspid isthmus; HF, heart failure; LA, left atrium; LVEF, left ventricular ejection fraction; MI, mitral isthmus; NA, not available; NS, nonsignificant; NYHA, New York Heart Association; PAF, paroxysmal atrial fibrillation; PV, pulmonary vein; PVI, pulmonary vein isolation; PW, posterior wall; QoL, quality of life; RNVG, radionuclide ventriculography; WACA, wide atrial circumferential ablation.

[a] AAD regimen nonspecified.

Data from Refs.[34–38]

SUMMARY

Catheter ablation of AF is a safe and effective non-pharmacologic strategy to achieve rhythm control in patients with HF. It may have positive effects in CRT patients with AF by controlling the heart rate and restoring AV synchrony, but no study has specifically addressed the incremental value of catheter ablation in AF patients with ventricular dyssynchrony. To note, AF ablation is beneficial in patients with HF regardless of CRT and it may be curative in those with tachyarrhythmia-related cardiomyopathy.

REFERENCES

1. Lloyd-Jones D, Adams R, Brown T, et al. Heart disease and stroke statistics. 2010 update: a report from the American Heart Association. Circulation 2010;121(7):e46–215.
2. Ehrlich J, Nattel S, Hohnloser S. Atrial fibrillation and congestive heart failure: specific considerations at the intersection of two common and important cardiac disease sets. J Cardiovasc Electrophysiol 2002;13(4):399–405.
3. Maisel WH, Stevenson LW. Atrial fibrillation in heart failure: epidemiology, pathophysiology, and rationale for therapy. Am J Cardiol 2003;91(6A): 2D–8D.
4. Cleland JG, Swedberg K, Follath F, et al. The Euro-Heart failure survey programme. A survey on the quality of care among patients with heart failure in Europe. Part 1: patient characteristics and diagnosis. Eur Heart J 2003;24(5):442–63.
5. Nieuwlaat R, Capucci A, Camm AJ, et al. Atrial fibrillation management: a prospective survey in ESC member countries: the Euro Heart Survey on Atrial Fibrillation. Eur Heart J 2005;26(22): 2422–34.
6. Wang TJ, Larson MG, Levy D, et al. Temporal relations of atrial fibrillation and congestive heart failure and their joint influence on mortality: the Framingham Heart Study. Circulation 2003; 107(23):2920–5.
7. Mamas MA, Caldwell JC, Chacko S, et al. A meta-analysis of the prognostic significance of atrial fibrillation in chronic heart failure. Eur J Heart Fail 2009; 11(7):676–83.
8. Heist EK, Ruskin JN. Atrial fibrillation and congestive heart failure: risk factors, mechanisms, and treatment. Prog Cardiovasc Dis 2006;48(4):256–69.
9. Shinbane JS, Wood MA, Jensen DN, et al. Tachycardia-induced cardiomyopathy: a review of animal models and clinical studies. J Am Coll Cardiol 1997;29(4):709–15.
10. Pozzoli M, Cioffi G, Traversi E, et al. Predictors of primary atrial fibrillation and concomitant clinical and hemodynamic changes in patients with chronic heart failure: a prospective study in 344 patients with baseline sinus rhythm. J Am Coll Cardiol 1998;32(1):197–204.
11. Li D, Fareh S, Leung T, et al. Promotion of atrial fibrillation by heart failure in dogs: atrial remodeling of a different sort. Circulation 1999;100(1):87–95.
12. Sanders P, Morton J, Davidson N, et al. Electrical remodeling of the atria in congestive heart failure: electrophysiological and electroanatomic mapping in humans. Circulation 2003;108(12):1461–8.
13. Gosselink AT, Blanksma P, Crijns H, et al. Left ventricular beat-to-beat performance in atrial fibrillation: contribution of frank-starling mechanism after short rather than long RR intervals. J Am Coll Cardiol 2000;26(6):1516–21.
14. Dickstein K, Bogale N, Priori S, et al. The European cardiac resynchronization therapy survey. Eur Heart J 2009;30(20):2450–60.
15. Tolosana J, Arnau A, Madrid A, et al. Cardiac resynchronization therapy in patients with permanent atrial fibrillation. Is it mandatory to ablate the atrioventricular junction to obtain a good response? Eur J Heart Fail 2012;14(6):635–41.
16. Brignole M, Auricchio A, Baron-Esquivias G, et al. 2013 ESC guidelines on cardiac pacing and cardiac resynchronization therapy: the task force on cardiac pacing and resynchronization therapy of the European Society of Cardiology (ESC). Developed in collaboration with the European Heart Rhythm Association (EHRA). Eur Heart J 2013; 34(29):2281–329.
17. Wilton SB, Leung AA, Ghali WA, et al. Outcomes of cardiac resynchronization therapy in patients with versus those without atrial fibrillation: a systematic review and meta-analysis. Heart Rhythm 2011;8(7): 1088–94.
18. Yin J, Hu H, Wang Y, et al. Effects of atrioventricular nodal ablation on permanent atrial fibrillation patients with cardiac resynchronization therapy: a systematic review and meta-analysis. Clin Cardiol 2014; 37(11):707–15.
19. Roy D, Talajic M, Nattel S, et al. Rhythm control versus rate control for atrial fibrillation and heart failure. N Engl J Med 2008;358(25):2667–77.
20. Chen MS, Marrouche NF, Khaykin Y, et al. Pulmonary vein isolation for the treatment of atrial fibrillation in patients with impaired systolic function. J Am Coll Cardiol 2004;43(6):1004–9.
21. Hsu LF, Jaïs P, Sanders P, et al. Catheter ablation for atrial fibrillation in congestive heart failure. N Engl J Med 2004;351(23):2373–83.
22. Tondo C, Mantica M, Russo G, et al. Pulmonary vein vestibule ablation for the control of atrial fibrillation in patients with impaired left ventricular function. Pacing Clin Electrophysiol 2006;29(9): 962–70.

23. Gentlesk PJ, Sauer WH, Gerstenfeld EP, et al. Reversal of left ventricular dysfunction following ablation of atrial fibrillation. J Cardiovasc Electrophysiol 2007;18(1):9–14.

24. Efremidis M, Sideris A, Xydonas S, et al. Ablation of atrial fibrillation in patients with heart failure: reversal of atrial and ventricular remodelling. Hellenic J Cardiol 2008;49(1):19–25.

25. Lutomsky BA, Rostock T, Koops A, et al. Catheter ablation of paroxysmal atrial fibrillation improves cardiac function: a prospective study on the impact of atrial fibrillation ablation on left ventricular function assessed by magnetic resonance imaging. Europace 2008;10(5):593–9.

26. De Potter T, Berruezo A, Mont L, et al. Left ventricular systolic dysfunction by itself does not influence outcome of atrial fibrillation ablation. Europace 2010;12(1):24–9.

27. Choi AD, Hematpour K, Kukin M, et al. Ablation vs. medical therapy in the setting of symptomatic atrial fibrillation and left ventricular dysfunction. Congest Heart Fail 2010;16(1):10–4.

28. Cha YM, Wokhlu A, Asirvatham SJ, et al. Success of ablation for atrial fibrillation in isolated left ventricular diastolic dysfunction: a comparison to systolic dysfunction and normal ventricular function. Circ Arrhythm Electrophysiol 2011;4(5):724–32.

29. Anselmino M, Grossi S, Scaglione M, et al. Long-term results of transcatheter atrial fibrillation ablation in patients with impaired left ventricular systolic function. J Cardiovasc Electrophysiol 2013;24(1):24–32.

30. Nedios S, Sommer P, Dagres N, et al. Long-term follow-up after atrial fibrillation ablation in patients with impaired left ventricular systolic function: the importance of rhythm and rate control. Heart Rhythm 2014;11(3):344–51.

31. Lobo TJ, Pachon CT, Pachon JC, et al. Atrial fibrillation ablation in systolic dysfunction: clinical and echocardiographic outcomes. Arq Bras Cardiol 2015;104(1):45–52.

32. Wilton SB, Fundytus A, Ghali WA, et al. Meta-analysis of the effectiveness and safety of catheter ablation of atrial fibrillation in patients with versus without left ventricular systolic dysfunction. Am J Cardiol 2010;106(9):1284–91.

33. Calvo N, Bisbal F, Guiu E, et al. Impact of atrial fibrillation-induced tachycardiomyopathy in patients undergoing pulmonary vein isolation. Int J Cardiol 2013;168(4):4093–7.

34. Khan MN, Jaïs P, Cummings J, et al. Pulmonary-vein isolation for atrial fibrillation in patients with heart failure. N Engl J Med 2008;359(17):1778–85.

35. MacDonald M, Connelly D, Hawkins N, et al. Radiofrequency ablation for persistent atrial fibrillation in patients with advanced heart failure and severe left ventricular systolic dysfunction: a randomised controlled trial. Heart 2011;97(9):740–7.

36. Jones DG, Haldar SK, Hussain W, et al. A randomized trial to assess catheter ablation versus rate control in the management of persistent atrial fibrillation in heart failure. J Am Coll Cardiol 2013;61(18):1894–903.

37. Hunter R, Berriman T, Diab I, et al. A randomized controlled trial of catheter ablation versus medical treatment of atrial fibrillation in heart failure (the CAMTAF trial). Circ Arrhythm Electrophysiol 2014;7(1):31–8.

38. Di Biase L, Mohanty P, Mohanty S, et al. Ablation vs. amiodarone for treatment of persistent atrial fibrillation in patients with congestive heart failure and an implanted device: results from the AATAC multicenter randomized trial. San Diego (CA): American College of Cardiology; 2015. Scientific Sessions, Available at: http://www.abstractsonline.com/pp8/#!/3658/presentation/37598.

39. Cappato R, Calkins H, Chen SA, et al. Updated worldwide survey on the methods, efficacy, and safety of catheter ablation for human atrial fibrillation. Circ Arrhythm Electrophysiol 2009;3(1):32–8.

40. Newby K, Zimerman L, Wharton J, et al. Radiofrequency ablation of atrial flutter and atrial tachycardias in patients with permanent indwelling catheters. Pacing Clin Electrophysiol 1996;19(11 Pt 1):1612–7.

41. Lakkireddy D, Patel D, Ryschon K, et al. Safety and efficacy of radiofrequency energy catheter ablation of atrial fibrillation in patients with pacemakers and implantable cardiac defibrillators. Heart Rhythm 2005;2(12):1309–16.

42. Di Biase L, Santangeli P, Bai R, et al. Impact of a new open irrigated catheter on the risk of fluid overload after ablation of long standing persistent atrial fibrillation: results from a prospective randomized study. J Am Coll Cardiol 2013;61(10):E320.

43. Anselmino M, Matta M, D'Ascenzo F, et al. Catheter ablation of atrial fibrillation in patients with left ventricular systolic dysfunction: a systematic review and meta-analysis. Circ Arrhythm Electrophysiol 2014;7(6):1011–8.

44. Dagres N, Varounis C, Gaspar T, et al. Catheter ablation for atrial fibrillation in patients with left ventricular systolic dysfunction. A systematic review and meta-analysis. J Card Fail 2011;17(11):964–70.

45. Trivedi C, Zhao Y, Di Biase L, et al. Relevance of non-PV triggers ablation to achieve long term freedom from atrial fibrillation in patients with low ejection fraction. Heart Rhythm 2014;11(5):S361–411.

46. Lee SH, Tai CT, Hsieh MH, et al. Predictors of early and late recurrence of atrial fibrillation after catheter

ablation of paroxysmal atrial fibrillation. J Interv Card Electrophysiol 2004;10(3):221–6.

47. Lo LW, Chiou CW, Lin YJ, et al. Differences in the atrial electrophysiological properties between vagal and sympathetic types of atrial fibrillation. J Cardiovasc Electrophysiol 2013;24(6):609–16.

48. Akkaya M, Higuchi K, Koopmann M, et al. Higher degree of left atrial structural remodeling in patients with atrial fibrillation and left ventricular systolic dysfunction. J Cardiovasc Electrophysiol 2013; 24(5):485–91.

49. Kalman S. Electrical remodeling of the atria as a consequence of atrial stretch. J Cardiovasc Electrophysiol 2001;12(1):51–5.

50. Kurotobi T, Iwakura K, Inoue K, et al. Multiple arrhythmogenic foci associated with the development of perpetuation of atrial fibrillation. Circ Arrhythm Electrophysiol 2009;3(1):39–45.

Response to CRT

The Role of Atrioventricular and Interventricular Optimization for Cardiac Resynchronization Therapy

Daniel B. Cobb, MD, Michael R. Gold, MD, PhD*

KEYWORDS

- Cardiac resynchronization therapy • Optimization • Heart failure • Implantable defibrillator
- AV delay

KEY POINTS

- Despite different attempts at patient selection and programming optimization, cardiac resynchronization therapy (CRT) nonresponder rates have remained relatively stable.
- Many different methods for atrioventricular (AV) and interventricular (VV) delay optimization have been developed, and all have demonstrated that optimized delays, regardless of the method, result in acute improvements in left ventricular diastolic and systolic function.
- As routine AV delay optimization was performed in most trials demonstrating efficacy of CRT, it is a reasonable strategy that does not appear to be harmful.
- Three large multicenter trials (FREEDOM, SMART-AV, and ADAPTIVE CRT) failed to show superiority of intracardiac electrogram–based optimization over nominal settings or echo techniques.
- At the present time, the benefit of routine use of AV and VV interval optimization is unclear and may be most useful in the population of CRT "nonresponders," although the benefit of this strategy also requires further study.

INTRODUCTION

Cardiac resynchronization therapy (CRT) is a cornerstone in the management of patients with heart failure (HF) with left ventricular (LV) systolic dysfunction and a ventricular conduction delay (**Table 1**).[1,2] Multiple randomized studies have demonstrated improvements in symptoms and cardiac function as well as reductions in morbidity and mortality in appropriately selected patients with moderate to severe HF despite optimal medical therapy.[3–7] More recent studies also have demonstrated benefit in patients with milder forms of HF, which has expanded the population eligible for device-based therapy.[8–10] Not all patients with HF respond to CRT, with as many as 30% of patients failing to show clinical improvement.[11] Given the inherent risks and costs of device implantation and maintenance, a reduction in the rate of CRT "nonresponders" is an important goal.

Patient selection and device optimization are 2 available strategies that can potentially increase the proportion of patients who respond to CRT. Using measures of mechanical dyssynchrony to aid in patient selection has been disappointing. The multicenter PROSPECT trial failed to identify

Division of Cardiology, Department of Medicine, Medical University of South Carolina, Charleston, SC, USA
* Corresponding author. Division of Cardiology, Medical University of South Carolina, 114 Doughty Street, MSC 592, Charleston, SC 29425.
E-mail address: goldmr@musc.edu

Card Electrophysiol Clin 7 (2015) 765–779
http://dx.doi.org/10.1016/j.ccep.2015.08.008
1877-9182/15/$ – see front matter © 2015 Elsevier Inc. All rights reserved.

Table 1
Summary of the various methods of AV and VV interval optimization

	AV Optimization	VV Optimization
Echocardiography	Mitral inflow (Ritter method, iterative method, "fast and simple") Aortic VTI	LV M-Mode (septal-posterior wall motion delay) Tissue Doppler imaging Aortic VTI
Alternative techniques	Impedance cardiography Finger photoplethysmography Acoustic cardiography Peak endocardial acceleration	Intracardiac echocardiography Electroanatomic mapping Radionuclide angiography Finger photoplethysmography Peak endocardial acceleration Surface electrocardiogram
Intracardiac electrogram-based algorithms	Boston Scientific SmartDelay St Jude Medical QuickOpt Medtronic adaptive algorithm	Boston Scientific Expert ease St Jude Medical QuickOpt Medtronic adaptive algorithm

Adapted from Brabham WW, Gold MR. The role of AV and VV optimization for CRT. J Arrhythm 2013;29:158; with permission.

any single echocardiographic marker of dyssynchrony that was predictive of response to CRT.[11] Even more concerning, the ECHO CRT studies showed that CRT increases mortality among patients with a reduced ejection fraction and mechanical dyssynchrony but a QRS duration less than 130 msec.[12]

Postimplantation device optimization includes individualized programming of the atrioventricular (AV) and interventricular (VV) delay to maximize the hemodynamic and, hopefully, clinical response to CRT. Early CRT devices simply allowed AV delay programming with simultaneous biventricular (BiV) pacing. Modern systems allow programming of both the individual AV and VV intervals. Considering additional variables such as the AV delay offset for atrial-sensed (AS) versus atrial-paced (AP) CRT and rate-adaptive AV delay modulation, the complexity of CRT programming is obvious. Given the multitude of options for CRT programming without a clearly defined gold standard, interpretation of the data becomes difficult. Additionally, the guidelines for CRT do not offer recommendations for device optimization, reflecting a clear lack of consensus on the issue.[1,2] Despite these limitations, AV and VV optimization may prove useful in select patients receiving CRT, and a working understanding of the methods and controversies involved is important for all physicians who manage these patients.

ATRIOVENTRICULAR OPTIMIZATION

The concept of AV synchrony seems simple, as preservation of both passive and active LV filling contribute to stroke volume and cardiac output. Interestingly, AV optimization may be more useful

to achieve interventricular and intraventricular electrical resynchronization than to optimize filling. Early studies involving patients with complete heart block and dual-chamber pacemakers confirmed variation in stroke volume with changes in programmed AV delay.[13] The vast majority of patients receiving CRT have preserved intrinsic AV nodal conduction but prolonged interventricular and intraventricular conduction. The effects of AV programming on LV systolic function can be measured by invasively monitoring dP/dT_{max}.[14] As a result, methods of AV delay optimization have been the focus of numerous studies using approaches to optimize either LV diastolic or systolic function, primarily through use of Doppler echocardiography (**Fig. 1**). Furthermore, all of the major trials of CRT in patients with HF, with the exception of the CONTAK-CD trial,[4] performed some method of AV delay optimization.

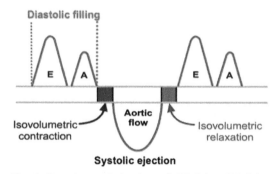

Fig. 1. Doppler optimization of AV delay. AV delay optimization techniques have focused on optimizing either LV diastolic (mitral inflow) or systolic (aortic outflow) function. (*Adapted from* Brabham WW, Gold MR. The role of AV and VV optimization for CRT. J Arrhythm 2013;29:154; with permission.)

Optimizing Left Ventricular Diastolic Filling

AV delay optimization based on LV diastolic function uses the filling pattern obtained through Doppler echocardiography of mitral inflow. Many different methods have been used and evaluated. Mitral inflow is dependent on timing of both left atrial and LV systole, and interatrial and interventricular conduction delays will affect optimal timing of ventricular pacing. A relatively short AV delay may result in truncation of the A wave, representing atrial systole, whereas a prolonged AV delay can also result in shortening of total diastolic filling time (**Fig. 2**).[15] One of the earliest and more commonly cited methods of AV delay optimization using mitral inflow is the Ritter method. This technique was originally validated in patients with dual-chamber pacemakers for heart block. The Ritter method involves measuring the interval from the QRS onset or pacing spike to the end of the A wave at relatively long and short AV delays. The difference between these two is then subtracted from the "long" AV delay to arrive at the optimal AV delay (**Fig. 3**). This technique is intended to optimize diastolic filling time without truncation of the A wave. AV delays derived using the Ritter method have been shown to correlate with improvements in stroke volume (derived from impedance cardiography) in comparison with nominal AV delays in patients with dual-chamber pacemakers.[13] This was the method of AV optimization used in the InSync III trial.[16]

Other strategies using the mitral inflow pattern include a "fast and simple" approach and the iterative method. The "fast and simple" method requires the presence of mitral regurgitation on the spectral Doppler pattern. The AV delay is set 5 to 10 ms below the longest AV delay, ensuring biventricular capture. The time interval from the end of the A wave to the onset of high-velocity mitral regurgitation (ie, LV contraction) is subtracted from the long AV delay to arrive at the optimal AV delay. AV delay intervals derived with this method have been shown to result in higher invasively measured cardiac output.[17]

The most common echocardiographic optimization technique is the iterative method; this was used in the CARE-HF[7] and the SMART-AV[18] trials and involves programming a relatively long AV interval with gradual shortening, typically in 20-ms steps. When truncation of the A wave is observed on the mitral inflow Doppler, the AV interval is gradually prolonged in 10-ms steps until the delay with maximal E and A wave separation is obtained (**Fig. 4**). However, use of this method did not result in improved clinical or echocardiographic outcomes over a nominal, fixed AV delay in CRT patients in the SMART-AV trial, as will be discussed later.[18] Additionally, the reproducibility and consistency of measurement of this technique has been challenged despite its relative ease of use compared with other techniques.[19]

Optimizing Left Ventricular Systolic Performance

Doppler-derived measures of LV systolic function also have been applied to AV delay optimization.

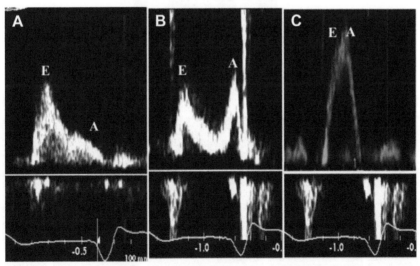

Fig. 2. Effect of AV delay on mitral inflow. AV delays that are either too short (*A*) or too long (*C*) will result in truncation of the A wave of mitral inflow or E and A wave fusion, respectively. (*B*) At the optimal AV delay, E and A wave separation results in maximum diastolic filling time without truncation of the A wave. (*Adapted from* Brabham WW, Gold MR. The role of AV and VV optimization for CRT. J Arrhythm 2013;29:155; with permission.)

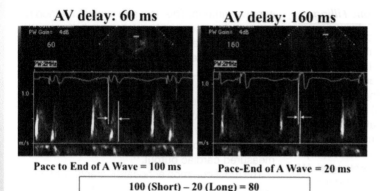

AV delay: 60 ms	AV delay: 160 ms
Pace to End of A Wave = 100 ms	Pace-End of A Wave = 20 ms

100 (Short) – 20 (Long) = 80
160 (Long AV delay) – 80 = 80 ms (optimal AVD)

Fig. 3. The Ritter method. The interval from the pacing spike to the end of the A wave on mitral inflow is measured at short and long AV delays. The difference in these time intervals is then subtracted from the long AV delay to calculate the optimal AV delay. (*Adapted from* Brabham WW, Gold MR. The role of AV and VV optimization for CRT. J Arrhythm 2013;29:155; with permission.)

In a study by Morales and colleagues,[20] a fixed AV delay of 120 ms was compared with a strategy of AV delay optimization by Doppler estimation of LV dP/dt_{max} from the mitral regurgitant jet. Although the study included only 26 patients, those who were optimized experienced more 6-month improvement in New York Heart Association (NYHA) class and ejection fraction than those with a fixed AV delay. Similar to the "fast and simple" method described previously, this method is limited by the requirement for a well-defined mitral regurgitant jet.

The aortic pulsed-wave Doppler velocity time integral (VTI) also has been used to optimize AV delay, as this method was shown to correlate with LV stroke volume.[21] This process is fairly simple, as one simply measures the aortic VTI over a range of AV delays. The AV delay is then considered optimized when the aortic VTI is greatest (**Fig. 5**). In 2 small, nonrandomized comparisons

No Pacing

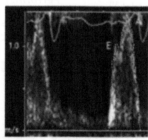

60 ms	80 ms	100 ms	120 ms	140 ms

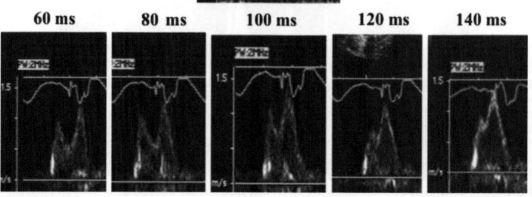

Fig. 4. The iterative method. Without pacing there is fusion of the E and A waves on mitral inflow. The AV delay is then gradually shortened, resulting in increased E and A wave separation until A wave truncation becomes apparent at a delay of 60 ms. The delay can then be prolonged in 10-ms steps to achieve maximal separation. (*Adapted from* Brabham WW, Gold MR. The role of AV and VV optimization for CRT. J Arrhythm 2013;29:156; with permission.)

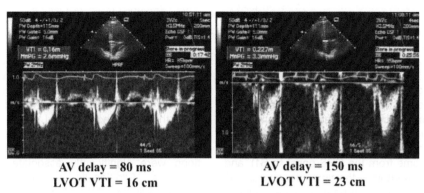

AV delay = 80 ms
LVOT VTI = 16 cm

AV delay = 150 ms
LVOT VTI = 23 cm

Fig. 5. Aortic VTI method. AV delay optimized to achieve the maximum stroke volume based on the aortic outflow tract VTI. In this case, the VTI increased from 16 to 23 cm with an increase in the AV delay from 80 to 150 ms. This also can be used in VV interval optimization (see text for details). (*Adapted from* Brabham WW, Gold MR. The role of AV and VV optimization for CRT. J Arrhythm 2013;29:156; with permission.)

of AV delay optimization by the aortic VTI method versus the Ritter method of mitral inflow, optimization by VTI was shown to result in a higher VTI.[22,23] This method also was compared with a fixed AV delay in a randomized study of 40 patients. Patients optimized using aortic VTI experienced greater 3-month improvement in NYHA class and quality of life. Importantly, they also reported stable optimal AV delays over time.[24]

Doppler measurements using mitral inflow VTI also have been used to optimize AV delay. In a study of 30 patients undergoing CRT implantation, AV delay was optimized based on the maximal increase in invasively measured LV dP/dt and compared with those derived from the maximal increase in mitral inflow E and A wave VTI, the iterative method, aortic VTI, and Ritter formula. These investigators found that the AV delay optimized using the mitral inflow VTI correlated best with the maximal increase in dP/dt (29 of 30 patients), whereas that derived from Ritter's formula showed no concordance.[25]

Other Methods of Atrioventricular Optimization

Echocardiography has been considered the "gold standard" for AV delay optimization, given its relative ease of use and widespread availability. Despite this, each of the previously described methods requires significant training, skill, time, and health care resources. As a result, several alternative noninvasive tools have been developed for AV delay optimization. In general, these include noninvasive measures of hemodynamic optimization and device-based intracardiac electrogram (IEGM) algorithms. Impedance cardiography (IC), for example, uses changes in transthoracic

impedance to estimate stroke volume.[13] In a study of 24 patients following CRT implantation, AV delay selected based on the maximal change in IC-derived stroke volume was comparable to that derived from the aortic VTI method ($\leq$20 ms difference in predicted AV delay in 88%).[26]

Finger photoplethysmography (FPPG) is one alternative noninvasive tool for hemodynamic assessment during AV delay optimization. FPPG measures changes in peripheral pulse pressure, which has been shown to correlate reasonably well with simultaneously measured central aortic pressure in 57 patients undergoing CRT.[27] In this group, the optimal AV delay, defined as that producing the greatest change in pulse pressure, was identical using either FPPG or central aortic pressure. Similarly, the Finometer (Finapres Medical Systems, Amsterdam, The Netherlands) is a device that provides continuous, noninvasive measurement of arterial pressure through a finger cuff photoelectric plethysmograph. In an initial study of 12 patients receiving CRT, this device predicted the optimal AV delay based on maximal increase in pulse pressure within 40 ms of that derived from aortic VTI.[28]

Peak endocardial acceleration (PEA) is a device-based algorithm that also has been evaluated for AV delay optimization. The algorithm uses an accelerometer incorporated into a pacing lead behind the pacing electrode, and it has been shown to correlate well with the optimal AV delay optimization using the Ritter method in patients with dual-chamber pacemakers and heart block.[29,30] The PEA algorithm also was evaluated for AV and VV optimization in patients receiving CRT. In the CLEAR trial, 238 patients receiving CRT were randomized to PEA-optimized AV/VV intervals or to "usual" optimization methods. At

1-year follow-up, response to CRT was significantly higher in the group optimized by PEA (76% vs 62%), although this benefit was largely restricted to improvements in subjective endpoints.[31]

Finally, acoustic cardiography is another novel technique for AV optimization. This technology integrates the surface electrocardiogram and heart sound data to measure the intensity of S3, the electromechanical activation time (EMAT, representing the time from the QRS onset to S1), and LV systolic time (LVST, the time interval from S1 to S2). Changes in each parameter can indicate worsening HF: an increase in S3 suggestive of increased LV filling pressure, prolongation of EMAT indicative of reduced LV contractility, and a reduced LVST suggestive of reduced systolic function. AV delay optimization using this method in 22 patients receiving CRT was comparable to the mitral inflow method.[32]

Intracardiac Electrogram-based Atrioventricular Optimization

Intracardiac electrogram (IEGM)-based AV delay algorithms are clearly desirable because these methods can be incorporated into device software for rapid optimization and potentially continuous modification. Such technology could reduce costs, time, and the possibility of user error introduced with more complex and user-dependent methods, such as echocardiography. Investigators from the PATH-CHF studies derived an algorithm based on the intrinsic AV delay and QRS width that accurately predicted the AV delay resulting in maximum dP/dt_{max},[33] which was subsequently used for AV delay programming in the COMPANION trial.[5] A further iteration of this algorithm (EEHF+) was later shown to be superior to aortic VTI and the Ritter method for optimizing dP/dt in 28 patients undergoing CRT implantation.[34] However, the pivotal SMART-AV trial ultimately cast doubt on the utility of routinely using this IEGM-based algorithm and AV delay optimization altogether. In the SMART-AV trial, 980 patients receiving CRT were randomized to a fixed AV delay of 120 ms, echocardiographically optimized AV delay via the iterative method, or AV delay programming using the SmartDelay algorithm (Boston Scientific, Natick, MA). At 6-month follow-up, there were no significant differences in improvement in LV volumes, ejection fraction, or clinical endpoints that included 6-minute walk distance, quality-of-life score, and NYHA classification.[18] However, a substudy of this trial was later performed to evaluate whether pacing at sites of long LV electrical delay increased the effectiveness of AV optimization (AVO) and CRT response. This substudy included 280 subjects who were randomized to either an electrogram-based AVO (SmartDelay) or nominal atrioventricular delay (120 ms). The QLV interval was defined as the time from onset of the QRS to the LV electrogram peak. CRT response was defined as a more than 15% reduction in LV end-systolic volume from implant to 6 months. Analysis from this substudy demonstrated that longer QLV durations were significantly associated with CRT response. Additionally, the benefit of AVO increased as the QLV prolonged.[35] This suggests that the QLV interval may predict response to CRT and that at long QLV intervals, AVO can increase the likelihood of a response to CRT.

Areas of Uncertainty in Atrioventricular Optimization

There are many issues in AVO that remain uncertain. Whereas most of the landmark trials of CRT incorporated some form of AV delay optimization at the time of implantation, definitive data supporting their superiority over an empiric, fixed AV delay are lacking. Most available data involve hemodynamic studies demonstrating an acute improvement with optimization. However, long-term randomized controlled studies of these methods focusing on clinical outcomes are lacking. With the exception of SMART-AV, comparative studies have been too small to draw meaningful conclusions. Indeed, SMART-AV suggests that empiric programming of a fixed AV delay results in similar clinical outcomes to an optimized AV delay, at least with the methods used in the trial. Given that this study examined AV delay in all patients referred for CRT, the results do not exclude the possibility of benefit in certain subgroups of patients such as CRT "nonresponders." One center, for example, has reported a reduction in adverse events through use of a CRT optimization clinic, in which device programming modification, including AV delay optimization, was deemed necessary in 47% of CRT "nonresponders."[36]

Other areas of uncertainty in AV delay programming include the stability of the optimal AV delay, atrial-paced/sensed offset, and rate-adaptive AV delay. Most studies report the acute hemodynamic effects of the optimal AV delay at implant or shortly thereafter, with few evaluating the long-term stability of the optimized AV delay. In 3 independent studies of AV delay optimization using mitral inflow Doppler at enrollment, repeat echocardiographically guided optimization at follow-up demonstrated significant differences from baseline values.[37–39] These findings suggest that the optimal AV delay is not constant and may in part explain the lack of long-term clinical benefit of optimization over an empiric AV delay in SMART-AV. Furthermore, if optimization is performed, the appropriate timing and method remain undefined.

Early studies in CRT primarily enrolled chronotropically competent patients with little need for atrial pacing. As a result, device programming generally used a VDD (ventricular pacing, dual chamber sensing, dual inhibit/trigger) pacing mode, with predominant or exclusive atrial sensing. Many patients with HF have both intrinsic and iatrogenic sinus node dysfunction, making atrial pacing clinically necessary and, at times, desirable. The optimal AV delay offset with AP has been shown to be patient specific and differ significantly from nominal device settings. In a comparison of IEGM AV delay optimization versus conventional Doppler methods in 28 patients, the mean optimized AP/AS offset was found to be 75 ms, and 88% of patients had an offset greater than the nominal 30 ms of the device. LV dP/dt was also found to be higher in this population.[34] A subsequent study of optimized AP/AS AV delays using dP/dt also demonstrated a 72-ms offset to achieve maximal hemodynamic response. Interestingly, the increase in dP/dt_{max} during AP was associated with reductions in echocardiographic measures of LV filling and stroke volume.[40] These results suggest that if AV delay optimization is performed, AS and AP AV delays should be determined individually. If not, an empirical AP/AS offset of 60 to 70 ms is reasonable. The utility of atrial support pacing in CRT has also been recently evaluated in the PEGASUS CRT trial.[41] In this study, 1433 patients were randomized to DDD40, DDD70, or DDDR40, with AV delay programming using the SmartDelay algorithm. Atrial pacing was more frequent in the DDD70 group (43%) than in the DDD40 (3%) or DDDR40 (4%), but there were no significant differences in mortality, HF events, NYHA functional class improvement, or arrhythmic burden. Despite a lack of benefit to atrial support pacing, the absence of observed harm is of clinical importance to safely allow such programming among patients with chronotropic incompetence.

Modern dual-chamber pacing systems universally incorporate some method of rate-adaptive delay shortening algorithms, as they have been shown to improve exercise capacity.[42] However, the utility of such an algorithm in CRT devices is controversial. One study of 36 patients determined the optimal AV delay during rapid atrial pacing and following exercise using the aortic VTI method. The optimal AV delay by VTI was paradoxically longer at faster heart rates.[43] However, 2 other studies have called this into question. Rafie and colleagues[44] observed that the optimal AV delay was shorter at higher atrial pacing rates, and clinical improvement was demonstrated with rate-adaptive AV delay programming. Shanmugam and colleagues[45] performed AV delay optimization using the iterative method in 52 patients at rest and with exercise and found that the optimal AV delay was shorter at higher heart rates. They also performed cardiopulmonary exercise testing in patients randomized to a rate-adaptive AV delay algorithm programmed on or off, and use of the algorithm resulted in significantly longer exercise times and higher peak oxygen consumption. Although the standard of care has been to disable this feature in CRT devices, these data suggest that it may in fact be beneficial. The RAVE study evaluated AV times with exercise and atrial pacing. This study will provide important data for the need for dynamic AV delay programming with IEGM-based timing algorithms.

INTERVENTRICULAR OPTIMIZATION

AV delay programming to ensure ventricular pre-excitation with optimal LV diastolic filling and systolic function is complex, as noted previously. These issues are even more apparent in studies of VV optimization. The landmark trials of CRT in HF all demonstrated a benefit of CRT using simultaneous BiV pacing in conjunction with AV delay optimization.[3,5,7,9,10,46] However, it stands to reason that individual variations in ventricular conduction delay in diseased myocardium should affect the timing of ventricular stimulation that results in optimal resynchronization. This could be targeted to improve response to CRT. Early hemodynamic data from 39 patients in the PATH-CHF studies demonstrated similar improvements in LV contractile function (dP/dt_{max}) with either simultaneous BiV or LV-only pacing.[47] In 41 patients from the same study population, AV optimized simultaneous BiV or LV-only pacing resulted in similar improvements in functional capacity and quality of life that was sustained at 12-month follow-up.[48] This suggests that the critical event in CRT is timing of LV stimulation. This is further supported by acute hemodynamic data from another prospective study showing that both the magnitude of response and the optimal AV delay were similar for BiV and LV-only pacing[49] Other studies have demonstrated acute hemodynamic improvements in invasively measured LV dP/dt with optimization of the VV interval over nominal simultaneous BiV pacing, with significant variation of this interval between patients.[25,50,51] Several noninvasive approaches to VV optimization have been proposed, each with its own limitations.

Dyssynchrony-Guided Interventricular Optimization

Similar to AVO, VV optimization has most often been performed with echocardiography in attempt to improve markers of cardiac dyssynchrony. Patients may display evidence of both VV and intraventricular dyssynchrony, which are related but slightly different entities. VV dyssynchrony results from a delay in LV contraction relative to right ventricular (RV) contraction, and it can be quantified as the difference in pre–ejection delay from the surface QRS to the onset of pulmonic and aortic systolic ejection visualized with pulsed Doppler echocardiography. Intraventricular dyssynchrony refers to delay in segmental wall motion, which can be quantified using LV septal to posterior wall motion delay, tissue Doppler imaging (TDI), and strain rate analysis using a variety of metrics. Bordachar and colleagues[52] evaluated the effect of sequential VV pacing on cardiac output (as measured by aortic VTI) and markers of VV and intraventricular dyssynchrony using pulsed Doppler and TDI in 41 patients receiving CRT. They found that improvements in intraventricular dyssynchrony correlated with an increase in cardiac output, whereas changes in VV dyssynchrony had no correlation. Furthermore, simultaneous BiV pacing was the optimal setting in only 15% of patients. This suggests that optimizing the VV delay using TDI markers of dyssynchrony will result in acute hemodynamic improvements over BiV pacing alone. Similar findings of the acute improvement in intraventricular dyssynchrony with sequential over simultaneous BiV pacing have been reported.[53] However, a 6-month follow-up study of this method of optimized sequential versus simultaneous pacing in 100 patients found no improvement in the rate of CRT responders.[54]

In a study by Abraham and colleagues,[55] 238 patients were randomized to simultaneous versus optimized sequential BiV pacing. The VV interval was adjusted to minimize the septal to posterior wall motion delay. At 6-month follow-up, significantly more patients had improved based on a clinical composite score with optimized sequential (75%) than with simultaneous BiV pacing (65%). However, there were no significant differences in the 6-minute walk distances, quality of life, or HF event rates. Importantly, 82% of patients in the optimized group had a VV interval other than 0 ms.

Even more so than AVO, VV optimization using echocardiographically derived markers of dyssynchrony is significantly limited by the time and

expertise required. For example, in the PROSPECT trial to evaluate the predictive value of echocardiographic markers of dyssynchrony for response to CRT, there was significant variability in TDI quality despite extensive training of study sites.[11] However the real world applicability of this optimization technique is uncertain. In a survey of AV/VV optimization practices at centers involving the FREEDOM trial of the St Jude QuickOpt algorithm (St Jude Medical, Inc, St Paul, MN), the reported use of TDI was only 13.6% among centers, which is likely an overestimate of its use among practices.[56]

Aortic Velocity Time Integral Method

Contrary to the previously described method, a more simple echocardiographic approach in principle involves optimization of the VV interval using aortic VTI, similar to AV delay optimization. In this method, the aortic VTI is measured at varying intervals of RV and LV preexcitation, and that producing the highest VTI is used as the optimal VV delay. In a study of 34 patients by Mortensen and colleagues,[57] VV optimization resulted in higher aortic VTI in comparison with simultaneous BiV pacing, although 3-month outcomes, as defined by NYHA classification and 6-minute walk distance, were similar among those who were or were not optimized. The InSync III trial[16] compared the aortic VTI method of VV optimization to simultaneous VV pacing in 422 patients using the MIRACLE[3] study population as the control group. The authors again demonstrated significant improvements in stroke volume and 6-minute walk distance with optimized VV pacing above simultaneous pacing alone, but there was no significant difference in improvement in NYHA class or quality of life. Subsequent studies also have failed to demonstrate an improvement in 6-month clinical outcomes with aortic VTI optimized VV intervals over simultaneous BiV pacing.[58,59]

Other Methods of Interventricular Optimization

Despite the limited data demonstrating improved clinical outcomes with echocardiographically guided VV optimization, several other approaches have been developed. These include real-time intracardiac echocardiography during CRT implantation,[60] electroanatomic mapping,[61] radionuclide angiography,[62] the Finometer,[63] PEA,[31] and optimization using the surface QRS.[64,65] Several device-based IEGM algorithms for VV optimization also have been developed and evaluated (**Table 2**).

The St Jude QuickOpt algorithm calculates the optimal AV delay and VV offset based on IEGMs

Table 2
Major trials of AV/VV delay optimization

	N	Technique	Result
Abraham et al (FREEDOM),[83] 2010	1525	Optimization at implant with standard of care vs QuickOpt AV/VV optimization every 3 mo	No difference in 12-mo clinical composite score
Ellenbogen et al (SMART-AV),[18] 2010	980	Fixed AV delay (120 ms), iterative method, or SmartDelay AV optimization	No difference in 6-mo change in LVESV, NYHA class, QOL, or 6-min walk
Martin et al (Adaptive CRT),[73] 2012	522	Echo optimized AV/VV delays (iterative and aortic VTI) vs Adaptive CRT algorithm	Adaptive CRT noninferior to echo optimization in clinical composite score (73.6 vs 72.5% improved)
Ritter et al (CLEAR),[31] 2012	238	Standard of care optimization (mostly echo) vs PEA AV/VV optimization algorithm	Significantly more improved in clinical composite score with PEA vs standard of care (76 vs 62%)

Abbreviations: AV, atrioventricular; CRT, cardiac resynchronization therapy; LVESV, left ventricular end systolic volume; NYHA, New York Heart Association; PEA, peak endocardial acceleration; QOL, quality of life; VTI, velocity time integral; VV, interventricular.

Adapted from Brabham WW, Gold MR. The role of AV and VV optimization for CRT. J Arrhythm 2013;29:159; with permission.

measured from the RA, RV, and LV leads. The AV delay is determined from the duration of the sensed atrial electrogram: if more than 100 ms, 30 ms is added to calculate the optimal AV delay and if less than 100 ms, 60 ms is added. For the paced AV delay offset, 50 ms is added to the sensed AV delay. The VV offset determination is more complex. The time interval between sensed local activation between the RV and LV leads is first measured (Δ). The difference in conduction delay to the RV lead during LV pacing and LV lead during RV pacing is then calculated (ε). The estimated optimal VV offset is then given by the formula $VV = 0.5(\Delta + \varepsilon)$, with positive values indicating LV preactivation and negative values indicating RV preactivation. This algorithm was initially evaluated in 11 patients and found to correlate well with the optimal VV delay obtained using the aortic VTI method.[66] However, subsequent validation studies have shown conflicting results, with some demonstrating a good correlation with echocardiographically optimized VV delays and others suggesting inferior performance of the algorithm.[67–70] More importantly, there are no prospective data on the effect of this algorithm on long-term clinical outcomes.

Another IEGM-based algorithm used in Boston Scientific devices has been evaluated as well. The optimal VV delay is estimated using the formula $VV = -0.33 \times (RV - LV \text{ electrical delay}) - 20$ ms. This was derived from unpublished data from PATH-CHF studies. The DECREASE-HF study

prospectively randomized 306 patients to a VV delay determined using this algorithm, simultaneous BiV pacing, or LV pacing alone. At 3- and 6-month follow-up, all patients showed improvements in LV volumes, stroke volume, and ejection fraction. With the exception of a greater decrease in LV end-systolic dimension with simultaneous pacing, there was no significant difference between groups.[71] As with the St Jude's QuickOpt, there are no long-term clinical outcome data using this algorithm.

A third IEGM-based algorithm developed by Medtronic (Medtronic, Inc, Minneapolis, MN) was evaluated in the Adaptive CRT trial. The algorithm provides continuous adjustment of the AV and VV intervals based on periodic measurement of the intrinsic AV interval (as measured from the RA and RV electrodes), the interval from the sensed atrial electrogram (EGM) to the end of a far-field P wave, and the interval from sensed RV EGM to the end of a far-field QRS complex. If the intrinsic AV interval is 200 ms or less and the heart rate is 100 beats per minute or less, LV-only pacing is provided at an AV delay to preempt intrinsic conduction by 40 ms or more. If the intrinsic AV interval is 200 ms or more or the heart rate 100 beats per minute or more, BiV pacing is provided at an AV delay that is longer than the duration of the far-field P wave but 50 ms or more before the intrinsic RV-sensed EGM. The VV offset is then determined based on the intrinsic AV delay and interval from the sensed RV EGM to the end of the QRS complex.[72] In Adaptive CRT, 522 patients were prospectively randomized to echocardiographically optimized CRT or continuous optimization using the IEGM-based algorithm. Aortic VTI correlated well at the optimal AV/VV settings in both arms, and at 6 months, patients managed with this algorithm had similar CRT response rates to those optimized echocardiographically, with no difference in HF events. Use of the algorithm also resulted in a 44% reduction in RV pacing at 6 months. In the subset of patients with normal AV conduction and left bundle branch block (LBBB), the algorithm resulted in more frequent LV-only pacing and significantly better response rates than echocardiographic optimization. This observation is consistent with either a benefit of LV only pacing or a deleterious effect of VV offset with biventricular pacing.[73] These data support the Adaptive algorithm as an alternative, noninferior method of AV/VV optimization to echocardiography. However, the study does not prove either optimization strategy superior to empiric AV/VV delay programming. Subsequently, an analysis of this trial was performed to assess whether synchronized LV pacing (sLVP) resulted in better clinical outcomes. Results of this analysis showed that greater than 50% sLVP pacing was independently associated with a decreased risk of death or HF hospitalization. This suggests that a higher percentage of LV-only pacing may be associated with superior clinical outcomes.[74] Recently, a reduction in readmissions for HF was demonstrated with this algorithm as well. Analysis of data from the Adaptive CRT trial demonstrated the 30-day readmission rate was 19.1% in patients optimized with Adaptive CRT compared with 35.7% in patients undergoing echocardiographic-guided optimization.[75]

Combined Atrioventricular and Interventricular Optimization Using 3-Dimensional Echocardiography

Few studies have looked at combined AV and VV optimization with regard to echocardiography. Previous work has shown that 3-dimensional (3D) echo optimization can lead to acutely improved LV systolic function and decreased dyssynchrony compared with empiric programming,[76] but long-term clinical implications were unclear. Sonne and colleagues[77] describe a novel technique of combining Doppler echocardiography and 3D echocardiography (3DE) for AV and VV optimization compared with conventional electrocardiogram (ECG) optimization. In this study, 77 patients were randomized to either echo-guided AV and VV interval optimization or ECG optimization. Echocardiographic optimization was performed the day after implant. AV delays were analyzed from 80 ms to 200 ms, with steps of 20 ms. Aortic flow was recorded as a VTI using continuous-wave Doppler. The AV delay with the highest VTI was programmed. VV intervals were analyzed at 5 different intervals: simultaneous LV and RV pacing, LV preactivation (LV +20, LV +40 ms), and RV preactivation (RV +20, RV +40 ms). For each interval, a complete 3D full volume was acquired and the device was programmed for other VV interval with the lowest systolic dyssynchrony index (SDI). The SDI is calculated as the SD of the time to minimal systolic volume in 16 segments (excluding the apical cap), corrected for the RR interval and expressed as a percentage. ECG AV delay optimization was achieved using a previously described technique.[78] The AV interval was programmed using a delay of 100 ms from the end of the P wave to peak/nadir of the paced ventricular complex. The optimal VV interval by surface ECG was programmed according to their institution convention as the VV interval with the most simultaneous appearance of the peak or nadir of the QRS interval in leads V1 to V6. Follow-up was obtained in all patients at 3 months and was assessed by NYHA functional class and 3DE. CRT response was defined as a reduction in NYHA by at least 1 class. After analysis, subjects undergoing combined echocardiographic optimization demonstrated a greater response to CRT compared with ECG-guided optimization (82% vs 58%, $P = .021$). Combined echocardiographic guidance also demonstrated a larger increase in ejection fraction and more pronounced reduction in SDI.[77]

QRS-Based Optimization of Cardiac Resynchronization

Many of the methods described previously used echocardiography or invasive hemodynamic measurements for optimization. Given the tedious methods, complexity of measurements, and technical expertise, investigators have begun to look at simpler and more widely available modalities. Arbelo and colleagues[79] describe a new method of QRS-based CRT optimization called fusion-optimized intervals (FOI), which uses fusion with intrinsic conduction and avoids echocardiographic AV and VV optimization. Their study included 76 patients who were implanted with a CRT device. Eligibility criteria were NYHA class II-IV on optimal medical therapy, LV ejection fraction less than 35%, and QRS width greater than or equal to 120 ms. Patients with atrial fibrillation or AV conduction disturbances (AV interval greater than or equal to 250 ms or complete AV block) were excluded.

In their method for optimization, the morning after CRT implantation, QRS measurements were performed in 3 different configurations: during spontaneous sinus rhythm, using the nominal device programming, and after optimization of the AV and VV intervals. To find the fusion band during atrial sensing, the AV interval was progressively shortened with LV pacing only. The AV interval that provided the narrowest QRS was selected and considered the fusion-optimized interval. This was again repeated during atrial pacing at 10 beats per minute above the sinus rate. Next the VV interval was adjusted during spontaneous sinus rhythm comparing the QRS duration in different configurations: simultaneous RV and LV pacing, LV preexcitation of 30 ms, and RV preexcitation of 30 ms. The VV interval that obtained the narrowest QRS was considered to be the fusion-optimized VV interval. The results were then validated 24 to 72 hours after the procedure using invasive measurements of +dP/dt$_{max}$ and echocardiographic TDI. Echocardiography was used to evaluate transmitral flow to assess the impact of AV delay LV filling time and A wave. TDI was used to assess measures of LV asynchrony.

Using the previously described methods, Arbelo and colleagues[79] report that baseline QRS was shortened more by FOI (59 ± 19 ms) than by nominal settings (40 ± 21 ms; P<.001). All echocardiographic asynchrony parameters were corrected by FOI. Additionally, baseline + dP/dt$_{max}$ improvement was greater in FOI than in nominal settings.[79] However, similar to many of the previously described methods, improvement was based on short-term hemodynamic or echocardiographic parameters and not long-term clinical outcomes.

Areas of Uncertainty in Interventricular Optimization

Although VV optimization using many of the previously described methods has been shown to acutely improve hemodynamics, long-term clinical improvement above that derived from simultaneous BiV pacing has not been proven. There are several possible explanations for this discrepancy in results. First, the methods used for VV optimization may be suboptimal to achieve adequate VV and intraventricular resynchronization. As previously discussed, the technical difficulty of Doppler optimization methods introduces the possibility of operator error. IEGM-based algorithms do not account for LV lead location, which can influence the degree of preexcitation required for maximum resynchronization.[80] Additionally, the sequence of AV and VV optimization may be of importance. In almost all studies of VV optimization, AV delay optimization was performed first followed by VV optimization. The utility of this strategy has been questioned by a study that determined the optimal AV/VV settings by testing 45 different combinations of AV and VV intervals. The optimal settings identified with this method were significantly different from a strategy of optimizing the AV or VV interval first.[81]

Second, the magnitude of hemodynamic improvement with optimized VV pacing may be too small to be clinically meaningful. In the study by Mortensen and colleagues,[57] for example, sequential pacing significantly increased stroke volume by 20% in comparison with simultaneous pacing, but the absolute increase was relatively small (12 mL). This may not be sufficient to result in measurable differences in clinical outcomes.

Third, it is has been repeatedly shown that the optimal VV delay, like the AV delay, varies over time[38,39,57,59] and with exertion.[82] Programming a fixed, although optimized VV interval at the time of implantation would then be similar to empiric programming at long-term follow-up. The FREEDOM trial attempted to address this problem by randomizing 1067 patients to routine CRT management or AV and VV optimization every 3 months using the QuickOpt algorithm. There was no observed difference in the response rates to CRT between the 2 management strategies.[83] As discussed previously, the Medtronic Adaptive IEGM-based algorithm provides virtually continuous AV/VV optimization, and it resulted in outcomes that were not inferior to fixed, although optimized AV/VV intervals.[73] Although these studies suggest that frequent AV/VV adjustment offers no benefit over optimization at implant, it is possible that the algorithms used were inadequate. It remains to be seen if continuous, hemodynamically optimized CRT could prove beneficial.

Finally, it may be that VV optimization has been applied to the wrong population of patients. Most CRT recipients appear to benefit from biventricular or LV pacing, particularly in the presence of an LBBB. Whereas VV optimization may not improve response rates in an unselected population of patients receiving CRT, focused application in patients with a suboptimal response or non-LBBB morphologies could potentially be beneficial. This question was addressed in a study of 65 patients identified as "nonresponders" who were randomized to simultaneous BiV pacing or VV optimization. Response rates were 18.9% higher at 9-month follow-up in the optimized group, although this difference was not statistically significant and 50% of patients in the control group became responders.[84]

SUMMARY

Despite different attempts at patient selection and programming optimization, CRT nonresponder rates have remained relatively stable. Many different methods for AV and VV delay optimization have been developed, and all have demonstrated that optimized delays, regardless of the method, result in acute improvements in LV diastolic and systolic function. Unfortunately, these functional improvements have not consistently translated into improvements in clinical outcomes or response rates to CRT. As routine AV delay optimization was performed in most trials demonstrating efficacy of CRT, it is a reasonable strategy that does not appear to be harmful. More recent data suggest, however, that an empiric AV delay of 120 ms is not inferior to available optimization methods. Moreover, 3 large multicenter trials (FREEDOM, SMART-AV, and ADAPTIVE CRT) failed to show superiority of IEGM-based optimization over nominal settings or echo techniques. This has led to the evaluation of other techniques for improving CRT outcome, such as placing LV leads in locations of late mechanical[76] or electrical activation.[77] Given the complexity and technical skill required, current techniques and available data make routine VV optimization impractical and unnecessary in most patients. At the present time, the benefit of routine use of AV and VV interval optimization is unclear and may be most useful in the population of CRT "nonresponders," although the benefit of this strategy also requires further study.

REFERENCES

1. Epstein AE, DiMarco JP, Ellenbogen KA, et al. ACC/AHA/HRS 2008 guidelines for device-based therapy of cardiac rhythm abnormalities: a report of the American College of Cardiology/American Heart Association Task Force on Practice Guidelines (writing committee to revise the ACC/AHA/NASPE 2002 guideline update for implantation of cardiac pacemakers and antiarrhythmia devices): developed in collaboration with the American Association for Thoracic Surgery and Society of Thoracic Surgeons. Circulation 2008;117(21):e350–408.

2. Vardas PE, Auricchio A, Blanc JJ, et al. Guidelines for cardiac pacing and cardiac resynchronization therapy: the task force for cardiac pacing and cardiac resynchronization therapy of the European Society of Cardiology. Developed in collaboration with the European Heart Rhythm Association. Eur Heart J 2007;28(18):2256–95.

3. Abraham WT, Fisher WG, Smith AL, et al. Cardiac resynchronization in chronic heart failure. N Engl J Med 2002;346(24):1845–53.

4. Higgins SL, Hummel JD, Niazi IK, et al. Cardiac resynchronization therapy for the treatment of heart failure in patients with intraventricular conduction delay and malignant ventricular tachyarrhythmias. J Am Coll Cardiol 2003;42(8):1454–9.

5. Bristow MR, Saxon LA, Boehmer J, et al. Cardiac-resynchronization therapy with or without an implantable defibrillator in advanced chronic heart failure. N Engl J Med 2004;350(21):2140–50.

6. McAlister FA, Ezekowitz JA, Wiebe N, et al. Systematic review: cardiac resynchronization in patients with symptomatic heart failure. Ann Intern Med 2004;141(5):381–90.

7. Cleland JG, Daubert JC, Erdmann E, et al. The effect of cardiac resynchronization on morbidity and mortality in heart failure. N Engl J Med 2005;352(15):1539–49.

8. Linde C, Abraham WT, Gold MR, et al. Randomized trial of cardiac resynchronization in mildly symptomatic heart failure patients and in asymptomatic patients with left ventricular dysfunction and previous heart failure symptoms. J Am Coll Cardiol 2008;52(23):1834–43.

9. Moss AJ, Hall WJ, Cannom DS, et al. Cardiac-resynchronization therapy for the prevention of heart-failure events. N Engl J Med 2009;361(14):1329–38.

10. Tang AS, Wells GA, Talajic M, et al. Cardiac-resynchronization therapy for mild-to-moderate heart failure. N Engl J Med 2010;363(25):2385–95.

11. Chung ES, Leon AR, Tavazzi L, et al. Results of the predictors of response to CRT (PROSPECT) trial. Circulation 2008;117(20):2608–16.

12. Ruschitzka F, Abraham WT, Singh JP, et al. Cardiac-resynchronization therapy in heart failure with a narrow QRS complex. N Engl J Med 2013;369(15):1395–405.

13. Kindermann M, Frohlig G, Doerr T, et al. Optimizing the AV delay in DDD pacemaker patients with high degree AV block: mitral valve Doppler versus impedance cardiography. Pacing Clin Electrophysiol 1997;20(10 Pt 1):2453–62.

14. Auricchio A, Stellbrink C, Block M, et al. Effect of pacing chamber and atrioventricular delay on acute systolic function of paced patients with congestive heart failure. The Pacing Therapies for Congestive Heart Failure Study Group. The Guidant Congestive Heart Failure Research Group. Circulation 1999;99(23):2993–3001.

15. Ishikawa T, Sumita S, Kimura K, et al. Prediction of optimal atrioventricular delay in patients with implanted DDD pacemakers. Pacing Clin Electrophysiol 1999;22(9):1365–71.

16. Leon AR, Abraham WT, Brozena S, et al. Cardiac resynchronization with sequential biventricular pacing for the treatment of moderate-to-severe heart failure. J Am Coll Cardiol 2005;46(12):2298–304.

17. Meluzin J, Novak M, Mullerova J, et al. A fast and simple echocardiographic method of determination of the optimal atrioventricular delay in patients after biventricular stimulation. Pacing Clin Electrophysiol 2004;27(1):58–64.

18. Ellenbogen KA, Gold MR, Meyer TE, et al. Primary results from the SmartDelay determined AV optimization: a comparison to other AV delay methods used in cardiac resynchronization therapy (SMART-AV) trial: a randomized trial comparing empirical, echocardiography-guided, and algorithmic atrioventricular delay programming in cardiac resynchronization therapy. Circulation 2010;122(25):2660–8.

19. Nijjer SS, Pabari PA, Stegemann B, et al. The limit of plausibility for predictors of response: application to biventricular pacing. JACC Cardiovasc Imaging 2012;5(10):1046–65.

20. Morales MA, Startari U, Panchetti L, et al. Atrioventricular delay optimization by Doppler-derived left ventricular dP/dt improves 6-month outcome of resynchronized patients. Pacing Clin Electrophysiol 2006;29(6):564–8.

21. Colocousis JS, Huntsman LL, Curreri PW. Estimation of stroke volume changes by ultrasonic Doppler. Circulation 1977;56(6):914–7.

22. Sawhney N, Waggoner AD, Faddis MN. AV delay optimization by aortic VTI is superior to the pulsed Doppler mitral inflow method for cardiac resynchronization therapy (abstr). Pacing Clin Electrophysiol 2003;26:1042.

23. Kerlan JE, Sawhney NS, Waggoner AD, et al. Prospective comparison of echocardiographic atrioventricular delay optimization methods for cardiac resynchronization therapy. Heart Rhythm 2006;3(2):148–54.

24. Sawhney NS, Waggoner AD, Garhwal S, et al. Randomized prospective trial of atrioventricular delay programming for cardiac resynchronization therapy. Heart Rhythm 2004;1(5):562–7.

25. Jansen AH, Bracke FA, van Dantzig JM, et al. Correlation of echo-Doppler optimization of atrioventricular delay in cardiac resynchronization therapy with invasive hemodynamics in patients with heart failure secondary to ischemic or idiopathic dilated cardiomyopathy. Am J Cardiol 2006;97(4):552–7.

26. Braun MU, Schnabel A, Rauwolf T, et al. Impedance cardiography as a noninvasive technique for atrioventricular interval optimization in cardiac resynchronization therapy. J Interv Card Electrophysiol 2005;13(3):223–9.

27. Butter C, Stellbrink C, Belalcazar A, et al. Cardiac resynchronization therapy optimization by finger plethysmography. Heart Rhythm 2004;1(5):568–75.

28. Whinnett ZI, Davies JE, Willson K, et al. Determination of optimal atrioventricular delay for cardiac resynchronization therapy using acute non-invasive blood pressure. Europace 2006;8(5):358–66.

29. Ritter P, Padeletti L, Gillio-Meina L, et al. Determination of the optimal atrioventricular delay in DDD pacing. Comparison between echo and peak endocardial acceleration measurements. Europace 1999;1(2):126–30.

30. Dupuis JM, Kobeissi A, Vitali L, et al. Programming optimal atrioventricular delay in dual chamber pacing using peak endocardial acceleration: comparison with a standard echocardiographic procedure. Pacing Clin Electrophysiol 2003;26(1 Pt 2):210–3.

31. Ritter P, Delnoy PP, Padeletti L, et al. A randomized pilot study of optimization of cardiac resynchronization therapy in sinus rhythm patients using a peak endocardial acceleration sensor vs. standard methods. Europace 2012;14(9):1324–33.

32. Hasan A, Abraham WT, Quinn-Tate L, et al. Optimization of cardiac resynchronization devices using acoustic cardiography: a comparison to echocardiography. Congest Heart Fail 2006;12(Suppl 1):25–31.

33. Auricchio A, Kramer A, Spinelli JC, et al. Can the optimum dosage of resynchronization therapy be derived from the intracardiac electrogram? J Am Coll Cardiol 2002;39(Suppl A) [abstract: 124A].

34. Gold MR, Niazi I, Giudici M, et al. A prospective comparison of AV delay programming methods for hemodynamic optimization during cardiac resynchronization therapy. J Cardiovasc Electrophysiol 2007;18(5):490–6.

35. Gold MR, Yu Y, Singh JP, et al. The effect of left ventricular electrical delay on AV optimization for cardiac resynchronization therapy. Heart Rhythm 2013;10(7):988–93.

36. Mullens W, Grimm RA, Verga T, et al. Insights from a cardiac resynchronization optimization clinic as part of a heart failure disease management program. J Am Coll Cardiol 2009;53(9):765–73.

37. Zhang Q, Fung JW, Chan YS, et al. The role of repeating optimization of atrioventricular interval during interim and long-term follow-up after cardiac resynchronization therapy. Int J Cardiol 2008;124(2):211–7.

38. O'Donnell D, Nadurata V, Hamer A, et al. Long-term variations in optimal programming of cardiac resynchronization therapy devices. Pacing Clin Electrophysiol 2005;28(Suppl 1):S24–6.

39. Valzania C, Biffi M, Martignani C, et al. Cardiac resynchronization therapy: variations in echo-guided optimized atrioventricular and interventricular delays during follow-up. Echocardiography 2007;24(9):933–9.

40. Gold MR, Niazi I, Giudici M, et al. Acute hemodynamic effects of atrial pacing with cardiac resynchronization therapy. J Cardiovasc Electrophysiol 2009;20(8):894–900.

41. Martin DO, Day JD, Lai PY, et al. Atrial support pacing in heart failure: results from the Multicenter PEGASUS CRT Trial. J Cardiovasc Electrophysiol 2012;23(12):1317–25.

42. Khairy P, Talajic M, Dominguez M, et al. Atrioventricular interval optimization and exercise tolerance.
Pacing Clin Electrophysiol 2001;24(10):1534–40.

43. Scharf C, Li P, Muntwyler J, et al. Rate-dependent AV
delay optimization in cardiac resynchronization therapy. Pacing Clin Electrophysiol 2005;28(4):279–84.

44. Rafie R, Qamruddin S, Ozhand A, et al. Shortening
of atrioventricular delay at increased atrial paced
heart rates improves diastolic filling and functional
class in patients with biventricular pacing. Cardiovasc Ultrasound 2012;10:2.

45. Shanmugam N, Prada-Delgado O, Campos AG,
et al. Rate-adaptive AV delay and exercise performance following cardiac resynchronization therapy.
Heart Rhythm 2012;9(11):1815–21. e1811.

46. Cazeau S, Leclercq C, Lavergne T, et al. Effects of
multisite biventricular pacing in patients with heart
failure and intraventricular conduction delay.
N Engl J Med 2001;344(12):873–80.

47. Auricchio A, Ding J, Spinelli JC, et al. Cardiac
resynchronization therapy restores optimal atrioventricular mechanical timing in heart failure patients
with ventricular conduction delay. J Am Coll Cardiol
2002;39(7):1163–9.

48. Auricchio A, Stellbrink C, Sack S, et al. Long-term
clinical effect of hemodynamically optimized cardiac
resynchronization therapy in patients with heart failure and ventricular conduction delay. J Am Coll Cardiol 2002;39(12):2026–33.

49. Gold MR, Niazi I, Giudici M, et al. A prospective,
randomized comparison of the acute hemodynamic
effects of biventricular and left ventricular pacing
with cardiac resynchronization therapy. Heart
Rhythm 2011;8(5):685–91.

50. Stellbrink C, Breithardt OA, Franke A, et al. Impact of
cardiac resynchronization therapy using hemodynamically optimized pacing on left ventricular remodeling in patients with congestive heart failure
and ventricular conduction disturbances. J Am Coll
Cardiol 2001;38(7):1957–65.

51. van Gelder BM, Bracke FA, Meijer A, et al. Effect of
optimizing the VV interval on left ventricular contractility in cardiac resynchronization therapy. Am J Cardiol 2004;93(12):1500–3.

52. Bordachar P, Lafitte S, Reuter S, et al. Echocardiographic parameters of ventricular dyssynchrony
validation in patients with heart failure using sequential biventricular pacing. J Am Coll Cardiol 2004;
44(11):2157–65.

53. Sogaard P, Egeblad H, Pedersen AK, et al. Sequential
versus simultaneous biventricular resynchronization
for severe heart failure: evaluation by tissue Doppler
imaging. Circulation 2002;106(16):2078–84.

54. Vidal B, Sitges M, Marigliano A, et al. Optimizing the
programation of cardiac resynchronization therapy
devices in patients with heart failure and left bundle
branch block. Am J Cardiol 2007;100(6):1002–6.

55. Abraham WT, Leon AR, St John Sutton MG, et al.
Randomized controlled trial comparing simultaneous versus optimized sequential interventricular
stimulation during cardiac resynchronization therapy. Am Heart J 2012;164(5):735–41.

56. Gras D, Gupta MS, Boulogne E, et al. Optimization
of AV and VV delays in the real-world CRT patient
population: an international survey on current clinical practice. Pacing Clin Electrophysiol 2009;
32(Suppl 1):S236–9.

57. Mortensen PT, Sogaard P, Mansour H, et al. Sequential
biventricular pacing: evaluation of safety and efficacy.
Pacing Clin Electrophysiol 2004;27(3):339–45.

58. Boriani G, Muller CP, Seidl KH, et al. Randomized
comparison of simultaneous biventricular stimulation
versus optimized interventricular delay in cardiac resynchronization therapy. The Resynchronization for
the HemodYnamic Treatment for Heart Failure Management II implantable cardioverter defibrillator
(RHYTHM II ICD) study. Am Heart J 2006;151(5):
1050–8.

59. Boriani G, Biffi M, Muller CP, et al. A prospective randomized evaluation of VV delay optimization in CRT-
D recipients: echocardiographic observations from
the RHYTHM II ICD study. Pacing Clin Electrophysiol
2009;32(Suppl 1):S120–5.

60. Saksena S, Simon AM, Mathew P, et al. Intracardiac
echocardiography-guided cardiac resynchronization therapy: technique and clinical application. Pacing Clin Electrophysiol 2009;32(8):1030–9.

61. Sperzel J, Brandt R, Hou W, et al. Intraoperative characterization of interventricular mechanical dyssynchrony using electroanatomic mapping system—a
feasibility study. J Interv Card Electrophysiol 2012;
35(2):189–96.

62. Burri H, Sunthorn H, Somsen A, et al. Optimizing
sequential biventricular pacing using radionuclide
ventriculography. Heart Rhythm 2005;2(9):960–5.

63. Whinnett ZI, Davies JE, Willson K, et al. Haemodynamic effects of changes in atrioventricular and
interventricular delay in cardiac resynchronisation
therapy show a consistent pattern: analysis of
shape, magnitude and relative importance of atrioventricular and interventricular delay. Heart 2006;
92(11):1628–34.

64. Vidal B, Tamborero D, Mont L, et al. Electrocardiographic optimization of interventricular delay in cardiac resynchronization therapy: a simple method to
optimize the device. J Cardiovasc Electrophysiol
2007;18(12):1252–7.

65. Bertini M, Ziacchi M, Biffi M, et al. Interventricular
delay interval optimization in cardiac resynchronization therapy guided by echocardiography versus
guided by electrocardiographic QRS interval width.
Am J Cardiol 2008;102(10):1373–7.

66. Min X, Meine M, Baker JH 2nd, et al. Estimation of
the optimal VV delay by an IEGM-based method in

cardiac resynchronization therapy. Pacing Clin Electrophysiol 2007;30(Suppl 1):S19–22.

67. Baker JH 2nd, McKenzie J 3rd, Beau S, et al. Acute evaluation of programmer-guided AV/PV and VV delay optimization comparing an IEGM method and echocardiogram for cardiac resynchronization therapy in heart failure patients and dual-chamber ICD implants. J Cardiovasc Electrophysiol 2007; 18(2):185–91.

68. van Gelder BM, Meijer A, Bracke FA. The optimized V-V interval determined by interventricular conduction times versus invasive measurement by LVdP/dtMAX. J Cardiovasc Electrophysiol 2008;19(9): 939–44.

69. Porciani MC, Rao CM, Mochi M, et al. A real-time three-dimensional echocardiographic validation of an intracardiac electrogram-based method for optimizing cardiac resynchronization therapy. Pacing Clin Electrophysiol 2008;31(1):56–63.

70. Kamdar R, Frain E, Warburton F, et al. A prospective comparison of echocardiography and device algorithms for atrioventricular and interventricular interval optimization in cardiac resynchronization therapy. Europace 2010;12(1):84–91.

71. Rao RK, Kumar UN, Schafer J, et al. Reduced ventricular volumes and improved systolic function with cardiac resynchronization therapy: a randomized trial comparing simultaneous biventricular pacing, sequential biventricular pacing, and left ventricular pacing. Circulation 2007;115(16):2136–44.

72. Krum H, Lemke B, Birnie D, et al. A novel algorithm for individualized cardiac resynchronization therapy: rationale and design of the adaptive cardiac resynchronization therapy trial. Am Heart J 2012; 163(5):747–52.e1.

73. Martin DO, Lemke B, Birnie D, et al. Investigation of a novel algorithm for synchronized left-ventricular pacing and ambulatory optimization of cardiac resynchronization therapy: results of the adaptive CRT trial. Heart Rhythm 2012;9(11):1807–14. e1801.

74. Birnie D, Lemke B, Aonuma K, et al. Clinical outcomes with synchronized left ventricular pacing: analysis of the adaptive CRT trial. Heart Rhythm 2013;10(9):1368–74.

75. Starling RC, Krum H, Bril S, et al. Impact of a novel adaptive optimization algorithm on 30-day readmissions: evidence from the adaptive CRT Trial. JACC Heart Fail 2015;3(7):565–72.

76. Sonne C, Bott-Flugel L, Hauck S, et al. Acute beneficial hemodynamic effects of a novel 3D-echocardiographic optimization protocol in cardiac resynchronization therapy. PLoS One 2012;7(2): e30964.

77. Sonne C, Bott-Flugel L, Hauck S, et al. Three-dimensional echocardiographic optimization improves outcome in cardiac resynchronization therapy compared to ECG optimization: a randomized comparison. Pacing Clin Electrophysiol 2014;37(3): 312–20.

78. Strohmer B, Pichler M, Froemmel M, et al. Evaluation of atrial conduction time at various sites of right atrial pacing and influence on atrioventricular delay optimization by surface electrocardiography. Pacing Clin Electrophysiol 2004;27(4):468–74.

79. Arbelo E, Tolosana JM, Trucco E, et al. Fusion-optimized intervals (FOI): a new method to achieve the narrowest QRS for optimization of the AV and VV intervals in patients undergoing cardiac resynchronization therapy. J Cardiovasc Electrophysiol 2014; 25(3):283–92.

80. Khan FZ, Virdee MS, Read PA, et al. Impact of VV optimization in relation to left ventricular lead position: an acute haemodynamic study. Europace 2011;13(6):845–52.

81. Zuber M, Toggweiler S, Roos M, et al. Comparison of different approaches for optimization of atrioventricular and interventricular delay in biventricular pacing. Europace 2008;10(3):367–73.

82. Bordachar P, Lafitte S, Reuter S, et al. Echocardiographic assessment during exercise of heart failure patients with cardiac resynchronization therapy. Am J Cardiol 2006;97(11):1622–5.

83. Abraham WT, Gras D, Yu CM, et al. Results from the FREEDOM trial—assess the safety and efficacy of frequent optimization of cardiac resynchronization therapy [abstract]. Heart Rhythm 2010;7(5):2–3.

84. Weiss R, Malik R, Wish M, et al. V-V optimization in cardiac resynchronization therapy nonresponders: RESPONSE-HF trial results. Heart Rhythm 2010; 7(5):S26.

What We Can Learn from "Super-responders"

Alessandro Proclemer, MD[a],*, Daniele Muser, MD[b], Domenico Facchin, MD[a]

KEYWORDS

- CRT • Left ventricular ejection fraction • Cardiac resynchronization therapy
- Left ventricular function

KEY POINTS

- In patients treated with cardiac resynchronization therapy (CRT) presenting an important improvement of left ventricular (LV) function, the long-term outcome is excellent.
- Super-responders have a low absolute risk of severe ventricular tachyarrhythmias; however, some cardiac events can occur several years after implantation despite normal or near-normal LV function.
- In patients with CRT with a defibrillator undergoing device replacement, a downgrading to CRT with a pacemaker should be considered with caution.

INTRODUCTION

Cardiac resynchronization therapy (CRT) has largely demonstrated to improve heart failure (HF) symptoms, left ventricular (LV) function and even survival in about 70% of patients with symptomatic HF, reduced LV ejection fraction (LVEF) and intraventricular conduction delays especially in patients with left bundle branch block (LBBB), regardless of HF etiology.[1,2] On this basis, current international guidelines suggest, as class IA recommendations, CRT implantation in patients with symptomatic HF (New York Heart Association [NYHA] class III and IV), QRS duration greater than 120 milliseconds, and severe reduction of LVEF ($\leq$35%). Even less symptomatic patients (NYHA class II) may benefit from CRT in terms of long-term survival in the presence of longer QRS duration ($\geq$150 ms).[3,4] In some patients ("super-responders"), we observe an exceptional clinical and instrumental improvement after CRT with the patient becoming almost asymptomatic (NYHA class I) with a normalization or near-normalization of the LVEF (>50%). In addition to an improvement of quality of life, super-response to CRT leads to a

decrease in the incidence of hospitalizations for HF symptoms, a decrease of the incidence of implantable cardioverter defibrillator (ICD) appropriate therapies, and eventually to a survival gain.[5]

The intended outcome for almost every patient undergoing CRT to become a "super-responder." Response to CRT depends on several factors, such as patient characteristics (ie, etiology, comorbidities) and anatomic features of the cardiac venous system and procedural aspects (ie, preprocedural planning, device selection), but the characteristics of super-responders to CRT are less well-studied than those of nonresponders and negative responders.

This review discusses the state of the art of knowledge in this field to help decision making in patients candidates to CRT and to analyze the long-term total and cardiac mortality, sudden death, and CRT with a defibrillator (CRT-D) intervention rate, as well as the evolution of echocardiographic parameters in patients with LVEF of greater than 50% after CRT implantation. Owing to "NYHA normalization" of LV function in super-responders, the need for a persistent defibrillator backup is also considered.

[a] University Hospital Santa Maria della Misericordia, Udine 33100, Italy; [b] Hospital of the University of Pennsylvania, 3400 Spruce Street, Philadelphia, PA 19104, USA
* Corresponding author.
E-mail address: proclemer.alessandro@aoud.sanita.fvg.it

Card Electrophysiol Clin 7 (2015) 781–788
http://dx.doi.org/10.1016/j.ccep.2015.08.019
1877-9182/15/$ – see front matter
© 2015 Elsevier Inc. All rights reserved.

DEFINITION OF SUPER-RESPONDERS TO CARDIAC RESYNCHRONIZATION THERAPY

Thus far, there is no full agreement concerning the definition of super-responders to CRT. Several clinical, instrumental, and combined criteria have been suggested.[6] Instrumental response to CRT is usually assessed by echocardiography quantifying reverse LV remodeling by changes in LV end systolic volume and/or LVEF at 3 to 6 months after CRT implantation. In these terms, an absolute normalization of LVEF ($\geq$50%) or improvement by almost 30% has been suggested as criteria for super-response.[5,7] Some studies suggests that LV reverse remodeling, more than the improvement in LVEF, is the best predictor of outcome.[8,9]

From a clinical point of view, response to CRT can be evaluated by improvement in NYHA functional class to II or I or better as quantified by the 6-minute walk test.[10,11] Probably the best definition of super-response to CRT is a combination of both clinical measures and imaging parameters[12]; thus, a clinical (NYHA class I or II) and echocardiographic (ie, LVEF $\geq$50%) definition of super-response should be encouraged as a standard definition.[13] However, an inconsistency exists between clinical and echocardiographic response in favor of the clinical response; less than 50% of patients who experience clinical improvement show significant LV reverse remodeling.[11,14] In the large trial Multicenter Automatic Defibrillator Implantation Trial With Cardiac Resynchronization Therapy (MADIT-CRT),[15] an absolute increase of LVEF of almost 18% was able to identify patients with better prognosis at follow-up, and for this reason it has been suggested as the more reliable parameter to evaluate response to CRT. In particular, a recent subanalysis of the MADIT-CRT population[16] demonstrated an improvement in LVEF from 29.5 $\pm$ 3.2% at baseline to 40.5 $\pm$ 5.9% at 12 months (P<.001). Of 752 patients, 55 (7.3%) achieved an LVEF of greater than 50%, whereas 594 patients (79%) achieved an LVEF of 36% to 50%, and the remaining 103 (13.7%) maintained a 35% or lower LVEF.

FROM BENCH TO BEDSIDE: CARDIAC RESYNCHRONIZATION THERAPY AND REVERSE REMODELING

The so-called ventricular remodeling is the pathophysiologic process that leads to a modification of LV geometry, dimensions, and structure after any type of myocardial injury. In the early stage of myocardial structural disease, LV remodeling represents a compensatory modification to maintain an adequate LVEF and systemic output thanks to the Frank–Starling rule. Unfortunately, as the remodeling continues, it sets up a vicious cycle leading to a progressive loss of contractility.

Ongoing HF is accompanied by a progressive dilation and loss of ellipsoidal shape by the LV in favor of a spherical one. The spherical shape increases wall stress as well as oxygen consumption. Moreover, it leads to a displacement of papillary muscles, leading to an incomplete cooptation of mitral leaflets that increases the severity of mitral regurgitation, which in turn increases the LV end diastolic filling pressure and depresses the ejection fraction, perpetuating further the vicious cycle.

This general principle makes it easy to understand how important action against ventricular remodeling can be. CRT shapes reverse remodeling, leading to a decrease in LV diameters and volume from the first months after implantation.[17] Within the first 6 to 12 months after implantation, there is a progressive LV reverse remodeling with a decrease in end diastolic and end systolic LV volumes, an improvement of LVEF with a decrease in the sphericity index, and a decrease in the severity of mitral regurgitation.[18,19] Reverse remodeling is observed regardless of the etiology of the dysfunction, although it tends to be more significant in patient affected by nonischemic cardiomyopathy.

Mechanisms of reverse remodeling are not fully understood, but probably involve wall stress and oxygen consumption reduction, lowering of sympathetic tone, and improvement of mitral regurgitation. CRT induces changes in the gene expression pattern of genes involved in contractile function and pathologic hypertrophy and modifies levels of HF biomarkers.[20] In super-responders, there is a decrease in absolute myocardial fibrosis, the apoptotic index, and of tumor necrosis factor-α levels.[21]

PREVALENCE AND PREDICTORS OF SUPER-RESPONSE TO CARDIAC RESYNCHRONIZATION THERAPY: LONG-TERM PROGNOSIS

Super-response to CRT has been reported to range between 7.3% and 40%.[14,16,22–24] Super-responders to CRT have shown not only a better quality of life owing to an amelioration of HF symptoms, but also a significant improvement in overall survival, a reduction in ICD appropriate therapy, and a decrease in hospitalizations for HF.[15] Mortality reduction goes along improvement of LVEF and reduction of LV volumes, confirming that the beneficial effect of CRT is largely attributable to reverse remodeling.[25]

Several studies have investigated predictors of super-response to CRT. Results show a considerable variability owing to the different criteria used to define super-response and different baseline inclusion criteria. **Table 1** summarizes the most important prospective trials evaluating predictors of super-response. The major part of them has included patients with severe HF symptoms (NYHA classes III and IV), low LVEF (<30%–35%), and basal QRS longer than 120 milliseconds. The definition of super-response ranged between normalization of LVEF (>50%), an absolute increment of almost 20%, a decrease in LV end diastolic diameter of almost 30%, and no events at follow-up (cardiovascular death, cardiac transplant, HF-related hospitalizations).

Nonischemic cardiomyopathy, QRS duration of more than 150 milliseconds, and duration of the QRS of greater than 40 milliseconds after CRT have been associated with a probability of normalization of LVEF of 75% within the first year of follow-up.[26] Time elapsed from HF symptoms onset has been correlated with improvement after CRT.[27] Patients that show a significant clinical (NYHA classes I or II) and echocardiographic improvement (relative increase of LVEF to the upper quartile) within 6 months after CRT are usually females with a body mass index of less than 30 kg/m^2 affected by nonischemic cardiomyopathy with a basal QRS of wider than 150 milliseconds, a complete left bundle branch block, and the absence of severe left atrium enlargement.[28] In the MADIT CRT trial patients, who obtained LVEF near-normalization more often had nonischemic cardiomyopathy, left bundle branch block QRS morphology, and no previous myocardial infarction.[16] In addition, all baseline echocardiographic parameters were significantly different between groups, including LV end-systolic volume, LV end-diastolic volume, and left atrial volume. In the majority of the studies evaluating the long-term outcome of super-responders, factors associated with LVEF normalization are also related to a reduced risk of ventricular tachyarrhythmias and patients who achieved LVEF normalization had an excellent prognosis, with a very low cumulative incidence of HF, sudden death, and cardiac mortality. Only inappropriate ICD therapy persisted with a rate similar to patients with subnormalization of LVEF. According to the MADIT CRT Trial, in the study by Van Bommel and colleagues,[29] none of the 42 patients with significant LVEF recovery received during a median follow-up of 3 years appropriate shocks, whereas 3 received more than 1 inappropriate shock. In contrast, in a single-center retrospective study the authors found that an LVEF of 35% or greater, 40% or greater, or 45% on follow-up

echocardiography did not predict the risk for appropriate ICD intervention.[30]

In our experience, only 1 of 62 super-responders died for cardiovascular reasons during a follow-up of more than 6 years.[31] In addition, major cardiac events (appropriate CRT-D intervention and hospital admissions owing to HF) were significantly less common than in the hyporesponder and nonresponder patients. An early identification of patients with cardiac events despite super-response to CRT seems to be extremely difficult and an incomplete reverse remodeling process could be considered the main cause of residual clinical events. According to these data, in patients with CRT-D undergoing device replacement, a downgrading to CRT-P should be considered with extreme caution.

A special subgroup of patients is represented by patients who develop progressive ventricular dysfunction secondary to chronic right ventricular pacing (pacing-induced cardiomyopathy). These patients showed an almost complete recovery of LVEF early after CRT implantation as consequence of the abolition of mechanical dyssynchrony that represent the primary etiology of the disease.[31] Sometimes patients could reach a complete LVEF recovery after up to 24 months, meaning that patients undergoing CRT should be followed for longer than 12 months.[31]

PATIENT SELECTION AND PROCEDURE PLANNING
Echocardiographic Evaluation

Several studies have investigated the power of echocardiography to predict which patients will develop a better response to CRT by assessing mechanical dyssynchrony with different approaches. M-mode anterior septum to posterior LV wall, tissue Doppler velocity imaging, speckle tracking based strain analysis, and real-time 3-dimensional echocardiography are all different modalities proposed.[29] However, despite echocardiography being able to evaluate mechanical dyssynchrony, none of these echocardiographic parameters have been shown to significantly predict the response to CRT, probably owing to the large intraobserver and interobserver variability.[32] The usefulness of mechanical dyssynchrony evaluation by echocardiography has largely been diminished after evidence that CRT implant in patients with systolic HF, mechanical dyssynchrony, but not electrical dyssynchrony (QRS <130 ms) not only does not decrease the rate of death or hospitalization for HF, but may actually increase mortality.[33] The adjunct value of echocardiography evaluation is in the optimization of LV lead

Table 1
Summary of studies evaluating super-response to CRT

Author	No. of Patients	NYHA Class	LVEF (%)	QRS (ms)	Others	Definition of "Super-Response"	Super-Responders (%)	Follow-up	Predictors of Super-response
				Inclusion Criteria					
Antonio	87	III-IV	35	120	QRS <120 ms + echo dyssynchrony	LVEF >45%, NYHA growth >1, LVESV reduction >15%	12	6 mo	HF onset <12 mo
Castellant	84	III-IV	35	140	LBBB, LVEDD ≥50 mm	LVEF ≥50%, NYHA I-II	13	6, 12, and 24 mo	Nonischemic etiology
Gasparini	517	II-IV	35	120	—	NYHA ≤ II, LVEF ≥50%	26	Every 3–6 mo	Nonischemic etiology, LVEDV <180 mL, FE 30%–35%
Castellant	51	III-IV	35	140	LBBB, LVEDD ≥ 60 mm, nonischemic cardiomyopathy	FE ≥ 50%, NYHA I-II	22	6, 12 and 24 mo	None
PROSPECT	286	III-IV	35	130	—	Relative reduction LVESD ≥30%	38	6 mo	Female gender, NYHA, QRS duration
Reant	186	III-IV	35	120	—	NYHA improvement >1 NYHA, LVEF ≥50%, LVESV reduction ≥15%	10	6 mo	Left atrial volume <55 mL, global longitudinal strain ≤12%
Rickard	233	II-IV	40	120	—	LVEF increasing ≥20%	14	>2 mo (11.6 ± 9)	LBBB

Study	n	NYHA			Definition	Super-responders (%)	Follow-up	Predictors
Adelstein	51	III-IV	35	—	Right ventricle pacing VP >90%, nonischemic cardiomyopathy	LVEF ≥50%	29	≥6 mo	LVESD <48 mm, LVEDD <58 mm, HF onset <24 mo
Qing	76	III-IV	35	35	LVEDD ≥55 mm	No events at follow-up (death/OCT/HF hospitalization), NYHA improvement >1, LVEF ≥50%	21	3 mo	LVEDD <68 mm
Serdoz	75	III-IV	35	35	HF onset earlier than 12 mo before	NYHA improvement >1, LVEF ≥50% without significant mortality at 1 y	17	Every 6 mo (17 ± 9)	Nonischemic cardiomyopathy, QRS within 144–186 ms, QRS shortening >40 ms
MADIT-CRT	752	I-II	30	30	—	LVEF increasing ≥14.5%	25	12 mo	Female gender, nonischemic cardiomyopathy, QRS >150 ms, LBBB, BMI <30 kg/m², no severe left atrial enlargement

Abbreviations: BMI, body mass index; CRT, cardiac resynchronization therapy; HF, heart failure; LBBB, left bundle branch block; LVEDD, left ventricular end diastolic diameter; LVEDV, left ventricular end diastolic volume; LVEF, left ventricular ejection fraction; LVESD, left ventricular end systolic diameter; LVESV, left ventricular end systolic volume; MADIT-CRT, Multicenter Automatic Defibrillator Implantation Trial With Cardiac Resynchronization Therapy; NYHA, New York Heart Association; OCT, orthotopic cardiac transplant; VP, ventricular pacing.

placement to increase the response to CRT. Patients who undergo image-guided CRT double their probability of developing a CRT response versus standard patients.[34–36]

Dobutamine Stress Echocardiography

The capacity of dobutamine stress test to assess myocardial viability in patients with severely depressed LVEF is well-known. However, few data are available about its predicting powerful in terms of response to CRT. It is supposed that an absolute increase of LVEF of almost 15% and a change in the wall motion score index of 0.7 or greater best predicts a super-response to CRT (defined as an increase in LVEF of >50% and a decrease in LV end-systolic diameter to <40 mm at 12 months of follow-up).[37,38]

CARDIAC MRI

Cardiac MRI is a rapidly growing imaging modality in all fields of cardiology owing to its capability of both functional and structural analysis of the heart. Cardiac MRI finds variable applications in the setting of CRT. Scar quantification by delayed enhancement imaging strongly correlates with clinical and instrumental response to CRT; patients with a total scar amount of less than 15% are better candidates for CRT.[12] Moreover, cardiac MRI offers a multimodal approach to evaluate best LV lead position. Cine displacement encoding with stimulated echoes provides high-quality strain for dyssynchrony and timing of onset of circumferential contraction, which, together to the electrical timing, could improve evaluation of the optimal LV lead position.[39]

COMPUTED TOMOGRAPHY

The use of computed tomography in the pre-CRT implant patient assessment is not widespread.[40] It can furnished data of great value in terms of procedure planning, especially concerning the definition of the anatomy of the cardiac venous system that matched with the cardiac MRI scar analysis can lead to optimal LV lead positioning. For instance, in the setting of a complex venous system anatomy with small or nonfavorably branched secondary vessels, the choice of a surgical approach could be better for transvenous lead implantation.[41]

Left Ventricular Only Versus Biventricular Pacing

The extent of CRT benefit on reverse LV remodeling that is owing to biventricular versus LV pacing is unclear. Despite only few randomized trials have

compared biventricular versus LV-only pacing in patients undergoing CRT, and it seems that LV-only pacing provides similar benefits to biventricular pacing in terms of all-cause mortality, need for transplantation, hospitalization, improvement in LVEF, and exercise tolerance. Moreover, in patients treated with CRT who are not pacemaker dependent, LV-only pacing is a strategy to increase battery longevity.[42]

Recovery or Remission?

Regardless the definition, super-response to CRT is characterized by an excellent long-term prognosis, either in terms of overall survival, life-threatening arrhythmic events, and quality of life (exercise tolerance improvement). Whether this is owing to a remission or a complete recovery remains an open question. A first prospective randomized experience shows that the majority (78%) of super-responders in whom the pacing function of CRT is deactivated deteriorates both in clinical and echocardiographic parameters at the 12-month follow-up. Furthermore, even adverse outcomes such as hospitalization for HF and appropriate device therapies increases in the follow-up of switched off patients.[13] As best medical treatment (beta-blockers, angiotensin-converting enzyme inhibitors, and potassium-spearing diuretics), CRT constitutes a lifelong treatment for the remission of cardiomyopathy when dyssynchrony is present.

SUMMARY

In patients treated with CRT presenting an important improvement of LV function (LVEF $\geq$ 0.50), the long-term outcome is excellent. Super-responders to CRT have in the majority of cases a low absolute risk of severe ventricular tachyarrhythmias, but some cardiac events, mainly CRT-D appropriate interventions, can occur several years after implantation despite the persistence of a normal or near-normal LV function. Early identification of these patients is difficult and a lesser degree of long-term reverse remodeling seems to be associated with a greater risk of adverse events. According to our data and other large experience, in patients with CRT-D undergoing device replacement a downgrading to CRT-P should be considered with caution.

REFERENCES

1. European Heart Rhythm Association, European Society of Cardiology, Heart Rhythm Society, et al. 2012 EHRA/HRS expert consensus statement on cardiac resynchronization therapy in heart failure:

implant and follow-up recommendations and management. Heart Rhythm 2012;9:1524–76.

2. European Society of Cardiology (ESC), European Heart Rhythm Association (EHRA), Brignole M, et al. 2013 ESC guidelines on cardiac pacing and cardiac resynchronization therapy: the task force on cardiac pacing and resynchronization therapy of the European Society of Cardiology (ESC). Developed in collaboration with the European Heart Rhythm Association (EHRA). Europace 2013;15: 1070–118.

3. Jessup M, Abraham WT, Casey DE, et al. 2009 focused update: ACCF/AHA guidelines for the diagnosis and management of heart failure in adults: a report of the American College of Cardiology Foundation/American Heart Association Task Force on Practice Guidelines: developed in collaboration with the International Society for Heart and Lung Transplantation. Circulation 2009;119:1977–2016.

4. Stevenson WG, Hernandez AF, Carson PE, et al. Indications for cardiac resynchronization therapy: 2011 update from the Heart Failure Society of America Guideline Committee. J Card Fail 2012;18:94–106.

5. Castellant P, Fatemi M, Bertault-Valls V, et al. Cardiac resynchronization therapy: "nonresponders" and "hyperresponders". Heart Rhythm 2008;5:193–7.

6. Fornwalt BK, Sprague WW, BeDell P, et al. Agreement is poor among current criteria used to define response to cardiac resynchronization therapy. Circulation 2010;121:1985–91.

7. Blanc J-J, Fatemi M, Bertault V, et al. Evaluation of left bundle branch block as a reversible cause of non-ischaemic dilated cardiomyopathy with severe heart failure. A new concept of left ventricular dyssynchrony-induced cardiomyopathy. Europace 2005;7:604–10.

8. Yu C-M. Left ventricular reverse remodeling but not clinical improvement predicts long-term survival after cardiac resynchronization therapy. Circulation 2005;112:1580–6.

9. Ypenburg C, van Bommel RJ, Borleffs CJW, et al. Long-term prognosis after cardiac resynchronization therapy is related to the extent of left ventricular reverse remodeling at midterm follow-up. J Am Coll Cardiol 2009;53:483–90.

10. Díaz-Infante E, Mont L, Leal J, et al. Predictors of lack of response to resynchronization therapy. Am J Cardiol 2005;95:1436–40.

11. Bleeker GB, Bax JJ, Fung JW-H, et al. Clinical versus echocardiographic parameters to assess response to cardiac resynchronization therapy. Am J Cardiol 2006;97:260–3.

12. White JA, Yee R, Yuan X, et al. Delayed enhancement magnetic resonance imaging predicts response to cardiac resynchronization therapy in patients with intraventricular dyssynchrony. J Am Coll Cardiol 2006;48:1953–60.

13. Cay S, Ozeke O, Ozcan F, et al. Mid-term clinical and echocardiographic evaluation of super responders with and without pacing: the preliminary results of a prospective, randomized, single-centre study. Europace 2015 [Internet]. Available at: http://europace.oxfordjournals.org/cgi/doi/10.1093/europace/euv129. Accessed July 13, 2015.

14. van Bommel RJ, Bax JJ, Abraham WT, et al. Characteristics of heart failure patients associated with good and poor response to cardiac resynchronization therapy: a PROSPECT (Predictors of Response to CRT) sub-analysis. Eur Heart J 2009;30:2470–7.

15. Moss AJ, Hall WJ, Cannom DS, et al, MADIT-CRT Trial Investigators. Cardiac-resynchronization therapy for the prevention of heart-failure events. N Engl J Med 2009;361:1329–38.

16. Ruwald MH, Solomon SD, Foster E, et al. Left ventricular ejection fraction normalization in cardiac resynchronization therapy and risk of ventricular arrhythmias and clinical outcomes: results from the Multicenter Automatic Defibrillator Implantation Trial With Cardiac Resynchronization Therapy (MADIT-CRT) trial. Circulation 2014;130:2278–86.

17. Chung ES, Leon AR, Tavazzi L, et al. Results of the Predictors of Response to CRT (PROSPECT) trial. Circulation 2008;117:2608–16.

18. St John Sutton MG, Plappert T, Abraham WT, et al, Multicenter InSync Randomized Clinical Evaluation (MIRACLE) Study Group. Effect of cardiac resynchronization therapy on left ventricular size and function in chronic heart failure. Circulation 2003;107:1985–90.

19. Abraham WT, Fisher WG, Smith AL, et al, MIRACLE Study Group. Multicenter Insync Randomized Clinical Evaluation. Cardiac resynchronization in chronic heart failure. N Engl J Med 2002;346:1845–53.

20. Vanderheyden M, Mullens W, Delrue L, et al. Myocardial gene expression in heart failure patients treated with cardiac resynchronization therapy responders versus nonresponders. J Am Coll Cardiol 2008;51:129–36.

21. Ascia D' C, Cittadini A, Monti MG, et al. Effects of biventricular pacing on interstitial remodelling, tumor necrosis factor-alpha expression, and apoptotic death in failing human myocardium. Eur Heart J 2006;27:201–6.

22. Stefan L, Sedláček K, Černá D, et al. Small left atrium and mild mitral regurgitation predict super-response to cardiac resynchronization therapy. Europace 2012;14:1608–14.

23. António N, Teixeira R, Coelho L, et al. Identification of "super-responders" to cardiac resynchronization therapy: the importance of symptom duration and left ventricular geometry. Europace 2009;11:343–9.

24. Tian Y, Zhang P, Li X, et al. True complete left bundle branch block morphology strongly predicts good response to cardiac resynchronization therapy. Europace 2013;15:1499–506.

25. Cleland JGF, Daubert J-C, Erdmann E, et al, Cardiac Resynchronization-Heart Failure (CARE-HF) Study Investigators. The effect of cardiac resynchronization on morbidity and mortality in heart failure. N Engl J Med 2005;352:1539–49.

26. Serdoz LV, Daleffe E, Merlo M, et al. Predictors for restoration of normal left ventricular function in response to cardiac resynchronization therapy measured at time of implantation. Am J Cardiol 2011;108:75–80.

27. Ellenbogen KA, Huizar JF. Foreseeing super-response to cardiac resynchronization therapy: a perspective for clinicians. J Am Coll Cardiol 2012; 59:2374–7.

28. Hsu JC, Solomon SD, Bourgoun M, et al, MADIT-CRT Executive Committee. Predictors of super-response to cardiac resynchronization therapy and associated improvement in clinical outcome: the MADIT-CRT (Multicenter Automatic Defibrillator Implantation Trial with Cardiac Resynchronization Therapy) study. J Am Coll Cardiol 2012;59:2366–73.

29. Van Bommel RJ, Ypenburg C, Borleffs CJW, et al. Value of tissue Doppler echocardiography in predicting response to cardiac resynchronization therapy in patients with heart failure. Am J Cardiol 2010;105:1153–8.

30. Steffel J, Milosevic G, Hürlimann A, et al. Characteristics and long-term outcome of echocardiographic super-responders to cardiac resynchronisation therapy: "real world" experience from a single tertiary care centre. Heart 2011;97:1668–74.

31. Zecchin M, Proclemer A, Magnani S, et al. Long-term outcome of "super-responder" patients to cardiac resynchronization therapy. Europace 2014;16: 363–71.

32. Yu C-M, Chau E, Sanderson JE, et al. Tissue Doppler echocardiographic evidence of reverse remodeling and improved synchronicity by simultaneously delaying regional contraction after biventricular pacing therapy in heart failure. Circulation 2002; 105:438–45.

33. Ruschitzka F, Abraham WT, Singh JP, et al, EchoCRT Study Group. Cardiac-resynchronization therapy in heart failure with a narrow QRS complex. N Engl J Med 2013;369:1395–405.

34. Khan FZ, Virdee MS, Palmer CR, et al. Targeted left ventricular lead placement to guide cardiac resynchronization therapy: the TARGET study: a randomized, controlled trial. J Am Coll Cardiol 2012;59: 1509–18.

35. Saba S, Marek J, Schwartzman D, et al. Echocardiography-guided left ventricular lead placement for cardiac resynchronization therapy: results of the Speckle Tracking Assisted Resynchronization Therapy for Electrode Region trial. Circ Heart Fail 2013; 6:427–34.

36. Bai R, Di Biase L, Mohanty P, et al. Positioning of left ventricular pacing lead guided by intracardiac echocardiography with vector velocity imaging during cardiac resynchronization therapy procedure. J Cardiovasc Electrophysiol 2011;22:1034–41.

37. Vukajlovic D, Milasinovic G, Angelkov L, et al. Contractile reserve assessed by dobutamine test identifies super-responders to cardiac resynchronization therapy. Arch Med Sci 2014;10:684–91.

38. Stankovic I, Aarones M, Smith H-J, et al. Dynamic relationship of left-ventricular dyssynchrony and contractile reserve in patients undergoing cardiac resynchronization therapy. Eur Heart J 2014;35: 48–55.

39. Bilchick KC, Kuruvilla S, Hamirani YS, et al. Impact of mechanical activation, scar, and electrical timing on cardiac resynchronization therapy response and clinical outcomes. J Am Coll Cardiol 2014;63: 1657–66.

40. Pison L, Proclemer A, Bongiorni MG, et al. Scientific Initiative Committee, European Heart Rhythm Association. Imaging techniques in electrophysiology and implantable device procedures: results of the European Heart Rhythm Association survey. Europace 2013;15:1333–6.

41. Giraldi F, Cattadori G, Roberto M, et al. Long-term effectiveness of cardiac resynchronization therapy in heart failure patients with unfavorable cardiac veins anatomy comparison of surgical versus hemodynamic procedure. J Am Coll Cardiol 2011; 58:483–90.

42. Santangeli P, Epstein A, Hutchinson M, et al. Comparative effectiveness of left ventricular versus biventricular pacing for cardiac resynchronization therapy: a meta-analysis of randomized controlled trials. J Am Coll Cardiol 2014;63. http://dx.doi.org/10.1016/S0735-1097(14)60317-X.

Cardiac Resynchronization Therapy
How to Decrease Nonresponders

José María Tolosana, MD, PhD, Lluís Mont, MD, PhD*

KEYWORDS

- Cardiac resynchronization therapy • Nonresponders • Heart failure

KEY POINTS

- Nonresponse to cardiac resynchronization therapy (CRT) therapy is still a major issue in therapy expansion.
- The description of fast, simple, cost-effective methods to optimize CRT could help in adapting pacing intervals to individual patients.
- A better understanding about the importance of appropriate patient selection, left ventricular lead placement, and device programming, together with a multidisciplinary approach and an optimal follow-up of the patients, may reduce the percentage of nonresponders.

BACKGROUND

Cardiac resynchronization therapy (CRT) in appropriately selected heart failure (HF) patients has been shown to induce left ventricular (LV) reverse remodeling and improve both functional capacity and quality of life, thus decreasing hospital admissions and mortality.[1] However, current CRT indications cover a broad spectrum of patients. Although CRT will improve symptoms and survival in most patients, about one-third (30%) of CRT recipients do not obtain clinical benefit from the therapy and are considered clinical nonresponders. The percentage reaches 40% when the criterion is echocardiographic response to CRT, defined as significant LV reverse remodeling.[2]

CRITERIA FOR RESPONSE TO CARDIAC RESYNCHRONIZATION THERAPY

To define clinical response, a rather imprecise criterion (improvement in New York Heart Association [NYHA] functional class) has been extensively used; more objective criteria, such as 10% or more increased distance in the 6-minute walking test, also have been applied. Several randomized studies have demonstrated the beneficial effects of CRT for patients in NYHA class III or ambulatory class IV, and more recently, in mild HF (class II with systolic dysfunction), and the indication for CRT has now been extended to patients in NYHA class II.[1] Patients with mild HF show less improvement in functional capacity, because it is already acceptable[3]; however, they clearly show LV remodeling. On the other hand, the magnitude of change in the left ventricular end-systolic volume has been correlated with a better survival rate and fewer hospital admissions.[4] Therefore, in class II patients, LV remodeling is a good marker of response.

FACTORS THAT MAY IMPROVE THE NUMBERS OF CARDIAC RESYNCHRONIZATION THERAPY RESPONDERS

The lack of response to CRT depends on multiple factors, starting with appropriate patient selection,

Hospital Clinic, Universitat de Barcelona, Villarroel 170, Barcelona, Catalonia 08036, Spain
* Corresponding author.
E-mail address: lmont@clinic.cat

Card Electrophysiol Clin 7 (2015) 789–796
http://dx.doi.org/10.1016/j.ccep.2015.08.009

followed by factors related to the implant procedure and to optimization of therapy, including appropriate drugs and programming, during follow-up (**Fig. 1**).

Patient Selection

Since the advent of CRT, numerous factors have been related to the success of the therapy. Several clinical and image-related characteristics help to identify patients with low probability to benefit from therapy. Improved patient selection using these important markers of response or nonresponse may reduce inappropriate indications, avoiding unnecessary patient risks and saving the costs associated with the therapy.

QRS morphology

Although patients with left bundle branch block (LBBB) clearly benefit from CRT, patients with wide QRS but right bundle branch block (RBBB) have a different activation pattern. Fewer than 25% of patients with RBBB demonstrated LV activation delay equivalent to LBBB results.[5] CRT was less effective in improving hemodynamics in an animal model of RBBB,[6] and recent clinical data from the MADIT-CRT[7] and RAFT[8] trials failed to demonstrate a reduction in hospital admissions and deaths in patients with RBBB treated with CRT.[9]

Subgroup analyses based on QRS morphology in the main randomized trials of CRT suggest that patients with complete LBBB (**Fig. 2**) receive greater benefit from CRT, compared with patients with nonspecific intraventricular conduction delay or with RBBB.[1]

QRS width

The lack of CRT benefit in patients with narrow QRS (<120 ms) is now widely accepted.[1] Most of the main randomized clinical trials included patients with wide QRS defined as QRS greater than 120 or 130 ms. However, a large meta-analysis did not report a significant reduction in death and hospital admissions in patients treated

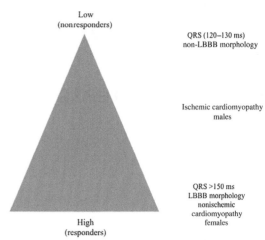

Fig. 2. Clinical factors and probability of response to CRT. (*Adapted from* Brignole M, Auricchio A, Baron-Esquivias G, et al. 2013 ESC Guidelines on cardiac pacing and cardiac resynchronization therapy: the task force on cardiac pacing and resynchronization therapy of the European Society of Cardiology (ESC). Developed in collaboration with the European Heart Rhythm Association (EHRA). Eur Heart J 2013;34(29):2302; with permission.)

with CRT who had a QRS of 120 to 149 ms, whereas CRT was more effective in reducing adverse clinical events in those patients with a QRS duration greater than 150 ms.[10] LV reverse remodeling and clinical responses increase progressively with increasing baseline QRS duration, but mainly in those patients with LBBB morphology.[11]

Heart failure cause

Patients with ischemic cardiomyopathy tend to have a poor response to CRT and show less improvement in LV reverse remodeling and left ventricular ejection fraction (LVEF).[12,13] The extent of myocardial scar tissue may be one of the key determinants of the poor response in these patients because slow conduction across the scar areas may reduce the efficacy of the therapy.[14]

On the other hand, the existence of large scar areas also limits the LV reverse remodeling.[15] It is likely that CRT mitigates the deleterious effects of dyssynchrony induced by the LBBB but cannot increase the contractility of necrotic areas (**Fig. 3**).

Gender differences

Subanalyses from randomized clinical trials and meta-analyses describe greater reductions in the risk of death or hospitalizations in women than in men. The degree of reverse cardiac remodeling also tended to be greater in women than in men.[16,17]

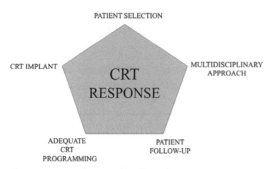

Fig. 1. Factors that could affect the response to CRT.

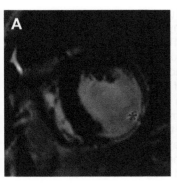 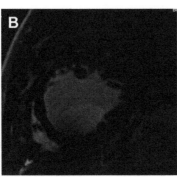

Fig. 3. cMRI axial view. (*A*) Dilated cardiomyopathy with a large posterolateral transmural scar (*red asterisk*). (*B*) Dilated cardiomyopathy without scar.

Men and women with HF are known to differ in comorbidities, risk factors, and response to medical treatment. Women had more nonischemic cause and LBBB morphology that has been associated with better CRT outcomes, compared with men. Moreover, women with dilated cardiomyopathy usually had less myocardial scar than their male counterparts.[18]

Atrial fibrillation

About 30% of patients with advanced HF will develop atrial fibrillation (AF). The prevalence of AF is directly related to worsening NYHA functional class.[19] However, despite the high prevalence of AF in CRT candidates, only 2% of the patients included in the main randomized trials were in AF.[1] Despite the lack of randomized studies in patients with AF, 23% of patients who received a CRT in Europe were in AF.[20]

In a meta-analysis that included 7945 patients from 33 observational studies, Wilton and colleagues[21] found that the 22% of patients in AF had a higher mortality and a greater risk of nonresponse to CRT than patients in sinus rhythm. Patients in AF have fast and irregular ventricular rates, which may interfere with complete biventricular pacing delivery. Therefore, strict control of the intrinsic heart rate is required in AF patients in order to achieve the maximum percentage of ventricular pacing.

Based on observational studies, some investigators[22] recommend systematic atrioventricular junction (AVJ) ablation in these patients to ensure 100% capture by pacing, while others support a conservative initial strategy, optimizing the medical treatment and programming the device to obtain a high percentage of ventricular pacing, and recommend reserving AVJ ablation only for patients with poor heart rate control.[23–26] Randomized trials may clarify the best strategy to follow in these patients.

Clinical parameters and comorbidities

Many clinical parameters and comorbidities help to identify patients with low probability of response

and an increased mortality risk. Numerous studies have found that a highly dilated left ventricle and severe mitral regurgitation indicate a lower probability of response.[12–28] Patients with very advanced disease have likely reached a point of no return and CRT may not reverse or stabilize HF in these patients.

The presence of multiple predictors of lower response and increased mortality has an additive effect.[29–33] Recently, the EAARN score,–an algorithm to calculate the risk of mortality in patients treated with CRT, has been reported. The score is based on preimplant risk factors (LVEF <22%; age ≥70 years, AF, renal dysfunction, and basal NYHA functional class IV).[34] The EAARN score demonstrated an excellent prognosis and low mortality in patients with 0 to 1 risk factors, whereas those patients with 3 risk factors or more had a high mortality despite the benefits of the therapy. Overall mortality was 21.4 per 100 person-years in the subgroup of patients with an EAARN score 3 or greater, compared with 7 per 100 person-years with an EAARN score of 0 or 1 (hazard ratio [HR] 4.04; confidence interval [CI] 95% 2.9–6.5, $P<.001$). This finding highlights the need to start CRT therapy at the earliest stages of the disease, avoiding unnecessary delay that could compromise response and survival.

Imaging as a tool for patient selection

The use of echocardiography to assess mechanical dyssynchrony and select patients for CRT has not yet been standardized. Many observational studies have shown that the presence of LV dyssynchrony is associated with an improvement in CRT response; nevertheless, these results were not supported by the large, multicenter, PROSPECT study. The echocardiographic parameters tested in that trial failed to predict the response to therapy with accuracy.[35]

Selection of patients for CRT based on LV mechanical dyssynchrony assessed with imaging techniques is not routinely recommended as a selection criterion for CRT.[1] One of the reasons to explain the lack of usefulness of echocardiographic methods is the complexity and heterogeneity of the parameters. A recent study has shown that when any of 4 simple criteria for dyssynchrony were present (septal flash, atrioventricular [AV] dyssynchrony, exaggerated right ventricular [RV]-LV response), the probability of response was high. The investigators suggest that CRT may only work when a correctable mechanism is present, and this mechanism can be identified by simple echocardiographic measurements.[36]

Although preimplant cardiac MRI (cMRI) is still uncommon in most practices, some studies have shown its benefit in assessing dyssynchrony and scar burden. Pacing in regions of scar detected by delayed enhancement MRI predicts lack of response to CRT.[15,37] Moreover, the presence, size, and heterogeneity of myocardial scar identified by cMRI predict appropriate ICD therapies in patients treated with CRT and may allow the identification of patients with a low risk of sudden cardiac death.[38] Large, randomized trials are needed to evaluate the use of cMRI in selecting patients for CRT.

Cardiac Resynchronization Therapy Implant Procedure, Left Ventricular Lead Localization, and Type of Leads

Lack of response to CRT is sometimes related to an inappropriate LV lead location. In one study that reviewed the reasons for lack of CRT response, suboptimal LV lead position was implicated in 21% of the patients.[39] Along with correct patient selection, the location of the LV lead also could improve the response to therapy.

Lead localization

In the absence of additional information regarding activation sequence, the greatest delay in mechanical contraction in patients with LBBB is frequently located in the LV posterolateral region. The REVERSE study showed that a lateral LV lead position was associated with better outcomes, in comparison with other locations.[40] On the other hand, data from the MADIT CRT trial demonstrated that an LV lead location in basal or midventricular positions was superior to apical positions. In that trial, LV apical lead position was associated with increased risk of HF (HR 1.72; 95% CI 1.09–2.71) and death (HR 2.91; 95% CI 1.42–5.97).[41]

The existence of individual variations in the conduction delay and the presence of myocardial scar may modify the site of latest activation. The TARGET trial randomized 220 HF patients to an LV nonapical position coincident with the latest activated areas (assessed with speckle-tracking echocardiography) or to a standard unguided LV lead position.[42] The first group had a greater proportion of clinical and echocardiographic responders at 6-month follow-up.

Knowledge of LV viability, scar distribution, and contraction patterns provided by MRI or echocardiography may help to optimize the LV lead position. In these cases, the use of myocardial imaging may individualize CRT and could help to place the LV in a vein adjacent to the latest activated region far away from the scar.[15–26,28–37]

Type of left ventricular lead

There is a great variability in coronary venous anatomy that complicates the placement of the LV lead in a target position. The standard bipolar leads have high rates of LV lead dislodgement, phrenic nerve stimulation, loss of capture, and increased LV pacing thresholds. The recent development of LV leads with different diameters and shapes may facilitate the placement of the lead in a correct position. One of the best advances in LV leads is the design of quadripolar leads, with 4 independent electrodes that allow the programming of additional vectors for LV pacing. Altogether, it is now easier to find a stable LV position with low pacing thresholds, minimizing the incidence of phrenic nerve stimulation.[43]

Recently, a single-center observational study described a lower rate of hospitalizations for HF and LV lead surgical revision in patients with quadripolar LV leads. The use of quadripolar leads facilitates targeting pacing at more proximal regions of the coronary venous branches, maintaining a more distal and stable lead position.[44]

Moreover, quadripolar leads enable multipoint pacing. This technology delivers 2 LV pulses from a single quadripolar lead (MultiPoint Pacing; St Jude Medical, Minneapolis, MN, USA). Early studies show promising results by improving hemodynamics and the rate of response to CRT.[45,46] However, the link between acute hemodynamic measures and long-term outcome is not yet proven. Whether multipoint pacing will translate into long-term clinical benefits remains unknown and will require testing in large randomized trials.[47]

Cardiac resynchronization therapy device optimization

Echocardiography has traditionally been considered the gold standard for CRT optimization. However, these methods include complex adjustments that require expertise and are time-consuming. Moreover, current literature suggests that routine

AV and interventricular (VV) delay optimization have no effect on CRT outcomes[48]; therefore, routine CRT optimization is not recommended in these patients.[1]

On the other hand, suboptimal programming of the AV or VV delays may limit the response to CRT. Therefore, optimization of the AV and VV intervals may be recommended to correct suboptimal device settings.[19]

Despite the lack of strong evidence in favor of optimization, many individual examples demonstrate the possibility to strongly improve response. Therefore, the description of fast, simple, cost-effective methods to optimize CRT could help in adapting pacing intervals to individual patients. In efforts to simplify CRT optimization, some automatic optimization algorithms based on intracardiac electrograms have been implemented, with conflicting results.[49–51]

Previous studies have linked QRS shortening to clinical response and echocardiographic improvement.[52,53] Therefore, shortening the paced QRS duration could be a simple and widely applicable optimization method.

The authors recently described a simple method of QRS-based optimization that is called fusion-optimized intervals (FOI), which uses fusion with intrinsic conduction to achieve the shortest possible QRS.[54] The idea behind fusion-guided biventricular pacing with the intrinsic rhythm is to allow partial or complete intrinsic depolarization of the VV septum (fusion pacing), which creates 3 activation fronts instead of 2 during pure biventricular pacing.

The FOI method is feasible and simple and can be easily performed after the implant. This method reduces the paced QRS duration and improves the acute hemodynamic response in comparison to nominal programming of the device.

The Medtronic Adaptive CRT algorithm uses intrinsic intervals to provide RV-synchronized LV pacing when AV conduction is normal, or biventricular pacing otherwise. A recent randomized study that evaluated this algorithm demonstrated that pacing with LV fusion was equivalent to echocardiographic optimization.[51–55]

Device Programming

Sustained and effective biventricular pacing is necessary to achieve response to CRT. Koplan and colleagues[56] demonstrated a 44% reduction in the composite end point of mortality and HF hospitalization in patients receiving 93% to 100% of biventricular pacing, compared with those receiving 92% or less. These results were reinforced by the published results of a series of 36,935 patients, showing the greatest reduction in mortality in patients with biventricular pacing greater than 98%.[57]

The main causes for lost ventricular pacing in patients treated with CRT were inappropriately long AV interval delay (34%) and atrial tachycardia, mainly AF (31%) or premature ventricular beats (17%).[58] Therefore, a great effort should be made to reach 100% of ventricular pacing, including aggressive suppression of atrial tachyarrhythmias by pharmacology, electrical cardioversion, catheter ablation, or AVJ ablation. Frequent premature ventricular beats also must be treated (drug therapy or ablation of the PVC foci) to ensure 100% of ventricular pacing.[59]

Remote Monitoring

Remote monitoring of CRT devices with regular transmissions of data such as atrial/ventricular arrhythmia burden, percentage of biventricular pacing, or heart rate histograms favors a faster detection and solution of problems that could worsen the response to CRT. In the IN-TIME[60] randomized trial, the automatic, daily, implant-based, multiparameter telemonitoring significantly improved clinical outcomes (all-cause mortality, hospitalization, change in NYHA class, and symptoms) for patients with HF.

Multidisciplinary Approach and Follow-Up

Patients who receive CRT often require care from cardiology subspecialties (electrophysiology, HF specialist, imaging). Unfortunately, the care delivered is often fragmented, with limited communication between the different subspecialties. A multidisciplinary approach to CRT patients, based on consensus among electrophysiology, cardiac imaging, and HF specialists, improves the benefits of the therapy.

Mullens and colleagues[39] identified the main causes of nonresponse in a series of 75 patients treated with CRT: suboptimal medical treatment, incorrect LV lead position or device programming, and presence of uncontrolled arrhythmias (AF or frequent premature ventricular beats). A multidisciplinary approach in these nonresponders led to significant improvements in LV function and reduction of adverse events.

Altman and colleagues[61] demonstrated that integrated multidisciplinary care improved outcomes in patients receiving CRT. There was a 38% relative risk reduction of death, heart transplant, or hospital admissions over 2 years in patients who received a multidisciplinary care approach versus standard clinical care.

SUMMARY

Nonresponse to CRT therapy is still a major issue in therapy expansion. It is due to many factors, some of them modifiable. A better understanding about the importance of appropriate patient selection, LV lead placement, and device programming, together with a multidisciplinary approach and an optimal follow-up of the patients, may reduce the percentage of nonresponders.

REFERENCES

1. Brignole M, Auricchio A, Baron-Esquivias G, et al, ESC Committee for Practice Guidelines (CPG). 2013 ESC Guidelines on cardiac pacing and cardiac resynchronization therapy: the Task Force on cardiac pacing and resynchronization therapy of the European Society of Cardiology (ESC). Developed in collaboration with the European Heart Rhythm Association (EHRA). Eur Heart J 2013; 34(29):2281–329.

2. YU CM, Hayes DL. Cardiac resynchronization therapy. Eur Heart J 2013;34(19):1396–403.

3. Landolina M, Lunati M, Gasparini M, et al, InSync/In-Sync ICD Italian Registry Investigators. Comparison of the effects of cardiac resynchronization therapy in patients with Class II vs. Class III-IV heart failure. Am J Cardiol 2007;100:1007–12.

4. Solomon S, Foster E, Bouroun M, et al, MADIT-CRT Investigators. Effects of cardiac resynchronization therapy on reverse remodeling and relation to outcome: multicenter automatic defibrillator implantation trial: cardiac resynchronization therapy. Circulation 2010;122:985–92.

5. Varma N. Left ventricular conduction delays and relation to QRS configuration in patients with left ventricular dysfunction. Am J Cardiol 2009;103:1578–85.

6. Byrne MJ, Helm RH, Daya S, et al. Diminished left ventricular dyssnchrony and impact of resynchronizaton in failing hearts with right vs left bundle branch block. J Am Coll Cardiol 2007;50:1484–90.

7. Zareba W, Klein H, Cygankiewicz I, et al, MADIT-CRT Investigators CRT-D. Effectiveness by QRS duration and morphology in the MADIT CRT patients. Circulation 2011;123(10):1061–72.

8. Tang AS, Wells GA, Talajic M, et al, Resynchronization-Defibrillation for Ambulatory Heart Failure Trial Investigators. Cardiac-resynchronization therapy for mild to moderate heart failure. N Engl J Med 2010;363:2385–95.

9. Sipahi I, Chou JC, Hyden M, et al. Effects of QRS morphology on clinical event reduction with cardiac resynchronization therapy: meta-analysis of randomized controlled trials. Am Heart J 2012;163(2):260–7.

10. Sipahi I, Carrigan TP, Rowland DY, et al. Impact of QRS duration on clinical event reduction with cardiac resynchronizaton therapy: meta-analysis of randomized controlled trials. Arch Intern Med 2011;171(16):1454–62.

11. Gold MR, Thébault C, Linde C, et al. Effect of QRS duration and morphology on cardiac resynchronization therapy outcomes in mild heart failure: results from the Resynchronization Reverses Remodeling in Systolic Left Ventricular Dysfunction (REVERSE) study. Circulation 2012;126(7):822–9.

12. Diaz- Infante E, Mont L, Leal J, et al, SCARS Investigators. Predictors of lack of response to resynchronization therapy. Am J Cardiol 2005;95:1436–40.

13. Shanks M, Delgado V, Ng AC, et al. Clinical and echocardiographic predictors of nonresponse to cardiac resynchronization therapy. Am Heart J 2011;161(3):552–7.

14. Sweney MO, Prinzen FW. Ventricular pump function and pacing: physiological and clinical integration. Circ Arrhythm Electrophysiol 2008;1:127–39.

15. Ypemburg C, Roes SD, Bleeker GB, et al. Effect of total scar burden on contrast-enhanced magnetic resonance imaging on response to cardiac resynchronization therapy. Am J Cardiol 2007;99:657–60.

16. Cheng YJ, Zhang J, Li WJ, et al. More favorable response to cardiac resynchronization therapy in women than in men. Circ Arrhythm Electrophysiol 2014;7(5):807–15.

17. Arshad A, Moss AJ, Foster E, et al, MADIT-CRT Executive Committee. Cardiac resynchronization therapy is more effective in women than in men: the MADIT-CRT (Multicenter Automatic Defibrillator Implantation Trial with Cardiac Resynchronization Therapy) trial. J Am Coll Cardiol 2011;57(7):813–20.

18. Loring Z, Strauss DG, Gerstenblith G. Cardiac MRI scar patterns differ by sex in an implantable cardioverter-defibrillator and cardiac resynchronization therapy cohort. Heart Rhythm 2013;10(5):659–65.

19. Daubert JC. Atrial fibrillation and heart failure. A mutually noxious association. Europace 2004;5:S1–4.

20. Dickstein K, Bogale N, Priori S, et al, Scientific Committee, National Coordinators. The European cardiac resynchronization therapy survey. Eur Heart J 2009; 30:2450–60.

21. Wilton S, Leung AA, Ghali WA, et al. Outcomes of cardiac resynchronization therapy in patients with vs. those without atrial fibrillation: a systematic review and meta-analysis. Heart Rhythm 2011;8(7): 1088–94.

22. Gasparini M, Auricchio A, Metra M. Long-term survival in pateints undergoing cardiac resynchronization therapy. The importance of performing atrio-ventricular junction ablation in patients with permanent atrial fibrillation. Eur Heart J 2008;29: 1644–52.

23. Tolosana JM, Hernandez Madrid A, Brugada J, et al, SPARE Investigators. Comparison of benefits and mortality in cardiac resynchronization therapy in

patients with atrial fibrillation vs. patients in sinus rhtym. Am J Cardiol 2008;102:444–9.

24. Delnoy PE, Ottervanger JP, Luttikhuis HO, et al. Comparison of usefulness of cardiac resynchronization therapy in patients with atrial fibrillation and heart failure vs. patients in sinus rhythm and heart failure. Am J Cardiol 2007;99:1252–7.

25. Khadjooi K, Foley PW, Chalil S, et al. Long-term effects of cardiac resynchronization therapy in patients with atrial fibrillation. Heart 2008;94: 879–83.

26. Tolosana JM, Arnau AM, Madrid AH, et al, SPARE II investigators (Spanish Atrial Resynchronization Study II). Cardiac resynchronization therapy in patients with permanent atrial fibrillation. Is it mandatory to ablate the atrioventricular junction to obtain a good response? Eur J Heart Fail 2012;14(6):635–41.

27. Ghio S, Freemantle N, Scelsi L, et al. Long-term left ventricular reverse remodelling with cardiac resynchronization therapy: results from the CARE HF trial. Eur J Heart Fail 2009;11(5):480–8.

28. Vidal B, Delgado V, Mont L, et al. Decreased likelihood of response to cardiac resynchronization in patients with severe heart failure. Eur J Heart Fail 2010;12:283–7.

29. Van Bomel RJ, Borleffs CJ, Ypengburg C, et al. Morbidity and mortality in heart failure patients treated with cardiac resynchronization therapy: influence of pre-implantation characteristics on long-term outcome. Eur Heart J 2010;31:2783–90.

30. Bogale N, Priori S, Cleland JG, et al, Scientific Committee, National Coordinators, and Investigators. The European CRT survey: 1 year (9-15 months) follow-up results. Eur J Heart Fail 2012;14:61–73.

31. Kronborg MB, Mortensen PT, Kirkfeldt RE, et al. Very long term follow-up of cardiac resynchronization therapy: clinical outcome and predictors of mortality. Eur J Heart Fail 2008;10:796–801.

32. Bai R, Di Biase L, Elayi C, et al. Mortality of heart failure patients after cardiac resynchronization therapy: identification of predictors. J Cardiovasc Electrophysiol 2008;19:1259–65.

33. Kreuz J, Horbeck F, Linhart M, et al. Independent predictors of mortality in patients with advanced heart failure treated by cardiac resynchronization therapy. Europace 2012;14:1596–601.

34. Khatib M, Tolosana JM, Trucco E, et al. EAARN score, a predictive score for mortality in patients receiving cardiac resynchronization therapy based on pre-implantation risk factors. Eur J Heart Fail 2014;16(7):802–9.

35. Chung ES, Leon AR, Tavazzi L, et al. Results of the predictors of response to CRT (PROSPECT) trial. Circulation 2008;117(20):2608–16.

36. Doltra A, Bijnens B, Tolosana JM, et al. Mechanical abnormalities detected with conventional echocardiography are associated with response and midterm survival in CRT. JACC Cardiovasc Imaging 2014; 7(10):969–79.

37. Adelstein EC, Saba S. Scar burden by myocardial perfusion imaging predicts echocardiographic response to cardiac resynchronization therapy in ischemic cardiomyopathy. Am Heart J 2007;153: 105–12.

38. Fernández-Armenta J, Berruezo A, Mont L, et al. Use of myocardial scar characterization to predict ventricular arrhythmia in cardiac resynchronization therapy. Europace 2012;14(11):1578–86.

39. Mullens W, Crimm RA, Verg T, et al. Insight from a cardiac resynchronization optimization clinic as part of a heart failure disease management program. J Am Coll Cardiol 2009;53:765–73.

40. Thebault C, Donal E, Meunier C, et al, REVERSE Study Group. Sites of left and right ventricular lead implantation and response to cardiac resynchronization therapy observations from the REVERSE trial. Eur Heart J 2012;33:2662–71.

41. Singh JP, Klein HU, Huang DT, et al. Left ventricular lead position and clinical outcome in the multicenter automatic defibrillator implantation trial-cardiac resynchronization therapy (MADIT-TRC) trial. Circulation 2011;123:1159–66.

42. Khan FZ, Virdee MS, Palmer CR, et al. Targeted left ventricular lead placement to guide cardiac resynchronization therapy: the TARGET study: a randomized, controlled trial. J Am Coll Cardiol 2012; 59:1509–18.

43. Forleo GB, Della Rocca DG, Papavasileiou LP, et al. Left ventricular pacing with a new quadripolar transvenous lead for CRT: early results of a prospective comparison with conventional implant outcomes. Heart Rhythm 2011;8(1):31–7.

44. Forleo GB, Di Biase L, Bharmi R, et al. Hospitalization rates and associated cost analysis of cardiac resynchronization therapy with an implantable defibrillator and quadripolar vs. bipolar left ventricular leads: a comparative effectiveness study. Europace 2015;17(1):101–7.

45. Rinaldi CA, Leclercq C, Kranig W, et al. Improvement in acute contractility and hemodynamics with multipoint pacing via left ventricular quadripolar pacing lead. J Interv Card Electrophysiol 2014; 40(1):7–80.

46. Pappone C, Ćalović Ž, Vicedomini G, et al. Improving cardiac resynchronization therapy response with multipoint left ventricular pacing: twelve-month follow-up study. Heart Rhythm 2015; 12(6):1250–8.

47. Rinaldi CA, Burri H, Thibault B, et al. A review of multisite pacing to achieve cardiac resynchronization therapy. Europace 2015;17(1):7–17.

48. Auger D, Hoke U, Bax JJ, et al. Effect of atrioventricular and ventriculoventricular delay optimization on clinical and echocardiographic outcomes of

patients treated with cardiac resynchronization therapy: a meta-analysis. Am Heart J 2013;166(1):20–9.

49. Ellenbogen KA, Gold MR, Meyer TE, et al. Primary results from the SmartDelay determined AV optimization: a comparison to other AV delay methods use in cardiac resynchronization therapy (SMART AV trial): a randomized trial comparing empirical, echocardiography guided and algorithmic atrioventricular delay programing in cardiac resynchronization therapy. Circulation 2010;122:2660–8.

50. Abrahan WT, Gras D, Yu CM, et al, FREEDOM Steering Committee. Rationale and design of a randomized clinical trial to assess the safety and efficacy of frequent optimization of cardiac resynchronization therapy: the Frequent Optimization Study Using the Quickopt Method (FREEDOM) trial. Am Heart J 2010;159(6):944–8.

51. Martin DO, Lemke B, Brinie D, et al, Adaptive CRT Study Investigators. Investigation of a novel algorithm for synchronized left-ventricular pacing and ambulatory optimization of cardiac resynchronization therapy: results of the Adaptive CRT trial. Heart Rhythm 2012;9:1807–14.

52. LecoQ G, Lecler C, Leray E, et al. Clinical and electrocardiographic predictors of a positive response to cardiac resynchronization therapy in advanced heart failure. Eur Heart J 2005;26:1094–100.

53. Hsin JM, Selzman KA, Leclercq C, et al. Paced left ventricular QRS width and ECG parameters predict outcomes after cardiac resynchronization therapy: PROSPECT-ECG sub-study. Circ Arrhythm Electrophysiol 2011;4:851–7.

54. Arbelo E, Tolosana JM, Trucco E, et al. Fusion-optimized intervals (FOI): a new method to achieve the narrowest QRS for optimization of the AV and VV

intervals in patients undergoing cardiac resynchronization therapy. J Cardiovasc Electrophysiol 2014; 25:283–92.

55. Krum H, Lemke B, Birnie D, et al. A novel algorithm for individualized cardiac resynchronization therapy: rationale and design of the adaptive cardiac resynchronization therapy trial. Am Heart J 2012; 163(5):747–52.

56. Koplan BA, Kaplan AJ, Weiner S, et al. Heart failure decompensation and all-cause mortality in relation to percent biventricular pacing in patient with heart failure: is a goal of 100% biventricular pacing necessary? J Am Coll Cardiol 2009;53:355–60.

57. Hayes DL, Boehmer J, Day J. Cardiac resynchronization therapy and relationship of percent biventricular pacing. Heart Rhythm 2011;8(9):1469–75.

58. Cheng A, Landman SR, Stadler RW. Reasons for loss of cardiac resynchronization therapy pacing: insights from 32 844 patients. Circ Arrhythm Electrophysiol 2012;5(5):884–8.

59. Lakkireddy D, Di Biase L, Ryschon K, et al. Radiofrequency ablation of premature ventricular ectopy improves the efficacy of cardiac resynchronization therapy in nonresponders. J Am Coll Cardiol 2012; 60(16):1531–9.

60. Hindricks G, Taborsky M, Glikson M, et al, IN-TIME Study Group. Implant-based multiparameter telemonitoring of patients with heart failure (IN-TIME): a randomised controlled trial. Lancet 2014;384(9943): 583–90.

61. Altman RK, Parks KA, Schlett CL, et al. Multidisciplinary care of patients receiving cardiac resynchronization therapy is associated with improved clinical outcomes. Eur Heart J 2012;33(17):2181–8.

Follow-up

Cardiac Resynchronization Therapy Follow-up
Role of Remote Monitoring

Cecilia Linde, MD, PhD*, Frieder Braunschweig, MD, PhD

KEYWORDS

- Cardiac resynchronization therapy • Follow-up • Hospitalizations • Heart failure • Mortality

KEY POINTS

- Remote monitoring is safe and allows more rapid detection of actionable events in implantable cardioverter-defibrillator (ICD) therapy, like technical failure and arrhythmias.
- Remote monitoring reduces the number of inappropriate and appropriate shocks and prolongs battery life of cardiac resynchronization therapy devices with defibrillation capabilities (CRT-D) compared with standard follow-up.
- Monitoring of device-derived parameters such as the percentage of biventricular stimulation, atrial and ventricular arrhythmia, hours of activity, and heart rate may improve the management of patients with heart failure.
- Pressure sensors for daily monitoring and transmission of pulmonary artery pressures compared with controls are linked to reduced need for heart failure hospitalizations in patients with heart failure with and without CRT-D therapy as indicated in the CHAMPION trial.
- The EHRA survey of implementation and reimbursement of remote monitoring for implantable devices in Europe indicated that physicians perceive remote monitoring as useful but that their use implies an increased workload. The biggest obstacle for wider use is lack of reimbursement.

INTRODUCTION

The prevalence of heart failure remains high despite recent advances in drug and device therapy.[1,2] This prevalence is largely related to increasing age in the population and better survival after myocardial infarction. The costs for heart failure care both in and out of hospital are substantial.[3] Cardiac resynchronization therapy (CRT) is an important treatment option for those patients with heart failure who have wide QRS complexes (about 30%)[4] and who remain symptomatic despite optimal medical therapy.[5] In clinical practice CRT devices are commonly supplied with defibrillation capabilities (CRT-D).[6] CRT is linked to a 30% relative risk (RR) reduction in the combination of heart failure hospitalizations and mortality and in mortality per se, as indicated in a recent case-based

Conflicts of Interest: C. Linde was principal investigator of REVERSE and MIRACLE EF, and cardiac resynchronization therapy studies sponsored by Medtronic; has received research grants, speaker honoraria, and consulting fees from Medtronic; and has received speaker honoraria and consulting fees from St. Jude Medical, Vifor, Cardio3 and Novartis. F. Braunschweig serves on adverse event committees of studies sponsored by Biotronik and Medtronic. He has received research grants, speaker honoraria and consulting fees from Medtronic, St. Jude Medical, Biosense Webster, and Boehringer Ingelheim.
Department of Cardiology, Karolinska University Hospital, Karolinska Institutet, Stockholm S-17176, Sweden
* Corresponding author.
E-mail address: cecilia.linde@ki.se

Card Electrophysiol Clin 7 (2015) 797–807
http://dx.doi.org/10.1016/j.ccep.2015.08.010

meta-analysis.[7] However, the risk for progressive deterioration, hospitalization, and death remains high even after CRT implantation because 30% of patients do not responding to CRT and because of the natural history of the underlying heart condition.

Therefore, structured follow-up with regular visits to device and heart failure specialists is mandatory to maintain stable clinical conditions. For this purpose, remote follow-up offers a valuable adjunct to in-clinic encounters. Apart from the possibility of ambulatory device checks and early notification of technical issues, CRT devices contain several features for arrhythmia detection and measurement of variables with relevance to heart failure management.[8] Monitoring of these variables enables clinicians to detect arrhythmias and changes in heart failure status early and to take appropriate therapeutic action. Furthermore, studies with implantable hemodynamic sensors indicate that monitoring of central pressures may further enhance the benefit from device-based monitoring. This article summarizes the current role of remote monitoring in CRT follow-up.

REMOTE MONITORING OF IMPLANTABLE DEVICES

Home monitoring of implantable devices was introduced in 2000 for the remote follow-up of pacemakers and was later expanded to implantable cardiac defibrillators (ICDs). Using an imbedded antenna, information on device function and other variables is transmitted to a local communication unit and then to a central data server that can be accessed by clinicians (**Fig. 1**). Early studies showed the feasibility and technical reliability of this approach.[9] Meanwhile, the option of remote monitoring is provided by all manufacturers of CRT and ICDs. Apart from technical device interrogation to detect lead fractures, insulation defects, or premature battery depletion, these systems provide alerts on critical clinical events such as arrhythmia onset or ICD shocks. Other advantages include the option to replace in-office device checkups with home monitoring, which is convenient for patients living in remote areas and has the potential to decrease the work burden in device clinics. In the 2013 European Society of Cardiology (ESC) guidelines on cardiac pacing and CRT, remote device follow-up received a class IIa recommendation.[5] It has been proposed that avoidance of traditional in-office visits for device monitoring translates into financial benefits for patients and health care organizations.

OBSERVATIONAL REGISTRIES

The ALTITUDE observational study[10] reported survival status in patients with ICD and CRT devices from a single manufacturer and compared patients traditionally followed at device clinics with those who transmitted remote data (on average 4 times monthly). For the 69,665 patients with ICDs and

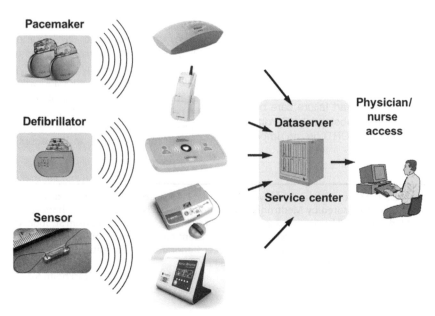

Fig. 1. Remote monitoring of implanted devices.

CRTs receiving remote follow-up via the network, 1-year and 5-year survival rates were significantly higher compared with 116,222 patients who received conventional device follow-up (50% relative reduction; $P<.0001$). Complete patient characteristics were not available but there was no difference in age, gender, device type or year, and socioeconomic background.

In a cohort of another manufacturer[11] a total of 269,471 patients including 61,475 with CRT-Ds and 7.906 with CRTS with pacemakers (CRT-Ps) (together 47%) was followed by remote monitoring with a varying degree of adherence. Remote monitoring was associated with improved survival (hazard ratio, 2.10; $P<.001$). Thus, these 2 large but nonrandomized studies support the use of remote device monitoring to improve patient outcomes. However, there was no information as to what clinical actions were taken based on information from remote monitoring.

CARDIAC RESYNCHRONIZATION THERAPY EFFECTIVENESS

A key parameter to assess the effectiveness of CRT delivery is the percentage of biventricular pacing, which can be reduced in patients with rapid ventricular response during atrial fibrillation or those with frequent ventricular extra beats, which may show ventricular pacemaker stimulation or lead to different degrees of fusion. Suboptimal programming of the sensed and paced atrioventricular (AV) intervals can also lead to loss of CRT.[12] Low CRT effectiveness is an important reason for nonresponse to treatment[13] and continuous surveillance of this parameter and alerts if CRT delivery is below a certain threshold allow appropriate interventions to be prescribed to improve CRT performance. Gasparini and colleagues[14] showed large and sustained long-term improvements of left ventricular function and functional capacity in patients having CRT with permanent atrial fibrillation only if optimal therapy delivery was ensured by AV junctional ablation. These findings were recently confirmed in a systematic review.[15] Other reports highlighted that ablation of ventricular ectopy can be helpful to improve CRT response.[16] The threshold for effective CRT delivery is very high and it is recommended that biventricular pacing should be kept as close as possible to 100%.[5] In a recent large cohort study the greatest CRT benefit was achieved in patients receiving an excess of 98% CRT pacing.[17]

A comprehensive table of predisposing factors or precursors for heart failure exacerbation or poor outcome is given in **Box 1**.

Box 1
Examples of predisposing factors or precursors for heart failure exacerbation or poor outcome

Factor/precursor

Onset of atrial tachycardia/atrial fibrillation (AT/AF)

High ventricular rate during AT/AF

Ventricular tachyarrhythmia

Increase in frequency of ventricular extra beats

Low percentage of biventricular pacing

Defibrillation shocks

Decreased patient activity

Low heart rate variability

Decreasing impedance

Increasing filling pressures

Increase in respiratory rate

Decrease in heart sound amplitude

Changes in external appliances linked to device monitoring (body weight, blood pressure)

RANDOMIZED STUDIES OF RESOURCE USE AND TIME TO CLINICAL DECISION

In light of the increasing number of patients with an implanted device, the reduction of resource use and clinic workload by replacing in-office visits with remote device interrogation is an attractive prospect. Furthermore, by early notification of device-related issues and arrhythmias, the time to treatment of these conditions can be markedly reduced. Nevertheless, the single-center evaluation by Al-Khatib and colleagues,[18] randomizing 151 patients with ICDs or CRT-Ds (18%) to remote monitoring or quarterly in-clinic interrogations, showed no reduction in cardiac-related resource use. The primary composite end point of cardiovascular hospitalization, emergency visits, and unscheduled device-related visits was not different after 1 year of follow-up (32% vs 34%).

An Italian multicenter trial randomized 200 patients with an ICD or CRT-D to remote monitoring or standard patient management.[19] After 16 months, emergency visits (−35%) and total health care visits (−21%) for heart failure, arrhythmias, or ICD-related events were significantly less frequent in the remote arm. Furthermore, the response time to ICD alert conditions was reduced by 23.4 days ($P<.001$). This reduction was associated with an improvement in quality of life, whereas the Clinical Composite Score remained unchanged.

In the CONNECT study, wireless remote monitoring with automatic alerts using the Medtronic CareLink system compared with standard in-office follow-up significantly reduced the time to clinical decision in response to clinical events and was associated with a significant reduction in mean length of stay for cardiovascular reasons. For patients assigned to the remote arm, automatic physician alerts were enabled concerning the atrial tachycardia/atrial fibrillation (AT/AF) burden (>12 h/d), ventricular rate during AT/AF (>120 beats/min for >6 hours AT/AF per day), 2 shocks or more delivered, and lead and device safety and integrity issues. There was no statistically difference in patient characteristics between the two groups. The mean age was 65 years, the mean left ventricular ejection fraction (LVEF) was 28%, and 71% of subjects were male. The median time from an event to clinical decision per patient was 4.6 days in the remote arm and 22 days in the in-office arm. This trial resulted in a significant 17.4-day reduction from the time an event occurred to a clinical decision ($P<.0001$). The mean length of stay during a cardiovascular hospitalization was reduced by 18% ($P<.002$) in the remote arm versus the in-office arm, meaning that the costs per hospitalization were significantly reduced.

CLINICAL OUTCOME TRIALS

In the IN-TIME study, 664 patients with chronic HF (New York Heart Association [NYHA] II–III) with either ICDs or CRT-Ds and with no permanent atrial fibrillation were randomly assigned to conventional or remote monitoring follow-up for 12 months.[20] The mean age was 65.5 years, 80% were male, the mean LVEF was 26%, and 58.7% received a CRT-D. The primary end point was the percentage worsened by the clinical composite end point developed by Packer and previously used in CRT studies.[21] Study device data were automatically transmitted (Biotronik Home Monitoring) to the investigators and, in parallel, to a central monitoring unit where trained nurses supported by physicians reviewed data. Predefined events were reported, such as atrial and ventricular tachyarrhythmias, frequency of ventricular extra beats, decrease in patient activity, and abnormal intracardiac electrocardiogram. Thereafter investigational sites were notified and had to confirm receipt of reports within 48 hours for patients assigned to remote monitoring. The clinical response to telemonitoring observations was done at the discretion of the investigators, who also completed a standardized telephone interview with the patient in case contact was established, asking about worsened overall condition or dyspnea, compliance with drug prescriptions, and increases in body weight. In the control group, no study participant had access to telemonitoring data until study completion.

At the end of the study 18.9% of 333 patients in the telemonitoring group and 90 (27%) of 331 patients in the control group ($P = .013$) had a worsened composite clinical score (odds ratio [OR], 0.63; 95% confidence interval [CI], 0.43–0.90). This difference was mainly driven by a lower mortality in the telemonitoring group (10 vs 27 deaths). The Kaplan-Meier estimate of 1-year all-cause mortality in the telemonitoring group was 3.4% versus 8.7% in the control group (hazard ratio [HR], 0.36; 95% CI, 0.17–0.74; **Fig. 2**).

The benefit of remote monitoring was similar in patients with ICDs and in those with CRT-Ds. Subgroup analysis revealed that patients with preexisting atrial fibrillation benefited more from telemonitoring than others and atrial tachyarrhythmia was also the most common reason for patient contact. This finding is not surprising because the most common cause of reduced percentage of biventricular pacing and inappropriate shocks is atrial tachyarrhythmias, which emphasizes the importance of early detection of atrial fibrillation. Atrial fibrillation may also be associated with fluid overload and as such may be an early sign of an upcoming heart failure event.

A preliminary report from MORE-CARE, a study in patients with CRT-Ds randomized to either a remote group with wireless automatic alerts on heart failure–related conditions or control showed that the median delay to clinical decisions was considerably reduced in the remote arm.[22] This reduction was associated with reduced in-hospital visits but no difference in all-cause hospitalizations.

META-ANALYSIS

Recently, Parthiban and colleagues[23] presented a meta-analysis of 9 randomized controlled remote monitoring trials in patients with ICDs and CRT-Ds, including a total of 6469 patients. On average, remote monitoring and office follow-up had similar mortality outcomes. However, a reduction in all-cause mortality was noted in the 3 trials using home monitoring with daily verification of transmission (OR, 0.65; $P = .021$). Although the odds of receiving any ICD shock were similar in the two groups, inappropriate shocks were reduced in remote monitoring patients (OR, 0.55; $P = .002$).

EXPERIENCE FROM TELEMONITORING IN HEART FAILURE

Many trials have investigated the potential benefit of remote patient management in heart failure by

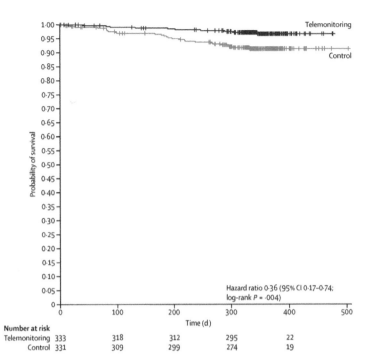

Fig. 2. The Kaplan-Meier curves of survival in the patients assigned to telemonitoring and control groups in the IN-TIME study. (*From* Hindricks G, Taborsky M, Glikson M, et al. Implant-based multiparameter telemonitoring of patients with heart failure (IN-TIME): a randomised controlled trial. Lancet 2014;384 (9943):586; with permission.)

telemonitoring of body weight, blood pressure, and symptoms, and/or structured telephone support (STS). Two meta-analyses have studied the potential value of such strategies.

In an abridged Cochrane analysis of 26 studies by Inglis and colleagues[24] encompassing a total of 8323 patients, 11 studies evaluated the value of telemonitoring (n = 2710) and 16 studies (n = 5613) evaluated STS. Only telemonitoring significantly reduced mortality (RR, 0.66; 95% CI, 0.54.0.81; P<.0001) (**Fig. 3**). Both strategies reduced heart failure hospitalizations, telemonitoring (RR, 0.79; 95% CI, 0.67–0.94; P = .008), and STS (RR, 0.77; 95% CI, 0.68–0.87; P<.0001). Also, both interventions improved quality of life, reduced costs, and were acceptable to patients.

The investigators concluded that the precise mechanism of external telemedicine devices or STS may be multifactorial. The benefit probably relates to the adherence to guidelines-indicated treatment, early identification of complications or disease progression, and a positive effect on patient psychology.

In a meta-analysis by Klersy and colleagues[25] of 21 randomized controlled studies comparing remote monitoring with usual care and including 5715 patients there was a significant reduction in the number of heart failure–related hospitalizations (RR, 0.77; 95% CI, 0.65–0.91; P<.001) and in all-cause hospitalizations (RR, 0.87; 95% CI, 0.79–0.96; P = .003) by remote monitoring, whereas

length of stay was not affected. The difference in costs between remote monitoring and usual care ranged between €300 and 1000.

However, because these studies applied a large variety of methods for monitoring, had different strategies for treatment interventions, and showed inconsistent results, it is difficult at present to draw clear conclusions as to the clinical value of telemonitoring. Accordingly, the recent ESC heart failure guidelines concluded that the optimum approach to noninvasive remote monitoring is uncertain and no guideline recommendation was given.[26] Similarly, no firm conclusion was drawn as to the effectiveness of STS.

HEALTH ECONOMY

By replacing in-office visits with remote monitoring, the costs of device clinics are expected to be reduced. However, the impact of remote monitoring on cost-effectiveness depends on several variables, such as its reimbursement and the effects on total health care consumption, quality of life, and survival. Health economy studies of remote monitoring evaluated these variables under different circumstances and thus came to varying conclusions.

Burri and colleagues[27] reported that remote monitoring is cost-effective in patients with ICDs and CRTs even using a conservative approach using a Markov model.

Structured telephone support

Study or Subgroup	Intervention Events	Total	Usual Care Events	Total	Weight	Risk Ratio M-H, Fixed, 95% CI
Barth 2001	0	17	0	17		Not estimable
Cleland 2005(Struct Tele)	27	173	20	85	7.8%	0.66 [0.40, 1.11]
DeBusk 2004	21	228	29	234	8.3%	0.74 [0.44, 1.26]
DeWalt 2006	3	62	4	65	1.1%	0.79 [0.18, 3.37]
Galbreath 2004	54	710	39	359	15.0%	0.70 [0.47, 1.04]
Gattis 1999 (PHARM)	3	90	5	91	1.4%	0.61 [0.15, 2.46]
GESICA 2005 (DIAL)	116	760	122	758	35.4%	0.95 [0.75, 1.20]
Laramee 2003	13	141	15	146	4.3%	0.90 [0.44, 1.82]
Mortara 2009 (Struct Tele)	9	106	9	160	2.1%	1.51 [0.62, 3.68]
Rainville 1999	1	19	4	19	1.2%	0.25 [0.03, 2.04]
Riegel 2002	16	130	32	228	6.7%	0.88 [0.50, 1.54]
Riegel 2006	6	70	8	65	2.4%	0.70 [0.26, 1.90]
Sisk 2006	22	203	22	203	6.4%	1.00 [0.57, 1.75]
Tsuyuki 2004	16	140	12	136	3.5%	1.30 [0.64, 2.64]
Wakefield 2008	25	99	11	49	4.3%	1.12 [0.60, 2.09]
Total (95% CI)		2948		2615	100.0%	0.88 [0.76, 1.01]
Total events	332		332			

Heterogeneity: Chi² = 8.48, df = 13 (P = .81); I² = 0%
Test for overall effect: Z = 1.78 (P = .08)

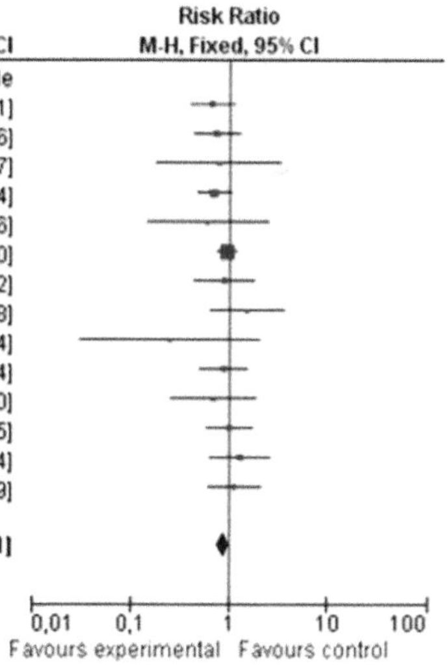

Telemonitoring

Study or Subgroup	Intervention Events	Total	Usual Care Events	Total	Weight	Risk Ratio M-H, Fixed, 95% CI
Antonicelli 2008	3	28	5	29	2.4%	0.62 [0.16, 2.36]
Balk 2008	9	101	8	113	3.6%	1.26 [0.50, 3.14]
Capomolla 2004	5	67	7	66	3.4%	0.70 [0.24, 2.11]
Cleland 2005 (Telemon)	28	168	20	85	12.8%	0.71 [0.42, 1.18]
de Lusignan 2001	2	10	3	10	1.4%	0.67 [0.14, 3.17]
Giordano 2009	21	230	32	230	15.5%	0.66 [0.39, 1.10]
Goldberg 2003 (WHARF)	11	138	26	142	12.4%	0.44 [0.22, 0.85]
Kielblock 2007	37	251	69	251	33.3%	0.54 [0.37, 0.77]
Mortara 2009 (Telemon)	15	195	9	160	4.8%	1.37 [0.61, 3.04]
Soran 2008	11	160	17	155	8.3%	0.63 [0.30, 1.29]
Woodend 2008	5	62	4	59	2.0%	1.19 [0.34, 4.22]
Total (95% CI)		1410		1300	100.0%	0.66 [0.54, 0.81]
Total events	147		200			

Heterogeneity: Chi² = 8.84, df = 10 (P = .55); I² = 0%
Test for overall effect: Z = 4.07 (P<.0001)

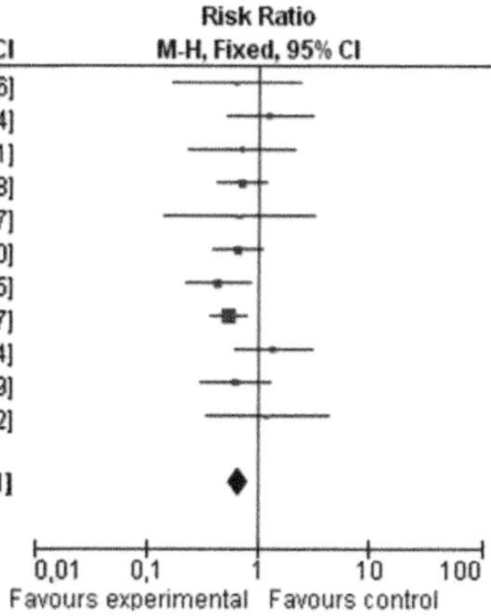

Fig. 3. Effect of STS and telemonitoring on heart failure on all-cause mortality. df, degrees of freedom. M-H, Mantel Haenzel methods. (*From* Inglis SC, Clark RA, McAlister FA, et al. Structured telephone support or telemonitoring programmes for patients with chronic heart failure. Cochrane Database Syst Rev 2010;(8):CD007228; with permission.)

The ECOST trial, randomizing 310 patients with ICDs to remote monitoring or ambulatory follow-up, found a reduction in non–hospital-related costs by €257 per patient-year with no difference in hospitalization costs.[28] It was concluded that remote management of patients with ICDs is cost saving from a French health insurance perspective. However, in the randomized EuroEco study (n = 312) Heidbuchel and colleagues[29] showed that follow-up–related costs for providers were not different for remote versus in-office follow-up. There were marked differences in reimbursement practices among the participating countries, which affected effective implementation of remote follow-up.

Taken together, these findings support a wider use of remote monitoring to reduce mortality and morbidity with a neutral or even beneficial effect on costs. In ICDs, technical problems and arrhythmias as detected early and battery life can be prolonged and number of hospital visits reduced. Recently this has also been shown for patients with DDD (dual pacing, dual chamber activity sensing, and dual response) pacemakers.[30]

Despite these favorable results, remote monitoring is not fully accepted as standard of care in patients with devices within the heterogeneous organizational, financial, and regulatory settings in Europe, as shown in a recent European Heart Rhythm Association Survey.[31] This survey indicated that doctors perceived remote monitoring as useful particularly for early detection of atrial fibrillation in pacemakers, lead failures in ICD therapy, and heart failure deterioration in patients having CRT (**Fig. 4**). However, in the centers using remote monitoring it was linked to an increase in workload. Reimbursement was a major barrier for wide implementation.

THORACIC IMPEDANCE

Thoracic impedance continuously measures impedance in the thoracic cavity against the device. Decrease in impedance may reflect volume increase in the lung. Decreases in thoracic impedance correlate with increased cardiac filling pressures[32] and precede overt heart failure,[33] making it theoretically possible to alert patients to contact their physicians for pending heart failure events in order for the physicians to take action to avoid heart failure hospitalization.[8] Frequent impedance decreases have also been associated with increased mortality risk.[34] However, the diagnostic performance of impedance-based fluid detection is low, particularly during the first months after device implantation.[35] In a controlled trial of 335 patients[36] the use of thoracic impedance with an audible patient alert tone in ICDs and CRT-Ds did not improve outcome and increased heart failure hospitalizations and outpatient visits. This finding led to further developments of how to use multiparameters from a device, including thoracic impedance to detect pending fluid overload.

INITIAL EXPERIENCE OF MULTIPARAMETERS TO DETECT PENDING HEART FAILURE EVENTS

The combination of atrial fibrillation burden, hours of activity per day, heart rate and heart rate variability, and impedance crossing is currently being

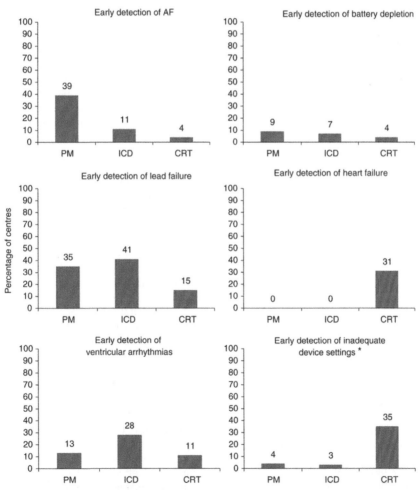

Fig. 4. Reported benefits of remote monitoring of ICDs, CRT, and pacemakers (PM). (*From* Mairesse GH, Braunschweig F, Klersy K, et al. * loss of biventricular capture. Implementation and reimbursement of remote monitoring for cardiac implantable electronic devices in Europe: a survey from the Health Economics Committee of the European Heart Rhythm Association. Europace 2015;17(5):815; with permission.)

assessed and is presumed to be more reliable to detect imminent heart failure deteriorations.[37,38] In the PARTNERS trial,[39] a combined heart failure device diagnostic algorithm was developed on an independent data set. The algorithm was considered positive if a patient had 2 of the following within a 1-month period: long atrial fibrillation duration, rapid ventricular rate during atrial fibrillation, high (>60) fluid index, low patient activity, abnormal autonomics (high night heart rate or low heart rate variability), or a notable device therapy (insufficient CRT pacing or ICD shocks), or only a very high (>100) fluid index. In 694 patients with CRT-Ds followed for 11.7 ± 2 months, 90 patients had 141 adjudicated heart failure hospitalizations. Patients with a positive combined heart failure diagnostic by this definition had a 5.5-fold increased risk for heart failure hospitalization with pulmonary signs or symptoms within the next months (HR, 5.5; 95% CI, 3.4–8.8; P<.0001) and the risk remained high after adjusting for clinical variables (**Fig. 5**). Although this was not a remote monitoring study (instead patients were followed at regular intervals of 3, 6, 9, and 12 months after enrollment), the combination of parameters could be used as part of remote monitoring. Cowie and colleagues[40] suggested a multiparameter-based heart failure score, which was effective in identifying patients at increased risk for heart failure hospitalization within 30 days.

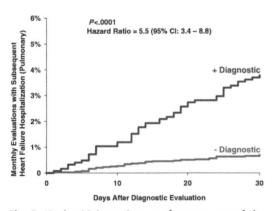

Fig. 5. Kaplan-Meier estimates of percentage of the monthly evaluations with a subsequent heart failure hospitalization because of sign/symptoms of pulmonary congestion. (*From* Whellan DJ, Ousdigian KT, Al-Khatib SM, et al. Combined heart failure device diagnostics identify patients at higher risk of subsequent heart failure hospitalizations: results from PARTNERS HF (Program to Access and Review Trending Information and Evaluate Correlation to Symptoms in Patients With Heart Failure) study. J Am Coll Cardiol 2010;55(17):1807; with permission.)

CONTINUOUS IMPLANTABLE HEMODYNAMIC MONITORING/PULMONARY ARTERY PRESSURE OR LEFT ATRIAL PRESSURE MONITORING

Most heart failure deteriorations are caused by fluid overload. It has become increasingly clear that fluid accumulation typically has already started and gradually increases weeks before clinical events, whereas clinical signs and symptoms develop first late in the course of decompensation. If physicians can detect early signs of deterioration only smaller adjustments of medication may be required to stop progression and avoid a heart failure hospitalization. The addition of hemodynamic telemonitoring to CRT may thus be expected to enhance therapy. Examples of such actions are adjustments of drug therapy and treatment of arrhythmias as soon as data are detected.

In the beginning of the 1990s an implantable hemodynamic monitor was created to guide heart failure treatment. It accurately and continuously measured central cardiac pressures[41] and early on was found to detect pending fluid overload in patients with heart failure.[42] This technology provided new knowledge and paved the way for the concept of remote monitoring in heart failure. However, in the randomized COMPASS trial the use of pressure monitoring to tailor heart failure medication failed to reduce the rate of total heart failure events (the primary end point) in patients with advanced heart failure.[43] Even though this was a negative study, the results from the Chronicle studies gave important hemodynamic data for how pressure increments precede clinical deterioration of heart failure by as much as 5 to 6 weeks in advance of a clinical event (and paved the way for the implantable left atrial pressure sensor studied in the HOMEOSTASIS trial[44] and the implantable pulmonary pressure sensor device studied in the CHAMPION study).[45]

In the HOMEOSTASIS trial an implantable left atrial sensor was used to tailor heart failure medication in patients in NYHA III to IV heart failure and acute decompensation. Following a 3-month blinded observation period, left atrial pressure was used to guide therapy. There was a lower short-term combined rate of heart failure hospitalization and all-cause mortality after left atrial pressure–guided therapy was initiated. Over the course of the treatment, patients also had significant improvements in quality of life, left atrial pressures, and left ventricular function.[44]

In the CHAMPION study,[45] patients in NYHA III and with a previous heart failure hospitalization were implanted with a wireless implantable hemodynamic monitoring system; a system with a radiofrequency sensor without batteries or leads placed in the distal part of the pulmonary artery. Medical therapy was guided by daily transmission of pulmonary artery pressure and compared with control with a follow-up of 15 months. A significant large reduction in hospitalization for heart failure of 39% compared with the control group was reported.

These studies indicate that the addition of central pressures or incorporation of the technology in CRT devices will further enhance CRT by anticipating and acting before clinical deterioration. Moreover, such devices will help to detect who is no longer responding to CRT and take action.

SUMMARY DISCUSSION

The follow-up of patients having CRT is a clinical challenge because the complex underlying heart disease, concurrent comorbidities, and technical device-related issues. Regular visits in a collaborative multidisciplinary setting are required to cover the different aspects of care in these patients. For this purpose, remote monitoring of implanted CRT-Ds or CRT-Ps offers several benefits and contributes in multiple ways to improved patient management.

Remote monitoring confers logistic advantages because of a lower burden of in-office visits and a reduced need for patient travel. However, these advantages are of secondary importance in relation to the clinical benefits in terms of superior device safety, improved arrhythmia diagnostics, and the potential for using the device-based diagnostic information for improved management of heart failure. Two observational studies in large US networks of remote device monitoring suggested that this strategy is associated with better survival.[10,11] Randomized comparisons of remote monitoring and traditional in-office follow-up suggested a reduction of hospitalization and a reduction in the number of inappropriate shocks.[46,47] However, the latter finding could not be generally confirmed in a recent meta-analysis.[23] This disparity between study findings may partly be explained by differences in how monitored events are reported to the clinicians and the strategies of transforming this information into clinical actions. Notably, remote monitoring studies ensuring a daily verification of transmissions resulted in improved survival.

Improvements in clinical outcomes are to a large extent associated with the early detection and clinical response to atrial and ventricular arrhythmias, technical device issues, and shock events, as shown in the TRUST and CONNECT trials.[47,48] Specific to the effectiveness of CRT, remote monitoring allows a close surveillance of the percentage of biventricular stimulation and, thus, guidance to ensure an optimal resynchronization effect, which is of essential importance in patients with atrial fibrillation or frequent ventricular ectopy.[14] In the In-Time study, implementing a dedicated service center and a detailed plan for clinical action taking and showing improvements in the heart failure composite score and survival, atrial or ventricular arrhythmias and percentage biventricular stimulation were the most frequent findings reported from remote monitoring leading to patient contact. These observations underline that a major challenge of remote monitoring is still the meaningful integration of remote diagnostic information into the routine work flow and its translation into appropriate clinical action. With the growing medical use of remote technology from implanted devices, telemonitoring, and smartphone applications, it can be expected that the understanding of how this modern technology can be used to effectively improve patient care will be improved. There are several algorithms that may specifically be useful in the management of heart failure; for example, impedance monitoring or monitoring of central filling pressures. Initial findings suggest that some of these methods may further add to better patient management. However, more results are needed and ways how to integrate this with implanted devices and there are several properly dimensioned randomized is ongoing.

In a recent editorial, Boriani[49] wrote that "Remote monitoring for disease management should be approached as a change in the paradigm of care provision, moving from empiric and 'reactive' in-hospital treatments and interventions to personalized out-of-hospital pro-active care, guided by continuous patient surveillance through RM [remote monitoring]."

In order to change the health care system to become more patient oriented and to modify and reverse disease progression, the obstacles to wide implementation of remote monitoring for CRT and other devices must be resolved.

REFERENCES

1. Mosterd A, Hoes AW. Clinical epidemiology of heart failure. Heart 2007;93(9):1137–46.
2. Zarrinkoub R, Wettermark B, Wandell P, et al. The epidemiology of heart failure, based on data for 2.1 million inhabitants in Sweden. Eur J Heart Fail 2013;15(9):995–1002.
3. Braunschweig F, Cowie MR, Auricchio A. What are the costs of heart failure? Europace 2011; 13(Suppl 2):ii13–7.

4. Lund LH, Jurga J, Edner M, et al. Prevalence, correlates, and prognostic significance of QRS prolongation in heart failure with reduced and preserved ejection fraction. Eur Heart J 2013;34(7):529–39.

5. Brignole M, Auricchio A, Baron-Esquivias G, et al. 2013 ESC guidelines on cardiac pacing and cardiac resynchronization therapy: the Task Force on Cardiac Pacing and Resynchronization Therapy of the European Society of Cardiology (ESC). Developed in collaboration with the European Heart Rhythm Association (EHRA). Europace 2013;15(8):1070–118.

6. Dickstein K, Bogale N, Priori S, et al. The European Cardiac Resynchronization Therapy Survey. Eur Heart J 2009;30(20):2450–60.

7. Cleland JG, Abraham WT, Linde C, et al. An individual patient meta-analysis of five randomized trials assessing the effects of cardiac resynchronization therapy on morbidity and mortality in patients with symptomatic heart failure. Eur Heart J 2013;34(46):3547–56.

8. Braunschweig F, Ford I, Conraads V, et al. Can monitoring of intrathoracic impedance reduce morbidity and mortality in patients with chronic heart failure? Rationale and design of the Diagnostic Outcome Trial in Heart Failure (DOT-HF). Eur J Heart Fail 2008;10(9):907–16.

9. Lazarus A. Remote, wireless, ambulatory monitoring of implantable pacemakers, cardioverter defibrillators, and cardiac resynchronization therapy systems: analysis of a worldwide database. Pacing Clin Electrophysiol 2007;30(Suppl 1):S2–12.

10. Saxon LA, Hayes DL, Gilliam FR, et al. Long-term outcome after ICD and CRT implantation and influence of remote device follow-up: the ALTITUDE survival study. Circulation 2010;122(23):2359–67.

11. Varma N, Piccini JP, Snell J, et al. The relationship between level of adherence to automatic wireless remote monitoring and survival in pacemaker and defibrillator patients. J Am Coll Cardiol 2015;65(24):2601–10.

12. Cheng A, Landman SR, Stadler RW. Reasons for loss of cardiac resynchronization therapy pacing: insights from 32 844 patients. Circ Arrhythm Electrophysiol 2012;5(5):884–8.

13. Mullens W, Grimm RA, Verga T, et al. Insights from a cardiac resynchronization optimization clinic as part of a heart failure disease management program. J Am Coll Cardiol 2009;53(9):765–73.

14. Gasparini M, Auricchio A, Regoli F, et al. Four-year efficacy of cardiac resynchronization therapy on exercise tolerance and disease progression: the importance of performing atrioventricular junction ablation in patients with atrial fibrillation. J Am Coll Cardiol 2006;48(4):734–43.

15. Ganesan AN, Brooks AG, Roberts-Thomson KC, et al. Role of AV nodal ablation in cardiac resynchronization in patients with coexistent atrial fibrillation

and heart failure a systematic review. J Am Coll Cardiol 2012;59(8):719–26.

16. Lakkireddy D, Di Biase L, Ryschon K, et al. Radiofrequency ablation of premature ventricular ectopy improves the efficacy of cardiac resynchronization therapy in nonresponders. J Am Coll Cardiol 2012;60(16):1531–9.

17. Hayes DL, Boehmer JP, Day JD, et al. Cardiac resynchronization therapy and the relationship of percent biventricular pacing to symptoms and survival. Heart Rhythm 2011;8(9):1469–75.

18. Al-Khatib SM, Piccini JP, Knight D, et al. Remote monitoring of implantable cardioverter defibrillators versus quarterly device interrogations in clinic: results from a randomized pilot clinical trial. J Cardiovasc Electrophysiol 2010;21(5):545–50.

19. Landolina M, Perego GB, Lunati M, et al. Remote monitoring reduces healthcare use and improves quality of care in heart failure patients with implantable defibrillators: the evolution of management strategies of heart failure patients with implantable defibrillators (EVOLVO) study. Circulation 2012;125(24):2985–92.

20. Hindricks G, Taborsky M, Glikson M, et al. Implant-based multiparameter telemonitoring of patients with heart failure (IN-TIME): a randomised controlled trial. Lancet 2014;384(9943):583–90.

21. Linde C, Abraham WT, Gold MR, et al. Randomized trial of cardiac resynchronization in mildly symptomatic heart failure patients and in asymptomatic patients with left ventricular dysfunction and previous heart failure symptoms. J Am Coll Cardiol 2008;52(23):1834–43.

22. Boriani G, Da Costa A, Ricci RP, et al. The MOnitoring Resynchronization dEvices and CARdiac patiEnts (MORE-CARE) randomized controlled trial: phase 1 results on dynamics of early intervention with remote monitoring. J Med Internet Res 2013;15(8):e167.

23. Parthiban N, Esterman A, Mahajan R, et al. Remote monitoring of implantable cardioverter-defibrillators: a systematic review and meta-analysis of clinical outcomes. J Am Coll Cardiol 2015;65(24):2591–600.

24. Inglis SC, Clark RA, McAlister FA, et al. Which components of heart failure programmes are effective? A systematic review and meta-analysis of the outcomes of structured telephone support or telemonitoring as the primary component of chronic heart failure management in 8323 patients: abridged Cochrane Review. Eur J Heart Fail 2011;13(9):1028–40.

25. Klersy C, De Silvestri A, Gabutti G, et al. Economic impact of remote patient monitoring: an integrated economic model derived from a meta-analysis of randomized controlled trials in heart failure. Eur J Heart Fail 2011;13(4):450–9.

26. McMurray JJ, Adamopoulos S, Anker SD, et al. ESC guidelines for the diagnosis and treatment of acute

and chronic heart failure 2012: the Task Force for the Diagnosis and Treatment of Acute and Chronic Heart Failure 2012 of the European Society of Cardiology. Developed in collaboration with the Heart Failure Association (HFA) of the ESC. Eur Heart J 2012; 33(14):1787–847.

27. Burri H, Sticherling C, Wright D, et al. Cost-consequence analysis of daily continuous remote monitoring of implantable cardiac defibrillator and resynchronization devices in the UK. Europace 2013;15(11):1601–8.

28. Guedon-Moreau L, Lacroix D, Sadoul N, et al. Costs of remote monitoring vs. ambulatory follow-ups of implanted cardioverter defibrillators in the randomized ECOST study. Europace 2014;16(8):1181–8.

29. Heidbuchel H, Hindricks G, Broadhurst P, et al. Euro-Eco (European Health Economic Trial on Home Monitoring in ICD Patients): a provider perspective in five European countries on costs and net financial impact of follow-up with or without remote monitoring. Eur Heart J 2015;36(3):158–69.

30. Mabo P, Victor F, Bazin P, et al. A randomized trial of long-term remote monitoring of pacemaker recipients (the COMPAS trial). Eur Heart J 2012;33(9): 1105–11.

31. Mairesse GH, Braunschweig F, Klersy K, et al. Implementation and reimbursement of remote monitoring for cardiac implantable electronic devices in Europe: a survey from the Health Economics Committee of the European Heart Rhythm Association. Europace 2015;17(5):814–8.

32. Vanderheyden M, Houben R, Verstreken S, et al. Continuous monitoring of intrathoracic impedance and right ventricular pressures in patients with heart failure. Circ Heart Fail 2010;3(3):370–7.

33. Yu CM, Wang L, Chau E, et al. Intrathoracic impedance monitoring in patients with heart failure: correlation with fluid status and feasibility of early warning preceding hospitalization. Circulation 2005;112(6):841–8.

34. Tang WH, Warman EN, Johnson JW, et al. Threshold crossing of device-based intrathoracic impedance trends identifies relatively increased mortality risk. Eur Heart J 2012;33(17):2189–96.

35. Conraads VM, Tavazzi L, Santini M, et al. Sensitivity and positive predictive value of implantable intrathoracic impedance monitoring as a predictor of heart failure hospitalizations: the SENSE-HF trial. Eur Heart J 2011;32(18):2266–73.

36. van Veldhuisen DJ, Braunschweig F, Conraads V, et al. Intrathoracic impedance monitoring, audible patient alerts, and outcome in patients with heart failure. Circulation 2011;124(16):1719–26.

37. Braunschweig F, Mortensen PT, Gras D, et al. Monitoring of physical activity and heart rate variability in patients with chronic heart failure using cardiac resynchronization devices. Am J Cardiol 2005;95(9): 1104–7.

38. Conraads VM, Spruit MA, Braunschweig F, et al. Physical activity measured with implanted devices predicts patient outcome in chronic heart failure. Circ Heart Fail 2014;7(2):279–87.

39. Whellan DJ, Ousdigian KT, Al-Khatib SM, et al. Combined heart failure device diagnostics identify patients at higher risk of subsequent heart failure hospitalizations: results from PARTNERS HF (Program to Access and Review Trending Information and Evaluate Correlation to Symptoms in Patients with Heart Failure) study. J Am Coll Cardiol 2010; 55(17):1803–10.

40. Cowie MR, Sarkar S, Koehler J, et al. Development and validation of an integrated diagnostic algorithm derived from parameters monitored in implantable devices for identifying patients at risk for heart failure hospitalization in an ambulatory setting. Eur Heart J 2013;34(31):2472–80.

41. Magalski A, Adamson P, Gadler F, et al. Continuous ambulatory right heart pressure measurements with an implantable hemodynamic monitor: a multicenter, 12-month follow-up study of patients with chronic heart failure. J Card Fail 2002;8(2):63–70.

42. Braunschweig F, Linde C, Eriksson MJ, et al. Continuous haemodynamic monitoring during withdrawal of diuretics in patients with congestive heart failure. Eur Heart J 2002;23(1):59–69.

43. Bourge RC, Abraham WT, Adamson PB, et al. Randomized controlled trial of an implantable continuous hemodynamic monitor in patients with advanced heart failure: the COMPASS-HF study. J Am Coll Cardiol 2008;51(11):1073–9.

44. Ritzema J, Troughton R, Melton I, et al. Physician-directed patient self-management of left atrial pressure in advanced chronic heart failure. Circulation 2010;121(9):1086–95.

45. Abraham WT, Adamson PB, Bourge RC, et al. Wireless pulmonary artery haemodynamic monitoring in chronic heart failure: a randomised controlled trial. Lancet 2011;377(9766):658–66.

46. Guedon-Moreau L, Lacroix D, Sadoul N, et al. A randomized study of remote follow-up of implantable cardioverter defibrillators: safety and efficacy report of the ECOST trial. Eur Heart J 2013;34(8):605–14.

47. Varma N, Epstein AE, Irimpen A, et al. Efficacy and safety of automatic remote monitoring for implantable cardioverter-defibrillator follow-up: the Lumos-T Safely Reduces Routine Office Device Follow-up (TRUST) trial. Circulation 2010;122(4):325.

48. Crossley GH, Boyle A, Vitense H, et al. The CONNECT (Clinical Evaluation of Remote Notification to Reduce Time to Clinical Decision) trial: the value of wireless remote monitoring with automatic clinician alerts. J Am Coll Cardiol 2011;57(10):1181–9.

49. Boriani G. Remote monitoring of cardiac implantable electrical devices in Europe: quo vadis? Europace 2015;17(5):674–6.

Moving?

Make sure your subscription moves with you!

To notify us of your new address, find your **Clinics Account Number** (located on your mailing label above your name), and contact customer service at:

Email: journalscustomerservice-usa@elsevier.com

800-654-2452 (subscribers in the U.S. & Canada)
314-447-8871 (subscribers outside of the U.S. & Canada)

Fax number: 314-447-8029

Elsevier Health Sciences Division
Subscription Customer Service
3251 Riverport Lane
Maryland Heights, MO 63043

*To ensure uninterrupted delivery of your subscription, please notify us at least 4 weeks in advance of move.